Quest for Conception

Quest for Conception

Gender, Infertility, and Egyptian Medical Traditions

Marcia C. Inhorn

University of Pennsylvania Press

Philadelphia

Cover photo: Infertile pilgrims ascending a cemetery path to a shrine of conception. (Photograph by Marcia Inhorn)

Printed in the United States of America

Library of Congress Cataloging-in-Publication Data
Inhorn, Marcia Claire, 1957–
Quest for conception: gender, infertility, and Egyptian medical traditions / Marcia C. Inhorn.
p. cm.
Includes bibliographical references and index.
ISBN 0–8122–3221–6 (cloth). — ISBN 0–8122–1528–1 (paper)
1. Infertility, Female—Treatment—Egypt. 2. Traditional medicine—Egypt. I. Title.
RG201.I544 1994
618.1'78'00962—dc20 94–10899
CIP

In Loving Memory of
My Infant Twin Daughters

Contents

Illustrations

Tables

Photographs

Abbreviations

AI	artificial insemination
AID	artificial insemination by donor
AIDS	acquired immune deficiency syndrome
AIH	artificial insemination by husband
CAPMAS	Central Agency for Public Mobilisation and Statistics
CFI	cervical-factor infertility
CHW	community health worker
CME	continuing medical education
D & C	dilatation and curettage
FSH	follicle-stimulating hormone
GIFT	gamete intrafallopian transfer
GnRH	gonadotropin-releasing hormone
HLA	human leukocyte antigen
hMG	human menopausal gonadotropin
HSG	hysterosalpingography
IUD	intrauterine device
IVF	in vitro fertilization
JAMA	*Journal of the American Medical Association*
MCH	maternal and child health
MFI	male-factor infertility
NRTs	new reproductive technologies
ob-gyn	obstetrical-gynecological
OFI	ovarian-factor infertility
ORTs	old reproductive technologies
PCO	polycystic ovary syndrome
PCT	postcoital test
PHC	primary health care
PID	pelvic inflammatory disease
PSA	public service announcement
STD	sexually transmitted disease
TBA	traditional birth attendant

TFI	tubal-factor infertility
UN	United Nations
USAID	US Agency for International Development
WHO	World Health Organization

Acknowledgments

This book and the study on which it is based would not have been possible without the intellectual, emotional, and practical support of many individuals—among them, informants, family members, friends, colleagues, teachers, research assistants, reviewers, and editors—and the financial and logistical support of a number of organizations and institutions both in Egypt and in the United States. Their assistance over the past eight years—beginning when I first ventured to Egypt, was made painfully aware of the plight of infertile Egyptian women, and subsequently planted the seeds of this study—has been invaluable.

Certainly, my most profound debt of gratitude is to the infertile Egyptian women who opened their hearts, homes, and voluminous medical records to me as willing informants in my study. During the course of extended interviews, visits, and long hours spent waiting together in dusty hospital corridors, these women revealed a tremendous amount about the experience of infertility in Egypt, much of which was heart-wrenching, demoralizing, and, at times, even shocking. Yet, I was continually impressed by the dignity, resourcefulness, and humor with which these women—some of whom had been "searching for children" for as long as two decades—faced their difficult situations. Without their willingness to disclose the most intimate and distressing details of their lives, to lead me down Alexandria's back alleys and across its desert outskirts to meet healers, herbalists, and hermaphroditic goats, and to sip sweet tea with me on lazy summer afternoons when I was feeling particularly tired and homesick, this study simply would not have been possible. To all of them, *alf isshok!* (a thousand thanks).

I also owe special thanks to the numerous individuals and organizations in Egypt who assisted me in various aspects of this study and who, through friendship, collegiality, and important favors, made my life in Egypt much easier. First and foremost, I must thank my four research assistants, Shayma' Hassouna, Rosie Kouzoukian, Hassanat Naguib, and Azza Hosam Shaker, who supported my research efforts and everyday life in Egypt in innumerable ways. Without their expert translation services and assistance in locating library materials, housing, well-stocked pharmacies, and the like, my life in Egypt certainly would have run less smoothly. In addition, I owe considerable thanks to those at the University of Alexandria's Shatby Hospital—particularly Drs. Mohammed Mehanna, Hassan Aly, Mohamad Rizk, and Soad Farid, as well as Emad Esmat, Hosam Farouk, Mohammed Hussein, Siham Zaki, and Khaled Zeitoun—who secured various permissions for me, recruited women for my study, drew crucial blood samples, participated in lively discussions about infertility and Egyptian biomedicine, and generally facilitated the semistructured interview portion of this study at Shatby Hospital. The help of Mustafa Abul Khair, one of several freelance taxi drivers at the hospital, was just as important. Mustafa drove me literally hundreds of miles through remote, sometimes roadless parts of northern Egypt to places where other drivers feared to venture. Without his kindness, acute sense of direction, and spirit of adventure, my peripatetic pilgrimages to healers and holy sites would not have been so easy.

In addition, the administrative and bureaucratic assistance provided by the staff of the Binational Fulbright Commission in Cairo—and especially its director, Ann Radwan—was invaluable during my fifteen-month tenure in Egypt. Likewise, throughout my study, I was provided with a Cairene "home away from home" by my friends Sandra Lane and Robert Rubinstein. To Sandy, I owe special thanks for a decade of unflagging friendship, delightful companionship during our first Egyptian fieldwork together, continuing scholarly stimulation, and open access to her extensive library. It was she who first told me about the developing infertility program at Shatby Hospital in Alexandria and thus directed me to a possible location for my fieldwork. In addition, she introduced me to the work of Dr. Gamal Serour, a Cairene infertility specialist who has provided me with important information on the epidemiological, social, and bioethical ramifications of infertility and the introduction of the new reproductive technologies in Egypt. I cannot begin to repay Sandy for all that she has done on my behalf.

Likewise, I am grateful to the family members and friends who journeyed to Egypt during the course of my study and who, without complaint, served as international porters of supplies and overstuffed, data-filled duffel bags. These include, most notably, my parents, Shirley and Stanley Inhorn, who not only purchased and moved many of those bags across the Atlantic, but also unselfishly cared for my obstreperous cats and generally "took care of business" for me while I was out of the country. Mia Fuller granted me the pleasure of two visits, during which time she accompanied me to the homes of many of my infertile friends, delighted them with professional-quality photographs of themselves, and always provided me with excellent companionship and advice throughout our Egyptian travels together. Molly Ryan's own research efforts with my informants while visiting me in Egypt resulted in a poignant National Public Radio piece, which highlighted the plight of infertile Egyptian women and my research findings. Visits from other friends, including Joan Ablon, Margaret Hutchinson, Molly Lee, Roland Moore, Marlowe Baldwin, and Ellen and Bill Ryan, were also much appreciated.

In the United States, I have benefited profoundly from associations with numerous institutions and individuals. During my years as a graduate student in the Joint Ph.D. Program in Medical Anthropology at the University of California, Berkeley, and the University of California, San Francisco, three individuals stand out as intellectual mentors and friends. As my adviser, Nelson Graburn not only encouraged all of my scholarly pursuits and early forays into academic publishing, but also provided excellent suggestions on numerous grant applications and manuscript drafts and generally guided me through the sometimes tortuous dissertation process. As fellow medical anthropologists, Joan Ablon and Frederick Dunn shared my interests in stigma, suffering, international health, and infectious disease and also served as excellent role models through their fieldwork, scholarship, and compassion. The contribution of all three of these individuals to my development as an anthropologist has been immense. Likewise, a special note of thanks must go to Catharine McClellan, my first anthropological teacher and mentor at the University of Wisconsin–Madison, without whose guiding hand I might never have decided to become an anthropologist.

Numerous others have contributed in large and small ways to the publication of this book, including the development of ideas presented herein, the facilitation of various aspects of the fieldwork (including language training and data collection) on which it is based, and the lengthy manuscript review and revision process. They include Anne Betteridge, Gay Becker, Peter Brown, Kimberly Buss, Janet Daling, Chandler Dawson, Jerrold Green, Fadia Hamid, John Hayes, Robert Kahler, Mary-Claire King, Ira Lapidus, William Longacre, Rani Marx, Beth Anne Mueller, Laura Nader, Mark Nichter, Maria Olujic, Maurice Salib, Carolyn Sargent, Julius Schachter, William Simmons, and Joseph Zeidan.

I feel especially fortunate to have worked with such an able editor, Patricia Smith, who, throughout the preparation of this manuscript, has provided an endless supply of enthusiastic encouragement, editorial advice, and good humor. I am also grateful to my two anonymous reviewers, whose suggestions for revision of the book were most helpful.

In addition, a number of organizations have provided crucial financial and logistical support for the research and publication of this book. Generous fellowships for fieldwork in Egypt were provided through the National Science Foundation Doctoral Dissertation Research Improvement Grant Program (#BNS-8814435); the Fulbright Institute of International Education Student Grant Program; and the Fulbright-Hays Doctoral Dissertation Research Abroad Grant Program. Post-fieldwork support for manuscript preparation was provided by the Soroptimist International Founder Region Fellowship Program; the WOSAC Council of the Department of Women's Studies, University of Arizona; and the Center for Middle Eastern Studies, University of Arizona. In addition, publication expenses were defrayed in part by a grant from the University of Arizona's Provost's Author Support Fund. I am grateful to all of these organizations and to the various individuals within them who made the funding of my research possible.

Finally, my heartfelt thanks go to two central persons in my life, Kristina Austin Nicholls, whose fine friendship over twenty-five eventful, sometimes turbulent years has never wavered, and to my husband, Kirk Hooks, whose unconditional love, generosity, kindness, and intellectual camaraderie have made the last three years of my life wondrous.

* * *

Chapter 5 is a revised and expanded version of my article, "*Kabsa* (a.k.a. *Mushāhara*) and Threatened Fertility in Egypt," to be published in *Social Science & Medicine.* Ideas presented in the Preface and Chapters 1 and 3 have been developed in different forms in the following articles: Marcia C. Inhorn and Kimberly A. Buss, "Infertility, Infection, and Iatrogenesis in Egypt: The Anthropological Epidemiology of Blocked Tubes," *Medical Anthropology* 15, no. 3 (1993):1–28; and Marcia Inhorn Millar and Sandra D. Lane, "Ethno-ophthalmology in the Egyptian Delta: An Historical Systems Approach to Ethnomedicine in the Middle East," *Social Science & Medicine* 26, no. 6 (1988):651–57. I am grateful to the editors and publishers of *Medical Anthropology* (Gordon and Breach Science Publishers S.A., Y-Parc, Chemin de la Sallaz, 1400 Yverdon, Switzerland) and *Social Science & Medicine* (Pergamon Press Ltd., Headington Hill Hall, Oxford OX3 OBW, United Kingdom) for their kind permission to draw from this work.

Notes on Transliteration

Because my research was carried out in colloquial Egyptian Arabic, I have attempted to transliterate words according to colloquial pronunciation, while generally following the transliteration system for vowels and consonants found in *The Hans Wehr Dictionary of Modern Written Arabic* (edited by J. M. Cowan, 1976). Thus, by virtue of this compromise, most words follow the *Wehr* English spellings simply because they are pronounced by Egyptian speakers this way. (This is especially true of medical terms.) Words that differ in colloquial pronunciation are transliterated according to that pronunciation. Most important, in Alexandrian Egyptian colloquial, "j" becomes a hard "g," and most "q" sounds are not vocalized and are represented by an apostrophe. The Arabic letter *hamza*, a glottal stop, is also represented by an apostrophe ('), while the letter *'ayn* is represented by an inverted, superscript comma ('). As in *Wehr*, stressed Arabic consonants are indicated by a dot below the letter and long vowels by a line above. However, I have not followed *Wehr* in that I spell out "kh," "sh," and "dh."

I have used Arabic plurals (e.g., *shuyūkh*, *dāyāt*), rather than adding a nonitalicized "s" as is often practiced (e.g., *shaikh*s, *dāyā*s). Place names and names of individuals are not necessarily written as pronounced, but rather as commonly transliterated by Egyptians themselves.

For simplicity's sake, I have made no attempt to transliterate all words of cultural significance, but only those that have particular bearing on the themes presented in this book. A glossary of these terms is provided at the back of the volume.

Preface: Hind's Story

"Since I was twelve, I suffered a lot. The first time I got married, God gave me a child and I was suffering with his sickness and my husband. And now that I have a good husband, I don't get a child. I did *a lot* of things to try to get pregnant. I'm sure after listening to each woman's problems, you'll see mine are the worst."

These are the words of Hind,[1] an infertile Egyptian woman who is "searching for children" by embarking on a desperate, relentless quest for therapy. The goal of her search is simple: to overcome her protracted state of infertility by becoming pregnant and delivering a living child. Yet, as we shall see in the story that follows, Hind's quest, which takes her down many therapeutic roads, proves to be a difficult journey, one filled with pain, suffering, and sadness.

The second of four daughters of a farmer who had migrated to Alexandria in search of work, Hind was widely considered within her *baladī*, or traditional, lower-income neighborhood to be a young, voluptuous beauty. By the age of ten, the budding Hind—whose body was already "big, boiling"—had two suitors, one of whom she loved and hoped to marry. But, despite Hind's protestations, her father married her as a twelve-year-old to another rural migrant, who Hind felt treated her like his "she-donkey." When concern arose over Hind's failure to conceive after five months of marriage, Hind's husband's sister brought her a small, miscarried fetus. She told Hind to place the fetus in a large pan of water and to bathe with this water at the time of the Islamic noon prayer over three consecutive Fridays. Lo and behold, Hind became pregnant after only a few months. However, her husband, prone to domestic violence, beat her with a boot in her pregnant belly, causing what Hind believed to be her future postpartum complications. When the baby was born, he had pus in his eyes and could not open them. Hind herself was "about to die": an excruciating, post-delivery pelvic infection had seized her abdomen, doubling her over with pain for a period of three months. When her father finally secured the money to take her to a doctor, the treatment caused "a lot of pus to come down and heat." With the doctor's strong medicine, Hind eventually recovered, but her infant son developed pus-filled boils over his entire body and, shortly after his first birthday, succumbed to a fatal respiratory infection and diarrhea. Abused and miserable, Hind pleaded with her father to help her obtain a divorce and was successful in convincing him—and, through him, her malicious husband—of the desirability of a dissolution of the ill-fated marriage. But, as a divorcée, Hind was a burden on her poor family, even though she served as a surrogate mother and wet nurse to her two infant sisters.

At the age of sixteen and against her will, Hind was married again—this time to a handsome young man named Rayda, who was also divorced and had no children. But their marriage, too, was plagued with troubles from the start. Because Rayda was an uneducated, unskilled laborer, he could not provide a stable income nor the key money necessary to secure a room, let alone a real apartment, for himself and his new bride Hind. Thus, Hind, whom Rayda forbade to work, was forced by economic circumstances to spend the next ten years of her second marriage living in the two-room apartment of her in-laws, located in a government housing project in central Alexandria. Not only was the tiny apartment cramped with furniture and seven human occupants, but it was also the site of perpetual discord between Hind and her mother-in-law, who was distraught by the continuing inability of her daughter-in-law to provide her eldest son Rayda with offspring.

Within two months of Hind's and Rayda's marriage, Hind's mother-in-law began telling Hind, "There is nothing" (i.e., no pregnancy). Soon, she began comparing Hind to other women in the neighborhood, saying, "This person became yellowish because she's pregnant. This woman gained weight because she's pregnant. And this other woman is tired because she delivered a baby. But you, you are like a house that is standing. You are like a man. You don't have children. You are like a tree that doesn't bear fruit." Feeling extremely pressured by her mother-in-law's incessant comments, Hind began "searching for children," a search that began with the doctor who had once treated her for her postpartum infection. He performed the painful procedure *kayy* (i.e., electrocautery of the cervix) on her and prescribed a year-long regimen of pills and vaginal suppositories. When these did not "cure" her presumed infertility, Hind took her neighbors' advice to make herself a *ṣūfa*, a vaginal suppository of sheep's wool dipped in black glycerin. Each evening for the three days immediately following her menstrual period, Hind "wore" the *ṣūfa*, removing it only during intercourse. In the morning, huge amounts of water gushed from Hind's vagina, indicating that she did, indeed, suffer from *ruṭūba*, or humidity, in her uterus. However, despite "drinking" the humidity, the *ṣūfa* did not make Hind pregnant.

So, after coaxing Rayda to give her money, Hind went to another doctor. This gynecologist performed a pelvic examination on Hind and prescribed "pills in a blue box"—namely, the fertility drug Clomid (clomiphene citrate), a drug that would be prescribed for Hind by at least seven other physicians. However, after Hind's first attempt at Clomid therapy failed to make her pregnant, she decided to undertake additional *wasfāt baladī*, or folk remedies, which she would try off and on again—and often simultaneously with medical therapies—over the course of her twelve-year therapeutic quest.

On one visit to a physician, Hind met another infertile woman who told her to go to the *ʿaṭṭār*, or herbalist, to buy a red and white stone called *dam al-akhawain*, or "blood of the two brothers." Hind was to crush this stone, boil it, and drink it with the boiled water, eating the crunchy remains. (She did not realize that this "stone" was actually a dark-red, resinous substance called *Dracaena cinnabari*, or "dragon's blood," derived from the dragon tree, *Dracaena draco.*) However, this "bloody" substance, which Hind dutifully ingested over several months, did not cause Hind's own bleeding (i.e., menstruation) to cease.

Thus, Hind's mother-in-law, who was becoming increasingly vexed with Hind's pregnancy delay, decided to intervene, bringing Hind three large pearls—one reddish, one greenish, and one yellowish. She told Hind to put the pearls in a pan of water and then bathe with this water at the time of the Friday noon prayer over three consecutive weeks. When this cure failed, her neighbors brought her a miscarried fetus that had been preserved in saltwater like a jar of pickled cucumbers and told Hind to immerse the pickled infant in water and then bathe herself with this water. Again, the cure failed, but Hind's resourceful neighbors encouraged her to go to a deserted Christian cemetery, to look for a child's bone there, and to step over this bone seven times. Hind did as she was told over three consecutive Fridays at the time of the Islamic noon prayer. In each case, Hind's in-laws and neighbors told her to perform these bathing and cemetery rituals because they strongly suspected that Hind had been subject in both marriages to *kabsa* (also known as *mushāhara*). In a state of *makbūsa* (also known as *mitshāhara*), Hind was deemed infertile because of reproductive "binding," which, in her case, probably resulted from some unclean woman entering her room during the first lunar month following one or both of her weddings and/or the birth of her son. Unless she found the appropriate means of unbinding herself, Hind would certainly continue to remain childless. Unfortunately for Hind, none of the *kabsa* rituals recommended for her during her second marriage were successful, although washing with a miscarried fetus had "unbound" her in her first, short-lived marriage.

Hind's mother-in-law, operating under the assumption that Hind might not be *makbūsa* after all, began suggesting other remedies, some of which she carried out on Hind's body. For example, she decided to perform *kasr*, or cupping, on Hind's back and abdomen to remove any humidity from her uterus and ovaries. First, she tied some salt in a piece of cloth, smeared the end of the bundle with cooking oil, then placed it on Hind's back and lit it. With the oily cloth ignited, she placed a small glass jar over the flame, extinguishing it and "catching" Hind's back. The repeated cuppings on Hind's back and abdomen caused some discomfort, but nowhere near that of the cuppings performed on her by a *dāya*, or traditional midwife, who undertook *kasr* with a large clay pot. The piece of pottery "held" Hind's back so strongly—like a suction cup—that each act of cupping was extremely painful. Each time the pot was removed, large amounts of steam, indicative of humidity in Hind's reproductive organs, emerged from beneath. The *dāya* repeated the cupping in several places on Hind's lower back, on her abdomen over her "tubes and ovaries," and on the front of her thighs and calves. Afterward, Hind was in excruciating pain, and her body became covered with large bruises. Realizing his wife's misery, Rayda became extremely upset at both Hind and his mother for attempting such a dangerous, nonsensical therapy.

However, Rayda's anger did not dissuade his mother from tormenting his wife with insults and relentless pressure to "find a cure." Although Hind's mother attempted to intervene—suggesting to Rayda's parents that it was their own son who was infertile, given his childlessness in his previous marriage and Hind's demonstrated reproductive success—Hind's mother-in-law could not be convinced that Rayda was to blame. Instead, her vituperative attacks on Hind, whom she called a *dhakar*, or male, increased over time, as did her pressure on Rayda to divorce Hind for a "fertile" wife.

By this point, Hind, fearing for her marriage, was becoming desperate. Earlier, Rayda had been "seduced" by a female coworker and had attempted to instigate a polygynous marriage, although he insisted to Hind that this had "nothing to do with children." When Hind told Rayda that she would rather be divorced again than to live with a cowife, Rayda rescinded his marriage offer to the other woman and renewed his commitment to Hind, telling her she was "precious" to him. Nevertheless, Rayda's desire for another wife bothered Hind tremendously; coupled with her mother-in-law's mistreatment of her and the old woman's pressure on her son to remarry, it made Hind's need for a child to "tie her husband" to her all the more pressing.

Indeed, Hind was willing to try almost any therapy in order to conceive. On one occasion, she went to a hospital "refrigerator" (i.e., the morgue) and, after providing the morgue attendant with a generous tip, was taken to a dead body covered with a sheet. The attendant told Hind to circumambulate the body seven times—much as the pilgrims on the *hajj* to Mecca circumambulate the holy stone called the *Kaʿba*. Upon Hind's final rotation, the attendant suddenly flung her onto the dead man's body, so that her head was on the dead man's head, from which fluids had leaked from his nostrils and mouth. This unexpected episode in the morgue shocked Hind—so much so that "since that day, I'm scared of anything." Yet, the point of the therapy was to do just that: to "countershock" Hind in case *khaḍḍa*, a shock or sudden fright, had caused her to become infertile. Earlier, Hind's father-in-law had tried to countershock her by placing a large, wriggling fish on her chest while she was sleeping, and Hind's brothers-in-law had thrown several mice and cats at her. However, Hind's infertility did not appear to be shock-related, because none of these countershocking strategies were successful.

With the household in an uproar over Hind's infertility, she began to seek spiritual intervention. First, Hind made a journey to the mosque and tomb of Shaikh Abū 'l-ʿAbbās al-Mursī, the famous dead *Ṣūfī* mystic and "pious one" who, by virtue of his *baraka*, or divine blessing, was able to intercede for pilgrims in their prayer-requests to God. Hind first prayed regularly, then requested from God that he give her a child, vowing to return to the mosque annually if he granted her wish. She also began talking to a number of other women pilgrims at the mosque. When Hind told them that she was infertile after having had a son who died, one of the women told her to go to a Muslim cemetery and find a gravekeeper who would be willing to let her dig up a baby buried face down. If Hind could turn the infant to the correct position on its back, this might serve to calm the *malaika*, or angels, who were angry at Hind for allowing her son to be buried face down in the earth, thus "giving his back to God." Hind also spoke to a *munaggima*, a female spiritist healer, who was known in the neighborhood for leading the *zār*, or spirit placation ceremony. The *munaggima* told Hind,

"You have a sister spirit who is upset with you, and you have to console her." She told Hind to wait until a Thursday evening and to light two candles, one behind the bathroom door and the other in front of the front doorstep, leaving the candles burning all night. On Friday at the time of the dawn prayer, Hind was to wipe the floor with licorice in water. She was to repeat the candle-burning ceremony the following two weeks, but each time placing only one candle on the side of the bed where she slept. In the morning, she was to wipe the floor with rose water, and the following week with henna. This, the *munaggima* assured her, would appease the *ukht taḥt il-arḍ*, Hind's "spirit-sister under the ground," who might be upset with Hind, thereby preventing her from becoming pregnant.

Hind could not bring herself to have a child dug up in the cemetery as she had been told by the woman at the mosque. But she did go home and perform the candlelight cleansing ceremony as directed by the *munaggima*. She waited several months to see if her spirit-sister would allow her to become pregnant, but the ceremony to appease the spirit had no effect.

Thus, Hind went to the mosque and tomb of Sitt Naima, a small, specialized mosque in Manshiyyah, the old quarter of Alexandria, known as a pilgrimage center for the infertile. There, Hind waited with a large crowd of other women until the Friday noon sermon for men was finished. Afterward, these women ascended the stairs, two by two, to the *shaikh* perched above the crowd. There, the *shaikh*, seated behind a pulled-back curtain, said prayers over each pair of women. After Hind finished her turn, she was told by the women organizing the proceedings to drink some of the ablution water from the front of the mosque and to rub a bit on her breast and abdomen. As Hind explained, "Sitt Naima is considered to be one of God's people, so it's blessed water from Sitt Naima. It has her *baraka* [blessing] in it." At the mosque, Hind also bathed her face and limbs with water in which the *mushāharāt*, or multicolored beads "from the Prophet" in Saudi Arabia, had been placed. Hoping that the *mushāharāt* would unbind her if she happened to be *makbūsa*, Hind returned on two consecutive Fridays to repeat the ritual. She was also told to go to a nearby cemetery with a doll made of henna, to bury it on the cemetery grounds, to urinate on the spot, and to leave the cemetery from a door other than the one she had entered. In addition, she was instructed to obtain some bones from the cemetery and to step over them seven times during the next three Friday noon prayers.

Not surprisingly, given Hind's previous lack of success, neither Shaikh Abū 'l-'Abbās al-Mursī's intercession, nor Sitt Naima's blessing, nor the *munaggima*'s strategy for spirit placation, nor the rituals to unbind *kabsa* were powerful enough to overcome Hind's infertility. Thus, Hind decided to seek the *baraka* of the "biggest physicians"—those working at the University of Alexandria women's hospital. Although Hind had already consulted numerous physicians about her case, none of them could tell her what was wrong with her, even though they had prescribed painful, invasive "therapies." These included *kayy*, or cervical electrocautery, and *nafq*, or tubal insufflation, a potentially life-threatening procedure in which carbon dioxide is insufflated, or pumped into the uterine cavity to supposedly "open up" blocked fallopian tubes. The problem was that none of these physicians had ever verified that Hind's fallopian tubes were, in fact, blocked, even though *nafq* had been carried out on Hind by four separate doctors. Thus, Hind hoped that, by going to the university hospital, she would finally learn something meaningful about her case.

Having preserved all of her medical records in immaculate condition under her mattress, Hind took them in a shopping bag to the hospital's outpatient clinic. There, the doctor in charge took one look at Hind's recent hysterosalpingogram (an X ray of her uterus and fallopian tubes), threw the X ray on the table, and told her, "Go home. Go home. Give up and leave your compensation to God." Hind was shocked and fainted, since "he meant I was not going to get pregnant at all." After they resuscitated Hind, the doctor told her, "I know it's very hard for you to accept, but that's the truth. I can't lie to you." Inconsolable and weeping, Hind ran into a neighbor who worked at the hospital, and he asked her what was wrong. She told him, and he took her to another physician. After examining Hind's X ray, the physician told Hind, "I think I can help you by doing an operation." Hind told the physician that she had already undergone many small operations and one big one. The doctor asked, "Did any of these gynecologists open your abdomen?" to which Hind replied, "No, they were from down [i.e., vaginal]." The doctor shouted, "The thieves! To open your tubes you need an operation to open your abdomen. They just stole your money and did nothing for you." He proceeded to perform a pelvic examination on Hind and to order a second X ray. He told her, "I want to see, honestly, if your tubes are blocked," and he promised her that she would be hospitalized only one day.

Unfortunately, one day turned into three months, in part because the X-ray machine was broken. Eventually, Hind underwent *il-manẓar*, or "the view" (i.e., diagnostic laparoscopy), to assess the state of her fallopian tubes and ovaries. The laparoscopy showed that Hind suffered from bilateral fallopian tubal obstruction, probably acquired nine years earlier as a result of her postpartum infection. The two "biggest professors" at the hospital advised Hind to have tubal surgery, which they would perform after they returned from the pilgrimage in Saudi Arabia. Hind immediately accepted their offer of free surgery (free because it was to be carried out in the university teaching hospital); however, when she told Rayda what she planned to do, he refused to sign the consent forms, fearing for Hind's life. Refusing to be dissuaded from her decision, Hind, although illiterate, "signed for him" (i.e., forged Rayda's signature).

While in the hospital awaiting surgery, Hind was seen by a young doctor, who told her, "Do you know the success rate of this operation? It's only 5 percent." Hind began to cry, but the doctor consoled her by saying, "Maybe you are one of the lucky 5 percent." Hind went ahead with the operation, marveling at the fact that "about thirty doctors were in the room."

Following the *'amalīya*, or operation, Hind was given powerful medicines to keep her fallopian tubes open. Yet, during a two-year postoperative period, Hind found that the surgery "brought no results." She returned to the hospital, where a doctor ordered yet another painful pelvic X ray with dye and then referred her to the newly created "infertility clinic." There, the young doctor in charge of Hind's case informed her that one of her fallopian tubes remained completely blocked and that the other one was open but badly damaged. Therefore, he did not consider her to be a good candidate for *il-ḥu'an*, or "the injections" (that is, artificial insemination using her husband's sperm). According to Hind, he told her, "The injection won't work with you, and I'm scheduling you for a tubes baby."

Despite her depression over the failure of her tubal surgery, Hind's hopes were restored by the possibility of having "*ṭifl l-anābīb*," or a "baby of the tubes" via in vitro fertilization (IVF). However, she feared Rayda's reaction to the subject. Rayda, frankly, had proved himself to be a devoted husband. No longer tolerating the fights between Hind and his mother, he had finally sided with Hind, moving her from his parents' centrally located apartment to a small apartment in the distant, rural outskirts of Alexandria. The move was extremely beneficial to their marriage, although Rayda continued to commute daily to visit his domineering mother.

However, when Hind told Rayda that she was being scheduled for a "baby of the tubes," he was extremely upset, asking her many difficult questions. How are babies made in tubes? Are they born in tubes? How would they ever know for sure that a tubes baby was their own child? How expensive is a tubes baby? Hind had no knowledge about how babies of the tubes were created or how much they cost. And, knowing how busy her doctor was, she feared asking him these questions, feeling that she would be imposing on his time.

Although Rayda, ultimately, left the choice for in vitro fertilization up to Hind, he did not want her to try yet another hopeless treatment. He told her, "I'm happy like this. Why should you go through this and suffer like this? If God wants to bring us children, he'll bring us. Without injections. Without treatment. Without operations. If he doesn't want to bring us, we are still happy like this. I will not one day ever think of remarrying or think that I want a baby at all." However, Hind convinced the reluctant Rayda to let her try IVF, even getting him to provide a semen sample for analysis after beseeching, "Look, I went through so many things. Do it for me this time."

Although eight months have passed since Hind was told about IVF, she is still far from undergoing the procedure at the hospital. Unfortunately, IVF is very expensive, and it will be affordable to Hind only if Rayda agrees to sell the television and stops smoking two packs of cigarettes a day. This, she concedes, will never happen. Thus, she must ponder some other way of obtaining the necessary cash. Although Hind is only thirty-one years old and has, theoretically, at least a decade of potentially fertile years ahead of her, she greatly fears that her overwhelming desire for a child—"just one child"—will never be satisfied. Although Rayda has been good to her and nearly convinces her that he will never "remarry for children," Hind still worries about his continuing commitment to her, given the ongoing pressures from his family to replace her with another wife. For Hind, the future is the source of uncertainty and fear. She hopes someday to be able to accrue the hundreds of Egyptian pounds necessary to create her own baby of the tubes, for she now feels that this may be the only solution to her recalcitrant infertility problem. Yet, whether or not she is able to undergo IVF, Hind vows that she will never stop "searching for children."

Part 1

Problem, Place, and Procreative Theory

1. The Infertility Problem in Egypt

Infertility: A Woman's Problem

In Egypt, infertility, or the inability to conceive, is a devastating problem for women, who attempt to rectify their socially tenuous situations by becoming pregnant and delivering a child. Yet, for many, pregnancy is not achieved easily, and in an attempt to facilitate conception — thereby overcoming the stigma of childlessness and solidifying their destabilized marriages — infertile women in Egypt usually embark upon a "quest for therapy" (Janzen 1978) involving remedies of quite disparate origins and natures. It would not be overstating the case to suggest that this "search for children," as Egyptian women themselves call it, is a near-universal phenomenon for infertile Egyptian women of all backgrounds — ethnic, educational, locational, social class, and so on. So powerful is their desire to have children and so mighty is the force of social pressure that comes to bear upon them that many infertile women may risk all that they have, including their lives, in the quest for conception.

This pilgrimage for pregnancy, a reproductive quest that shares many of the features of other instrumental, healing pilgrimages (Morinis 1992), is the subject of this book. In the preface, we follow the conceptive quest of Hind, an infertile Egyptian woman of the urban lower class, whose peripatetic pilgrimage from doctor to healer to holy site is in some ways typical of those of her fellow sufferers and therefore serves to illustrate many of the themes to be explored further in the chapters that follow. Most important, Hind's case demonstrates that in Egypt infertility is essentially a woman's problem. Not only are women typically blamed for the reproductive failing, but they must bear the burden of overcoming it through a therapeutic quest that is sometimes traumatic and often unfruitful. Furthermore, women face the tyranny of social judgment regarding infertility, for they are cast as being less than other women, as depriving their husbands and husbands' families of offspring, and as endangering other people's children through their uncontrollable envy.

Among the urban poor, who are the focus of this book, infertile women's greatest immediate threat comes from husbands, who have the right under Islamic law to replace an infertile wife through outright divorce or polygynous remarriage. Such replacement is usually urged by husbands' extended family members, who view a wife who thwarts her husband's procreativity as, at best, "useless" and, at worst, a threat to the social reproduction of the patrilineage at large. Thus, in Egypt, infertile women tend to face tremendous social pressures, ranging from duress within the marriage, to stigmatization within the extended family network, to outright ostracism within the larger community of fertile women.[1] Indeed, of all of the types of persons that one could be, there are very few less desirable social identities than that of the infertile woman, or *Umm Il-Ghayyib*, "Mother of the Missing One," as Egyptians are apt to call her, giving this particular identity all of the classic features of a stigma. Goffman (1963:3) defined a stigma as "an attribute that makes [her] different from others in the category of persons available for [her] to be, and of a less desirable kind—in the extreme, a person who is quite thoroughly bad, or dangerous, or weak. [She] is thus reduced in our minds from a whole and usual person to a tainted, discounted one. Such an attribute is a stigma, especially when its discrediting effect is very extensive."

In urban areas of Egypt, the overarching emphasis on the importance of motherhood and the resultant stigmatizing effect of infertility are also intimately tied to recent, rapid rural-to-urban migration and the accompanying loss of women's other productive roles in the household economy. In the poor, urban, *baladī* neighborhoods to be described in Chapter 2, women spend much of their time indoors in apartments that often consist of only one, incommodious room. There, children are their primary concern and the focus of their daily activities. For infertile women, however, daily existence often revolves around cooking, eating, listening to the radio or television, and sleeping. Many infertile women complain that their lives are "boring" and "unaccomplished," and they sense, too, that their husbands are dissatisfied with the monotony of a childless household.

Yet, among poor urban women, alternatives to motherhood and domesticity are largely absent. Women's work outside the home is viewed by many poor urban Egyptians, and especially by men of this social class, as "shameful" and degrading to women as well as to their husbands, who are seen as poor providers when their wives must venture into the outside world of wage labor. Thus, most women, influenced by their husbands' perceptions, prefer to remain *sittāt il-bait*, or housewives, an occupation that poor women generally do not question. However, when children are absent from the household, an infertile housewife remains "unoccupied"; without children to bring "joy to the home"—and, by extension, the marital relationship—women lead lives that are marked by loneliness, isolation, and deepening states of depression and despair.

Furthermore, most Egyptian women are unable to fulfill their motherhood needs through adoption, a solution to infertility that is found throughout much of the non-Muslim world. Islam disallows adoption, although it specifies in great detail how orphans are to be treated (Esposito 1982, 1991). The permanent, legal fostering of abandoned infants who do not assume their foster fathers' name *is* available in Egypt. However, among most poor Egyptians, such permanent fostering of illegitimate or otherwise abandoned children—which, for all intents and purposes, is tantamount to adoption as it is known in the West—is unacceptable for a host of cultural reasons (Inhorn n.d.).

Thus, biological parenthood—having a child of one's own—is the only tenable option for most poor urban Egyptians. However, the "biology" of parenthood in Egypt can be seen to vary considerably from that which most Westerners assume to be universal. Instead of a child "belonging" equally to both parents—who, in the duogenetic theory of procreation found in the West, are seen as contributing equally to the hereditary substance of their offspring—children in Egypt are seen by many poor urban adults as being "created" primarily by their fathers. In other words, in the popular, monogenetic theory of procreation found throughout Egypt, as well as in Turkey (Delaney 1991) and perhaps many other parts of the Middle East, men are seen as creating preformed fetuses through spermatogenesis; these fetuses are then carried in men's sperm, or "worms," as sperm are referred to among the urban poor, to women's wombs through the act of sexual intercourse. In other words, if men's "worms carry the kids," as Egyptians are apt to put it, then women's wombs are seen as mere vessels, or receptacles, for men's most essential, substantive input.

This monogenetic theory of procreation, which will be elaborated in greater detail in Chapter 3, has multiple implications for gender relations in contemporary urban Egypt (Inhorn n.d.). In Egypt, patriarchy—or relations of relative power and authority of men over women, which are institutionalized on many societal levels and maintained through mechanisms of male domination and control—can be seen to be legitimated in large part by the perceived procreative potency of "patriarchs," or men whose familial supremacy comes by virtue of their fatherhood. Among the

Egyptian poor, fathering is more than a social act, for it involves what many view as the exclusive biological act of creating the lives of one's children.

As Delaney (1991) has so forcefully argued, monogenetic theory also receives substantial symbolic support from the three major monotheistic religions, Judaism, Christianity, and Islam, which arose in the Middle East. In the cosmologies of these religions, the universe and all earthly life are ultimately created by a male God. In Egypt and other parts of the Muslim world, the creative power of Allah, the one God, who is gendered male, is symbolically associated with the procreative powers of earthly males, whose ties to the divine are apparent in the realm of religious practice.

Thus, in this androcentric procreative scenario, Egyptian women are strictly marginalized as reproducers, and the products of their bodies are even seen as polluting to men and the fetuses that men create. Moreover, women are blamed for endangering masculine procreativity by virtue of wombs that fail to facilitate this most important act of male creation. Given that men are seen as engendering offspring, it is certainly ironic that women are blamed for failures in the reproductive realm. However, as will be described in detail in Chapters 3 and 8, women's reproductive bodies are seen as more complicated than those of men and, hence, more prone to mechanistic failures of the "reproductive equipment." Although the dissemination of biomedical knowledge through the advent of semen analysis in Egypt has led to widespread recognition that men, too, may be infertile because of "weak worms," most Egyptians see women's reproductive bodies as the site of numerous potential problems, a view that has been perpetuated by Western-based biomedicine in the Egyptian setting.

To wit, in biomedical infertility management, it is Egyptian women's bodies — not men's — that tend to be subjected to invasive, agonizing methods of surveillance and control. In fact, Foucault's (1977) notion of "biopower," in which human bodies become the site of ideological control and are disciplined, punished, and in other ways manipulated through "technologies of the body" designed to create, ultimately, politically docile bodies/individuals, seems quite appropriate to this discussion.[2] For, as we shall see, Egyptian biomedicine, the institutionalized source of biopower in this setting, has created, through subtle, hegemonic coercion and consent (Gramsci 1971), a class of docile, subordinated infertile women, ready to subject themselves to most forms of biogynecological bodily invasion through their belief in the inherent superiority of high-tech biomedical "fixes." That mostly male biogynecologists willingly invade women's bodies, surgically and vaginally, in the pursuit of blatantly patriarchal and capitalist ends will become exceedingly apparent in Chapter 9 in the discussion of "untherapeutic therapeutics" rampant in the Egyptian biogynecological setting.[3]

Although this book is not intended as an invective against Egyptian biomedicine, it will become apparent in Chapters 8 through 11 that I am highly critical of many of the ways in which women's reproductive bodies are manipulated by Egyptian biogynecologists. Yet, as an outsider to Egyptian biomedical culture, I do not stand alone in my "cultural critique," to use Ehrenreich's (1978) term, of Egyptian biogynecology. Rather, as we shall see in Chapters 8 and 9, this critique comes from within the Egyptian biogynecological community itself and involves the subversive discourse of primarily younger, often university-based physicians, who rail against the inefficacious and even iatrogenic practices of many community-based biogynecologists, who perform irrational, useless, but highly invasive procedures on infertile women largely "for money." Thus, a critical analysis of Egyptian biogynecology as a hegemonic, neocolonial, capitalist enterprise—one affected by the "smothering dominance" of the technological imperative (Barger-Lux and Heaney 1986; Turshen 1991), but diminished by a crucial lag in the reproduction of appropriate technical knowledge—is certainly necessary and will be found in Chapters 8 and 9. This will be followed by an indigenous critique of the "old," outmoded, but pertinacious biogynecological technologies themselves as they are applied to infertile women's bodies. In Chapters 10 and 11, the transfer to Egypt of the "new" reproductive technologies—artificial insemination by husband (AIH) and in vitro fertilization (IVF)—will be examined in some detail, focusing on the "local moral worlds" (Kleinman 1992) of infertile Muslim women who are forced to grapple with the difficult therapeutic decision-making process.

Indeed, in their biomedical quests for conception, infertile Egyptian women must make many difficult, often morally based decisions: Should I keep taking these drugs despite their frightening side effects? Should I undergo yet another abdominal surgery? Should I inform my husband of his low sperm count? Should I pawn my wedding ring so that I can undergo a therapy that may be unsuccessful? That women make numerous decisions of this nature over the course of months and years indicates that they are more than mere bodies, more than passive, corporeal subjects. In contrast to Orientalist stereotypes of Middle Easterners as inordinately fatalistic and prone to immobilizing predestination beliefs,[4] Egyptian women display a remarkable degree of activism and agency in their quests for conception—often without the intervention of supportive "therapy management groups" (Janzen 1978, 1987). Namely, because of increasing nuclearization and isolation of the urban Egyptian family, because of the stigmatization of infertility, and because of the tenacity of many infertility problems, therapy management groups consisting of spouses, families, friends, and neighbors tend to collapse over time, and infertile women are often left to go it alone. That many infertile women are stubbornly persistent in their therapeutic quests—venturing to new doctors, new healers, new shrines on their own, amid the negative scrutiny of their neighbors (who condemn any woman who "comes and goes" too much)—is a testament to infertile women's activism and their ability to make important decisions for themselves. Furthermore, some infertile women demonstrate striking resistance to male subordination, actively defying their husbands' instructions not to undertake unorthodox ethnogynecological cures and withstanding various forms of biomedical coercion. Not only do many women insist upon curative eclecticism, capitalizing on the ambiguities and indeterminacies of medical pluralism and often opting for the gynocentric comfort of the indigenous, ethnomedical realm, but they also criticize and challenge the biomedical system through multiple strategies of counter-hegemonic resistance. These include "doctor shopping," noncompliance with unpleasant therapeutic regimens, seeking of second opinions and popular health information, and open criticism of doctors' treatments, greed, inability to communicate, and lack of ethnogynecological savvy. Through their actions and their subordinate discourse on "useless" therapies, operations that "bring no results," and doctors who fail to understand their problems, infertile Egyptian women take a stand against their biomedical subjectivity and demonstrate what Becker and Nachtigall (1991) have called the "nebulous power" of infertile patients in the biomedical system.

Egyptian Gynecologies

Thus, despite their desperation to be cured, many infertile Egyptian women refuse to allow biogynecology to take over their lives, resorting instead to multiple strategies of diagnosis and cure. In Egypt, rather than there being only one hegemonic form of gynecology, we may speak of multiple "gyneco*logies*," or multiple philosophies regarding the appropriate diagnostic and therapeutic treatment of women's reproductive bodies. For heuristic purposes, it is easiest to divide these gynecologies into two major categories, biogynecology and ethnogynecology. But, as we shall see in the chapters that follow, such a dualistic and seemingly dialectically opposed representation of the Egyptian gynecological realm is nothing if not simplistic. Instead, within the historically pluralistic health-care setting described in Chapter 3, numerous healing philosophies are still present, despite the dynamic supplantation of older medical systems by newer ones throughout a 5,000-year or more medical history in Egypt (Gran 1979; Millar and Lane 1988). Thus, the numerous gynecologies present in Egypt today must be historically contextualized and seen as emerging from a number of literate medical traditions in this region.

Furthermore, the multifaceted array of etiological, diagnostic, and therapeutic beliefs and practices regarding the nature and treatment of infertility—a vast armamentarium to be described in some detail in Chapters 4 through 11—must be seen as a reflection of two important and related phenomena: first, the pluralistic health-care environment still existing in present-day Egypt, which is a result of the syncretism of the aforementioned millenia-old medical traditions in this region; and, second, the resultant multiplicity of causal and therapeutic beliefs held by Egyptian patients and healers of various types.

In Chapters 4 and 8, the various ethno- and biogynecologists involved in treating infertile women will be introduced, as will the medical philosophies that they uphold and may attempt to inculcate in their patients. Special attention will be paid in this discussion to four key issues of medical anthropological concern:

1. *Competing belief systems and their hegemony.* What are the competing belief systems regarding infertility causation? Who holds them? Is any one system hegemonic in Egypt?
2. *Cognitive dissonance.* Can individuals, either patients or healers, hold simultaneously contrasting belief systems regarding infertility causation? If so, does this cause "cognitive dissonance" (Festinger 1957), or do these individuals accommodate conflicting beliefs without experiencing cognitive confusion?
3. *Diagnosis as part of the therapeutic process.* Is the quest for etiological understanding considered an essential part of the therapeutic process by both patients and healers? How willing are these parties to undertake diagnostic measures in the quest for this information?
4. *Diagnostic information as sacred knowledge.* Is information gained through the diagnostic quest considered "sacred" by either patients or healers? How willing are healers to impart this information to

their patients, and is such disclosure considered mandatory? Do patients consider such disclosure to be within their rights?

However, my attempt is to go beyond analyses of emic, meaning-based models of infertility causation to provide a broader analytical construction of the proximate, medial, and ultimate causes of infertility—an analysis of what I call "causal proximity." That is, are the causes of infertility suggested by these models located within the individual body, the social body, or the body politic (Lock and Scheper-Hughes 1990; Scheper-Hughes and Lock 1987)? As I will argue, ethnogynecological and biogynecological models of infertility causation in Egypt are largely concerned with proximate causes of infertility, which, by definition, are endogenous and are considered to be corporeally located within individual bodies. However, as we shall see, some ethnogynecological explanations are concerned with social relations and the effects of social actions on fertility; hence, these constructions of causation can be defined as exogenous and of medial proximity. For infertile Egyptian women, however, the question "Why me?" always involves contemplation of the ultimate wisdom of God; thus, questions of causation—not only of infertility, but of all illness and misfortune—also have an ultimate, divine dimension that receives supportive consensus within the larger political community of Muslim believers.

For infertile Egyptian women, questions of causation of one's own misfortune always involve a significant degree of a posteriori interpretation of these multiple levels of causation. The result is often the presentation of creative illness narratives linking one's body to one's social relations to one's submission to God's authority. Despite most women's lack of formal religious education, women are clear about their relationship to God and are proud of their personal piety and faith. The importance of Islam in infertile Egyptian women's lives must not be underestimated; not only does it play a major role in women's interpretations and emotional acceptance of their infertility problems, but it guides women's therapeutic praxis, from the timing and location of healing rituals, to the use of symbolic appurtenances, to the visiting and vowing at sacred pilgrimage centers. These issues will be explored in greater detail in Chapters 4 through 7.

The Political Epidemiology of Infertility

Although this book is largely devoted to Egyptian gynecologies and the interpretation of indigenous beliefs surrounding infertility causation, diagnosis, and cure, it is important to look at other ways of explaining infertility in Egypt, even if these explanations are not indigenously based. Two explanatory perspectives that can help to shed light on the infertility problem in Egypt are the political-economic and the epidemiological ones—disparate perspectives that can be usefully merged into a "political epidemiology" of infertility.

The political economy of health, as the orientation is often called within medical anthropology and sociology (Doyal 1979; McKinlay 1984; Morsy 1990), is devoted to explicating the historical, political, and economic origins of disease and distress and the particular set of macrostructural relations underlying the social production of illness and suffering. In doing so, it attempts to discover ultimate origins of disease, which are often linked to significant power differentials between social classes and core and peripheral nations, resulting in global and regional inequalities in access to basic resources necessary to ensure well-being.

The political-economic perspective has been touted as the "missing link" in anthropological studies of health and illness (Morsy 1979), one that draws attention to "historically specific social forces, relations, and processes surrounding sickness and health care . . . of collective health conditions as they relate to social, economic, political, and ideological processes" (Morsy 1990:44). Morsy, the leading proponent of political-economic medical anthropology (or "PEMA," as she calls it) in health studies of the Middle East, notes in a seminal essay devoted to this subject:

> Reference to poverty is not a substitute for examining the structural constraints associated with particular productive systems and related exploitative relations and state imposed policies which foster ill-health and which limit access to health care. Moreover, poverty in the Middle East is not synonymous with the underdevelopment of the region. In examining the relationship between problems of health care and poverty, the latter should not be assumed to be an original condition. It is necessary to explain such problems in relation to developing historical systems of social production and the related *process* of underdevelopment in the Middle East. In short, amelioration of health problems requires the consideration of these problems in their specific historical and political-economic contexts. What is needed is the construction of analytical models which would *explain* cross-cultural variations in the provision of health care services and guide the formulation of realistic health care policies. (1981:162)

In much of the Middle East, including Egypt, problems of poverty and poor health can clearly be shown to be tied to colonial and postcolonial political histories; concomitant capitalist penetration; resultant underdevelopment, social stratification, and the creation of urban and rural elites; and widespread impoverishment of the agrarian and urban underclass segments of society (Morsy 1993). Although these problems can be found throughout much of the postcolonial developing world, Egypt clearly has been subject to all of these pressures and has been recently dubbed by one Middle Eastern political analyst as "the stalled society" (Ansari 1986).

Although it is quite easy to link many of Egypt's most pressing public health concerns, including malnutrition, schistosomiasis, hepatitis, neonatal tetanus, infant diarrhea and acute respiratory infections, tuberculosis, generally high maternal and infant mortality rates, and relatively low life expectancy (Alubo 1990; Carney 1984; Institute of Medicine 1979), to processes of underdevelopment, it is more difficult to see how the problem of infertility is linked to political and economic factors. Yet, as I will attempt to show here, the contemporary problem of infertility in Egypt is directly tied to historically situated political and economic transformations in the country as a whole, which have significantly affected the epidemiological distribution and determinants of disease in the Egyptian body politic.

Epidemiology, like the political economy of health, is concerned with the origins and patterns of disease within given populations (Kelsey, Thompson, and Evans 1986; Mausner and Kramer 1985). The branch of epidemiology concerned with discovering the underlying causes of diseases in various populations is called "analytical epidemiology" and is focused primarily on populations' exposures to disease-causing risk factors. However, as Turshen (1984) has noted in her critique of epidemiology, the discipline remains narrowly focused on a limited, triadic model of "agent, host, and environment," a model that "ignore[s] the economic basis of human behavior, neglect[s] the unequal power relations between classes of individuals, and reject[s] historical evidence of the political evolution of class society" (1984:13). Thus, the epidemiological model "does not explain why epidemics occur at certain historical moments . . . [and] does not reveal the conditions that produce disease and therefore cannot prevent the occurrence of illness" (Turshen 1984:15).

Turshen is correct in assessing epidemiology as an essentially ahistorical and depoliticized discipline. However, I contend that epidemiology can be made both political and historical, as it has at times in its past (Trostle 1986), through a merging of epidemiological analysis with political-economic interpretation. In the political epidemiology of infertility offered here, I intend to show how the epidemiological distribution and determinants of infertility among the Egyptian urban poor are linked to broader political-economic transformations that have metamorphosed the Middle Eastern region during the past half-century. These transformations have included rapid urbanization, uncontrolled industrialization, unhealthy competition, un- and underemployment, and resultant economically motivated labor migration, all of which can be shown to be tied to urban infertility problems.

* * *

To begin, however, one must first ask the basic question: Why worry about infertility among the Egyptian urban poor? Aside from the issue of human suffering, one of the most compelling reasons pertains to global patterns of increasing infertility, especially on the continent of Africa. In terms of its epidemiological distribution, infertility is a public health problem that appears to vary widely in prevalence—from rates of childlessness among married women as low as 1 percent in Thailand and Korea to those as high as 42.5 percent for different districts in Sudan (Belsey and Ware 1986). However, it is now recognized that Africa is different, epidemiologically speaking, from the rest of the world (including both non-African developing countries and developed countries), because of a threatening, high-prevalence "infertility belt" stretching across Central Africa from southwestern Sudan (Egypt's southern neighbor) to Gabon (Belsey 1976; Belsey and Ware 1986; Caldwell and Caldwell 1983; Cates, Farley, and Rowe 1985; Collet et al. 1988; Mtimavalye and Belsey 1987; Muir and Belsey 1980; World Health Organization 1975, 1987a). In some Central African populations, infertility problems may be present in 30 to 50 percent of all couples attempting to conceive, resulting primarily from infection-induced scarring and occlusion of the fallopian tubes (World Health Organization 1987a). Coupled with the epidemic of acquired immune deficiency syndrome (AIDS) throughout many parts of Central and Southern Africa, such high rates of infectious infertility pose the threat of further depopulation.

These troubling levels of infectious infertility in Africa have generated concern in the international health community, including the World Health Organization (WHO), which has attempted to obtain baseline statistical information on country- and regionwide infertility prevalence patterns throughout Africa (Farley and Belsey 1988; World Health Organization 1987a). Although Egypt is located just north of the Central African infertility belt and is estimated to have a less startling infertility level of 8 percent among couples who have never conceived,[5] Egyptian infertility investigators suspect that this figure is an underestimate, judging from the relatively high levels of infection-induced tubal-factor infertility found among Egyptian women in various clinical studies (Abdullah, Zarzoor, and Ali 1982; Inhorn and Buss 1993; Serour, El Ghar, and Mansour 1991). For example, in one major study of nearly fifteen hundred infertile couples in Cairo, Serour, El Ghar, and Mansour, preeminent Egyptian infertility investigators, found tubal-factor infertility to be present among 42 percent of all couples, making it the leading cause of infertility in the study sample. As they noted:

> All . . . studies show that tubal obstruction or pathology is the commonest cause of infertility in Egypt. This is in agreement with other workers who reported . . . similar and sometimes much higher rates in other developing countries. The high incidence of tubal factor in this study is due to the increased rate of post-partum and post-abortive infections, folk methods for treatment of infertility, post-operative adhesions following pelvic surgery, pelvic tuberculosis, non-sexually transmitted organisms and sexually transmitted diseases (STDs) [such] as gonorrhoea, chlamydial infection and mycoplasmas and possible bilharziasis. As most of the deliveries in Egypt are attended by the traditional birth attendant (DAYA) it is likely that post-partum infection will be an important cause of secondary infertility in Egypt. (1991:47)

In my own smaller-scale, case-control study of infertility in Alexandria, Egypt, 46 percent of infertile cases who were evaluated for tubal pathology had evidence of tubal-factor infertility. Given this high percentage, I attempted to assess the various factors, including all those mentioned by the Cairene investigators, that might place these lower-class, urban Egyptian women at risk of sterilizing tubal infection. Although the results of my epidemiological study have been reported in some detail elsewhere (Inhorn and Buss 1993; Inhorn and Buss 1994), it is important to note here that the three most important categories of risk for tubal-factor infertility in the study sample were: (1) the iatrogenic effects of the various invasive infertility treatments to be discussed in Chapter 9 of this book; (2) the "ethnoiatrogenic" effects of female circumcision, a widespread practice among the Egyptian urban and rural poor; and (3) the sterilizing effects of sexually transmitted diseases (STDs), primarily genital chlamydial infections.

To a large extent, problems of both biomedical iatrogenesis and STDs are attributable to political-economic transformations that have metamorphosed Egyptian society over the past four decades, particularly since the

1952 military revolt that resulted in the overthrow of the monarch, King Farouk, and brought President Gamal Abdel Nasser to power. The revolution instigated a number of fundamental and far-reaching changes in Egyptian society. Among the most basic were land reform, Egyptianization of assets, and the nationalization of the Suez Canal Company (Gadalla and Rizk 1988). The Land Reform Act, instituted by the socialist Nasser in part to wrest power from the urban, landed bourgeoisie, increased the private land ownership of the *fallāḥīn* (peasants who were mostly landless sharecroppers before the revolution), by redistributing land in excess of two hundred *fadādīn*[6] (Ansari 1986; Gadalla and Rizk 1988). However, when Anwar Sadat came to power in 1970, reversals in socialist policy that had begun on a limited basis during Nasser's presidency were accelerated and carried out at the expense of the small peasants who had been the main beneficiaries of the agrarian reforms (Ansari 1986). Sadat offered political rehabilitation to prerevolutionary elites and desequestered land that had been confiscated under Nasser's socialist decrees. Sadat's open-door policy, which laid the cornerstone for a free-market economy, was the culmination of Sadat's efforts to lift the restrictions instigated under Nasser and to attract foreign investment to Egypt, especially from the West.

However, as Ansari (1986:5) describes it, this rapid reversal from a socialist to a free-market economy resulted in "the emergence of a mixed economy that combined the worst features of both systems." According to Ansari, "Egypt today gives the impression of affluent urban society amid massive poverty. Growth in the commercial and construction sectors contrasts sharply with the increasing impoverishment of the majority of the people. Industrialization has lagged behind, while importation of goods, including one-half of Egypt's food requirements, has continued apace, thus putting a heavy burden on the country's foreign exchange earnings and pushing its external debt even higher" (1986:5).

In addition, the 1967 war, which resulted in Egypt's loss of the Sinai Peninsula to Israel and Israel's occupation of the East Bank of the Suez Canal, was also responsible in part for the undermining of Egypt's economy and was largely responsible for the major influx of migrants from the war zone to Cairo (Abu-Lughod 1985). This, along with the failure of agricultural land reforms and the relocation of Nubians accompanying the construction of the Aswan Dam, led to massive demographic changes in the country, particularly rapid urbanization as a result of rural-to-urban migration. Furthermore, as Abu-Lughod (1985) notes, outmigration from Egypt, which had been relatively minimal before the early 1950s, increased dramatically following the 1967 war and involved the export of Egypt's trained manpower (including physicians), as well as its unskilled labor force.

Moreover, following the economic boom years of the 1970s when the government's open-door policy encouraged foreign investment in Egypt, when revenues from oil and the Suez Canal were high, and when many Egyptian male workers were able to send home remittances from neighboring petro-rich countries, Egypt experienced a relatively acute economic upheaval. A steep drop in oil prices in 1986, followed by the Gulf War in the early 1990s, put many Egyptian overseas laborers out of work, reducing remittances to Egypt and escalating the ranks of the landless unemployed, who flocked to urban areas.

Thus, over the past four decades, Egypt has experienced three types of large-scale population movement: internal, rural-to-urban migration; external outmigration; and return migration of large portions of the external labor force. With respect to the first, between 1960 and 1982, the Egyptian urban population increased from 38 to 45 percent, largely as a result of migration of Egyptians from rural to urban areas (Seifelnasr 1986; Gadalla and Rizk 1988). Three Egyptian governorates, Cairo, Giza (adjoining Cairo), and Alexandria, accounted for 55 percent of the total urban Egyptian population as of 1986 and attracted about 67 percent of the total inmigrants (Seifelnasr 1986). Today, the metropolitan area of Cairo alone has more than ten million residents; accommodates more than 20 percent of the total population of Egypt; increases in size by 350,000 each year; has population densities as high as 300,000 people per square mile; and is expected to reach seventeen to twenty million by the turn of the century, making it a true primate city (CAPMAS 1988; Schiffer 1988).

As a result of this rural-to-urban population movement, all aspects of the urban Egyptian infrastructure and economy, including housing, roads, water, sanitation, communication, electricity, and education and health facilities, have been taxed. Urban housing in particular is in notoriously short supply, causing inflated down payments on vacant units, which usually consist of only one or two rooms (Schiffer 1988). In addition, housing in Egypt, both urban and rural, is often of substandard quality. For example, in urban areas of Egypt, 7 percent of the population in 1985 was without safe water; 5 percent was without adequate sanitation; and 23 percent was without electricity (United Nations 1991). In Cairo as of 1988, 35 percent of the city's housing was deemed by the Egyptian government as unsafe for human occupancy because of serious structural problems. (The

Cairene earthquake of 1992, in which many houses collapsed in poor neighborhoods, serves as a grim reminder of this problem.)

As for external migration, it was negligible until the early 1970s (CAPMAS 1988). But, by the time the Egyptian census was taken in 1976, more than 1.4 million Egyptians were living abroad (CAPMAS 1988; Gadalla and Rizk 1988). By 1986, the official number of Egyptians working or living in other Arab countries (particularly the neighboring oil-producing countries of the Arab Gulf, Libya, and Iraq) was estimated at 2.25 million, approximately 5 percent of the total Egyptian population of 42.2 million (CAPMAS 1988; Gadalla and Rizk 1988). Furthermore, whereas internal migration in Egypt during this period often involved the movement of families (including women and children), this external migration of Egyptians to oil-rich Arab nations was comprised almost exclusively of adult males. Abu-Lughod (1985) describes this external migration to the "oil zones" as follows:

> For political as much as for economic reasons . . . capital does not flow into other regions of the Middle East which have large population surpluses but little capital (e.g., Egypt), but rather has been drained off for "recycling" in the developed world, which depends upon oil imports. Instead of capital being brought to labor, labor has gravitated to capital in the form of migrations to the oil-wealthy countries. Since this labor is not viewed as being within the same market as that of the "citizens" of these countries, all sorts of barriers are developing; these will eventually lead either to the substitution of "native" labor or to the formal crystallization of the migrants into a permanent undercaste. (1985:184)

Although largely proletarianized, Egyptian migrants to the oil-producing countries of the Middle East have found wage scales on the order of ten or more times those in Egypt to be worth the hardships of participation in migrant life. For example, in 1980, per capita income in Egypt was only $580 compared to $11,260 in labor-importing Saudi Arabia. As a result of its low per capita income, Egypt has been ranked on the lower end of the lower-middle-income group of nations, according to the classificatory system developed by the World Bank (Carney 1984; Faour 1989).

Because of its meager resource base compared to its oil-rich neighbors, Egypt can be described as a poor Arab nation, with a large, impoverished rural and urban underclass. As suggested by Ansari (1986), Egypt's pyramidal class structure is quite apparent, with a small, educated, mostly urban elite; a relatively small but growing, educated middle class; and a large population base of mostly lower- and lower-middle-class citizens in both rural and urban areas. Likewise, the population structure, like that of many other Third World countries, is pyramidal as well, with a large percentage of the total population consisting of dependent children under fifteen years of age. Thus, economic "providers" in Egypt constitute only 30 percent of the total population (Gadalla and Rizk 1988), due in part to the age structure of Egyptian society and the limited participation of women (officially 9 percent as of 1990) in the work force (United Nations 1991).

As a result of these various factors, wages in Egypt are not only low in general, but, in the public sector, are both low and tied to educational certificates that many Egyptians do not hold. The result is an inefficient public-service sector staffed by poorly paid employees who therefore manifest little incentive to increase productivity; and a swollen private sector that cannot possibly employ the multitudes of unskilled, semiskilled, and highly skilled professional laborers who seek private employment (Institute of Medicine 1979). Currently, the major urban centers—Cairo, with more than half of the total urban population, and Alexandria, with nearly a quarter of it—suffer from a serious shortage of jobs (Schiffer 1988). As a result, many Egyptian men, who constitute the bulk of the labor force, seek to supplement their incomes with second or third jobs in the Egyptian private sector or choose the often more lucrative avenue of labor abroad.

Given the contemporary economic climate in Egypt, which, to summarize, is marked by low wages, spiraling inflation, un- and underemployment, inflated housing prices, and occasional "bread riots" over the increasing cost of subsidized foodstuffs (El-Sokkari 1984; Ansari 1986), it is not surprising that many Egyptian men choose or are forced to migrate, either within or outside of Egypt. For example, among the 190 women who participated in this study (see Appendixes 1 and 2), 30 percent of their husbands had migrated abroad—79 percent of these during the postmarital period and, in almost every case, without their wives.

Studies from around the world and from Africa in particular have shown that male labor migration brings with it a variety of social ills, one of the primary ones being infertility-producing—and even life-threatening—STDs, including AIDS (Inhorn and Brown 1990). Given strict cultural norms regarding women's premarital virginity and marital fidelity, Egyptian women themselves are unlikely sources of sexually transmitted infection. Rather, their husbands, many of whom migrate for extended periods, may contract gonorrhea, genital chlamydial and other sterilizing infections primarily from prostitutes, who serve as a major reservoir of infection.

Although information about prostitution in the religiously conservative nations of the Middle East is limited, prostitution is known to exist in most Arab countries, including the urban areas of Egypt (Inhorn and Buss 1993). Thus, the migration-prostitution-STD triad found in sub-Saharan Africa and other parts of the Third World is probably operative in Egypt as well. That it is linked to STD-induced tubal-factor infertility is also likely, based on studies that are beginning to emerge from both rural and urban Egypt showing rates of various STDs similar to those found in the West.[7] As one concerned Egyptian biogynecologist lamented:

> [Sexually transmitted disease] is, I think, the major factor [in tubal-factor infertility]. Many of these husbands get some sort of practice before marriage. Many times, it is a eunuch [i.e., homosexual] practice! He may take some sort of antibiotic or chemotherapy, but this is not enough to overcome the infection, and he can't go to a doctor and tell him he is practicing [i.e., premarital or extramarital sex], so the infection becomes chronic in his prostate. A real factor in primary infertility in our community is husbands who have chronic prostatitis. The first night [i.e., the wedding night], they inject the pus, or organism, into the vagina of their wives, causing ascending infection, which destroys the tubes. After some time, the doctor discovers the cause [i.e., tubal-factor infertility]. The man can be treated and sometimes he is okay. So he's the origin. And many of the wives lost their fertility and their marital life while they were just innocent and didn't know. . . . If a father is responsible for his newly married daughter, he should ask for a semen analysis to be sure [about STDs], because [her husband] can destroy her tubes from the first night.

In addition to husbands "destroying the tubes" of their wives, physicians may unwittingly *cause* tubal-factor infertility among their patients through invasive procedures that lead to pelvic infection. According to many university-based Egyptian biogynecologists, iatrogenic potential in Egypt is great, with many Egyptian women being subjected to multiple reproductive procedures that may be complicated by tubal-infertility-producing infection. In biomedical (as well as ethnomedical) settings in Egypt, the idea of sterile technique, based on Western notions of germ theory, is often lacking. Instead, techniques are often septic, or infection-producing.

In the area of reproductive health, most Egyptian women over the course of their lifetimes are subjected to one or more potentially septic procedures. In the ethnogynecological realm, these may include female circumcisions; traditionally induced abortions; deliveries by midwives; and a variety of vaginally invasive procedures used by healers to treat infertility (to be described in Chapters 5 and 6). Although Egyptian biogynecologists are often quick to point to *dāyāt*, traditional midwives, as the primary contributors to problems of sepsis in women, many university-based Egyptian biogynecologists also acknowledge the significant problem of sepsis produced in biomedical settings. Included among the possible biomedical sources of sepsis cited by them are hospital and clinic (public and private) deliveries, both vaginal and caesarean; intrauterine fetal deaths and miscarriages followed by dilatation and curettage (D & C); so-called criminal abortions by physicians (abortions are illegal in Egypt); intrauterine device insertions; and unindicated abdominal surgeries, especially appendectomies and urinary tract operations undertaken for the complications of schistosomiasis. In addition, many of these physicians point to the septic potential of practices used in the putative *treatment* of infertility in Egypt—practices to be described in detail in Chapter 9.

According to these physicians, there are two major reasons why these invasive procedures continue to be practiced on a widespread basis throughout the country. First, invasive procedures are performed by many physicians as money-making ventures in an economic climate of stiff competition for paying clientele. Because of the aforementioned economic problems in Egypt, because of an ill-coordinated national health policy that has led to the training of excessive numbers of Egyptian physicians, most of whom want to practice in urban areas (Institute of Medicine 1979), and because women desperate to become pregnant are often willing to subject their bodies to costly invasive procedures and may even request these procedures from physicians, Egyptian physicians may feel that they are under considerable pressure to perform invasive reproductive procedures as a source of significant income and as a means of attracting patients. Second, as we shall see in Chapter 9, many physicians perform such procedures because they deem them standard practice, even when the procedures are outdated and potentially harmful to patients. Thus, as it now stands, women in Egypt who go to physicians, in some cases hoping to become pregnant, may be at significant risk of irreparable, infertility-producing tubal damage through procedures currently used to treat them. The irony of this situation is not lost on many university-based Egyptian biogynecologists, who decry the current state of affairs in their country. However, as they also acknowledge, the current climate of irrationality and iatrogenesis in Egyptian biogynecology, and infertility management in particular, is unlikely to change substantially without radical transformations in Egyptian biomedical education and the elimination of the physician glut in urban areas that has promoted truly unhealthy competition.

In addition to problems of tubal-factor infertility, ovarian-factor infertility, the second leading cause of female infertility in Egypt (Serour, El Ghar, and Mansour 1991), is clearly linked to changes in dietary practices accompanying rural-to-urban migration and resultant high rates of female obesity among poor urban women. Studies in the West have shown that women who are even mildly obese may be anovulatory, as are women who are excessively underweight (Bates 1984; Green, Weiss, and Daling 1988; Hartz et al. 1979; Kissebah, Freedman, and Peiris 1989).

The tendency toward obesity among poor urban Egyptian women appears to be related to three major factors. First, mild female obesity is a cultural ideal in Egypt, one to which many women aspire. As in many other cultures, leanness is a sign of poverty and excessive manual labor and is not something which Egyptians, men or women, wish upon themselves. Among women, informal pubertal "fattening" may occur, in part to signify the transition from girlhood to adulthood and accompanying marriageability. Women who remain thin after marriage often view this as a problem, as do their husbands, who desire a plump wife to "fill their eyes." However, it is also important to note that many women who begin marriage with "ideal," mildly obese body types end up expanding after marriage from mild to moderate or severe obesity.

Second, obesity among poor urban women is clearly related to traditional diets rich in starches (such as rice, pita bread, macaroni), refined sugar, and saturated animal fats used as cooking oil. Among the urban poor, diets are low in proteins from dairy products and meats, fruits, and a variety of vegetables, all of which are unaffordable on a regular basis. Indeed, among the poorest families, the diet may consist almost exclusively of rice, fava beans, and bread. Furthermore, vegetable products, when prepared, are often brimming in saturated palm oil or a clarified beef fat called *samna*. Thus, the urban poor diet is high-fat, high-starch, and usually low in other important nutrients.

Third, among poor urban women, the loss of productive roles has been accompanied by a substantial reduction in household physical labor. Urban homes consisting of only one or two small rooms allow very little room for movement, and although cleaning, washing, marketing, and cooking involve some physical exertion, sustained aerobic exercise is essentially lacking for most women in the urban environment. This situation contrasts significantly with that of rural areas, where women participate in agricultural labor, walk great distances to do their marketing, to fetch water, and so on, and undertake sometimes excessive physical labor within the household itself. Yet, the transition from the traditional labor-intensive agrarian to the physically restrictive urban Egyptian life-style has not been accompanied by a substantial change in diet or diminution in caloric intake. Diets among the rural poor are not markedly different from those among the urban poor; yet, the amount of exercise is vastly diminished among the latter, especially among women.

Moreover, among poor urban *infertile* women, the tendency toward obesity is even more pronounced. Egyptian biogynecologists, noticing this tendency, believe that infertile women "eat out of boredom." To a certain extent, this may be true, in that infertile women may look for comfort in food rather than the children who are missing from their lives. Furthermore, infertile women without children may simply have more disposable income with which to purchase a greater quantity and variety of foodstuffs. And, once this food is prepared, there are fewer mouths to feed in infertile households.

Although a combination of factors is certainly responsible for urban Egyptian female obesity, many urban Egyptian women suffer from the obesity-linked chronic "diseases of modernization," including hypertension, diabetes, and heart disease. These, in turn, lead to substantial morbidity and reduced longevity (Galal 1992). Obesity, too, is related to the significant problem of ovarian-factor infertility in Egypt, with large numbers of overweight urban women suffering from sometimes intractable amenorrhea, other menstrual irregularities, anovulation, and polycystic ovary syndrome (Inhorn 1991; Serour, El Ghar, and Mansour 1991).

It is important to point out that these are not the only causes of infertility in Egypt; for example, male-factor infertility can be shown to be related to men's heavy smoking and various unhealthful occupational exposures (Inhorn and Buss 1994). Nevertheless, from this discussion of female infertility, it can be seen that the infertility problem in Egypt is, in fact, a political-economic one, which, in order to be fully understood, must be assessed epidemiologically and situated historically, politically, and economically. When such merging of perspectives takes place, it is apparent that the leading causes of female infertility in Egypt—tubal- and ovarian-factor infertility—are tied to historically recent processes of underdevelopment, which have resulted in economic impoverishment of the majority of the Egyptian populace, accompanying survival-oriented movements of the Egyptian body politic, and the introduction of health problems linked to these population movements and, more specifically, to attempts by Egyptian male heads of households to ensure their families' economic survival in an inauspicious environment.

Although the ultimate causes of infertility in Egypt can be viewed in this way, the "political epidemiology of infertility" offered here is not an indigenous perspective. As I have noted elsewhere (Inhorn and Buss 1993), neither epidemiology nor the political economy of health are well-developed orientations in either academic or biomedical circles in Egypt. Rather, as we shall see, Egyptians of all stripes, be they patients, traditional healers, or physicians, seek *their* ultimate explanations of infertility from God, who controls *both* fertility and infertility, problems that are related.

The Fertility-Infertility Dialectic and Other Lacunae

Understanding the infertility experience in a poor country such as Egypt may shed significant light on issues of *fertility*. Fertility and infertility exist in a dialectical relationship of contrast, such that understanding one leads to a much greater understanding of the other. Infertility, in particular, provides a convenient lens through which fertility-related beliefs and behaviors can be explored; these include, among other things, ideas about conception and how it is prevented both intentionally and unintentionally; understandings of, attitudes toward, and practices of contraception; beliefs about the importance of motherhood, fatherhood, and children themselves; and perceptions of risk and risk-taking regarding the body and its reproductive processes.

Because such information is crucial in designing culturally sensitive family planning programs, it is ironic that infertility has generally been viewed as an inconsequential problem on the national policy level in countries around the world (Schroeder 1988). Rather, attention is directed almost entirely to issues of fertility and especially to their articulation with the problem of poverty. To wit, in the now burgeoning literature on Middle Eastern fertility trends and family planning initiatives, information on infertility is often inserted as an interesting but irrelevant aside.[8] From a reading of this literature, it would appear that most of the Middle Eastern, as well as Western, intellectuals writing about the topic of Middle Eastern fertility have largely accepted what George (1977) has called the "population myth"—namely, that the major problem facing a Third World country such as Egypt is its high birth rate, leading to overpopulation and poverty. However, in his penetrating critique of United States development industry involvement in Egypt, Mitchell (1991) deconstructs the Egyptian overpopulation myth, arguing, in effect, that livestock—not humans—are "overpopulating" the country, in response to Western development industry pressures to increase meat consumption among the urban elite by converting large tracts of arable land into fodder for livestock production.

Unfortunately, in accepting the notion that Egyptians and other Middle Easterners are "hyperfertile" and in need of reproductive regulation, both Western and indigenous scholars and population policymakers have largely disregarded the problem of infertility, the human suffering engendered by it, and what it can tell us about fertility trends and reproductive desires. The case of Egypt stands out in this regard. Egypt has been considered the quintessential example of the purported nexus between excessive fertility and overpopulation in the Middle East and, as such, has been the experimental site of early and repeated population control efforts (Gadalla 1978; Stycos et al. 1988). Yet, as the first Middle Eastern Muslim country to initiate a statewide family planning campaign, Egypt has achieved little success over thirty years in controlling population growth (Stycos et al. 1988). Over the past decade, Egypt's annual population growth rate has actually *increased* rather substantially from 2.2 percent during the period from 1965 to 1980 to 2.7 percent during the 1980s (Mitchell 1991).

Furthermore, distinctly absent from Egypt's family planning strategy is any attempt to provide services for those who desire children but are unable to have them. Given the national policy obsession with population control, infertility is clearly not considered a priority in Egypt, although women seeking services at maternal and child health clinics and other government-sponsored facilities throughout the country often come in search of infertility treatment. In fact, in their assessment of health-care utilization in Ismailia, Egypt, Abu-Zeid and Dann (1985) noted that infertile patients far exceed other categories of patients in terms of average health-care expenditures, suggesting that their needs are not being met in "free" government health-care facilities. Frankly, at the present time, infertility services in Egypt are not coordinated in any manner and are available primarily through private sources, be they hospitals, clinics, or private practitioners (biogynecologists or ethnogynecologists), who offer care on a fee-for-service basis. What is not known — but what is crucial information in the development of population policy — is what happens to infertile couples who eventually conceive with such treatment. Do they go on to limit their family sizes? Or, given their previous frustrations and fears of contraceptive-related secondary infertility, do they go on to have large family sizes — larger than if their infertility had been systematically handled early on?

It is important to note that the lack of national policy and coordinated services for infertility is not limited to Egypt or the rest of the developing world. In the United States, critics have pointed to the problem of differential access to infertility care and the fact that little has been done on a policy level to rectify this situation (Holbrook 1990; Schroeder 1988). As it now stands in the United States, only the affluent, who can afford costly infertility services out of pocket, tend to receive optimal treatment, given the tendency of health insurance companies to view infertility services as elective. Because most studies of infertility carried out in the West have focused on patients seeking treatment, little is known about the untold numbers of women and their husbands who are unable to afford biomedical infertility interventions, which are only occasionally paid for by insurance policies among those who happen to be covered.

As in the United States, infertility diagnostic and treatment services in Egypt tend to be costly over time, given that they are paid for out of pocket and involve expensive drugs and surgical interventions. Hence, affording these services tends to be particularly problematic for the Egyptian poor, whose poverty limits options in other areas of life as well. Although some callous observers argue that "poor people who can't afford treatment shouldn't be having children in the first place," it is fair to say that Egyptians' relatively strong desires for children cross class lines and are perhaps even more intense among the poor.

Understanding why poor Egyptians want children is particularly important, given that the lower class constitutes the bulk of the Egyptian populace. The desire for children and the level of childbearing among the urban poor is, in many ways, tied to (if not directly determined by) membership in the urban underclass, which, as discussed, is rapidly growing with rural-to-urban migration. Although pronatalism among the urban poor is beyond the scope of this discussion and is explored elsewhere in detail (Inhorn n.d.), suffice it to say here that children become one's primary capital, less a means of production in the urban environment than a form of symbolic capital and perpetuity after death. With widespread anomie and alienation in the urban environment, the Egyptian poor look to their children as compensation for all that is lacking in their lives of hardship and despair. This may be especially true of poor urban men, whose children stand as proof of their virility and masculine procreativity and who may, as a result, exert significant pressure upon their wives to bear many children (El-Mouelhy 1990; Inhorn 1994a). Furthermore, the loss of women's productivity in the urban household economy and the consequent obsessive focus on *re*productivity among poor urban women in Egypt should not be underestimated in discussions of both fertility and infertility.

That the fertility-infertility dialectic has been neglected by population policymakers is not surprising, given that infertility has also been underprivileged as a topic of serious scholarly investigation. In the Egyptian social scientific literature, for example, there are numerous passing references to the social problems posed by infertility and even occasional presentations of case histories of infertile women.[9] However, amid the serious coverage of a variety of reproductive topics—including female circumcision (Assaad 1980; Gordon 1991; Kennedy 1970; Meinardus 1967), birth (Morsy 1982), midwifery (El-Hamamsy 1973; El Malatawy 1985; Khattab 1983; Morsy 1982; Nadim 1980; Sukkary 1981), indigenous fertility regulation (Sukkary-Stolba 1985), nonindigenous fertility regulation (DeClerque et al. 1986; Fox 1988; Gadalla, McCarthy, and Campbell 1985; Gadalla, Nosseir, and Gillespie 1980; Stokes, Schutjer, and Poindexter 1983), and breastfeeding (Harrison et al. 1993)—in-depth, analytical investigation of infertility in Egypt has been wholly neglected.

That infertility has been ignored in the social scientific literature on Egypt is frankly not surprising, when one considers the Eurocentric focus of infertility scholarship in general. Social scientific study of infertility has been oriented almost exclusively to the problems of affluent Western women (primarily those in America, Western Europe, and Australia)—so much so that infertility appears from this literature to be an exclusively Western, bourgeois concern. In some senses, Western feminist social scientists are particularly guilty of wearing cross-cultural blinders. Despite burgeoning and intellectually provocative literature on the patriarchal perils of the new reproductive technologies,[10] discussion of the human suffering engendered by infertility in the often emphatically pronatalist societies of the non-Western world, as well as that engendered by the misappropriation and misapplication of technology in these settings, has been woefully absent in feminist studies.

Similarly, with a few notable exceptions,[11] medical anthropologists have been rather silent on the topic of infertility and other issues of reproduction gone awry (e.g., miscarriage, ectopic pregnancy, stillbirth). In my view, this is remarkable, given the fascination within medical anthropology with what Browner and Sargent (1990:217) have called "paradigms of maternity," or "the socially and culturally constructed forces that shape maternal roles, childbirth, and related reproductive activities and that link culturally constituted notions of femininity and maternal behavior." In their excellent review of the anthropological literature on human reproduction, they summarize the multifarious, recent research on almost every aspect of the human reproductive life cycle—from the management of menstruation and menopause, to obstetrical events, to fertility regulation. Yet, as they note in their conclusion on "directions for future research," very little attention has been paid to issues of ethnicity and social class and their impact on women's reproductive desires and behavior; on the role of men in all aspects of human reproduction; and on the firsthand experiences of infertile women subjected to the new reproductive technologies. Likewise, in their recent review of the largely anthropological literature on the "politics of reproduction," Ginsburg and Rapp (1991) note that the female life cycle has been "revisited" in the now abundant academic discourse on fertility control, adolescence and teen pregnancy, birth, motherhood and nurturance, and the meanings of menopause. But what of those women whose unfolding life cycle is thwarted? As in the aforementioned literature review by Browner and Sargent, the problems of infertile women are indexed only in passing under discussion of the new reproductive technologies. This is less a problem of the reviews themselves than of the state of the current medical anthropological literature, in which scant reference has been made to the multidimensional problems of the infertile and especially infertile women, who, as it now stands, remain a "muted" group (Ardener 1978).

Furthermore, the medical anthropological literature on the Middle Eastern region[12] is (1) relatively sparse, especially in comparison to works from Asia, Latin America, and the West; (2) scattered in various, often obscure, collected volumes and journals; (3) diverse in subject matter and thus lacking comparative, synthesizing, analytical traditions; (4) largely descriptive rather than theoretical; and (5) plagued by "socioculturalism" and "reductionism" in its focus on local-level belief systems at the expense of power relations, class differences in health care, and the impact of colonialism and neocolonialism on health (Morsy 1981). There are also very few major works in Middle Eastern medical anthropology. Perhaps this is why Abu-Lughod's (1989) recent review of "zones of theory" in Middle Eastern anthropology lacks explicit reference to medical anthropology, including in her overview of "unexplored areas." Morsy's very recent volume, *Gender, Sickness, & Healing in Rural Egypt: Ethnography in Historical Context* comprises the first bonafide medical anthropological ethnography on the Muslim Middle East. The few other book-length works devoted to medical anthropological themes have not been written by medical anthropologists per se and focus primarily on the exotic world of the spirit possessed (Crapanzano 1973; Boddy 1989) and drug users (Kennedy 1987). (Morsy's book is also devoted in part to spirit possession.) Indeed, spirit possession and female circumcision — two areas of overemphasis in the limited Middle Eastern medical anthropological literature (Pillsbury 1978) — have become "theoretical metonyms" (Appadurai, cited in Abu-Lughod 1989), standing for the entire corpus of belief and practice pertaining to health and illness in the Middle East. That this could not be further from the truth should become apparent in this examination of infertility in Egypt, where, for example, spirit possession and hence the *zār* ceremonies necessary to placate the spirits of the possessed have little bearing on the lived experiences of poor urban infertile women in their health-seeking quests. (This is not to say that infertile women in the urban Egyptian environment do not interact with the spirit world. But, as we shall see, their interactions with spirits do not normally involve possession.)

The unfortunate upshot of the rather limited focuses of Middle Eastern medical anthropological scholarship is that certain realms of belief and experience have been privileged to the exclusion of important others. For example, in her early review of traditional health care in the Middle East, Pillsbury (1978) was forced to gather largely anecdotal and only partial information from a small number of Middle Eastern countries because, as she lamented, relatively little was known at that time about traditional medicine in the Middle East. Unfortunately, over the past decade and a half, little has changed. There are still no comprehensive studies of ethnomedicine or medical pluralism from any part of the Middle East, despite the rich, historical medical traditions found throughout this region. Furthermore, the recent spate of suggestive historical works, all of which examine the rise of various medical traditions, are devoted exclusively to Egypt and, as histories, do not extend into the contemporary period (Dols 1984; Gallagher 1990; Kuhnke 1990; Sonbol 1991).

Beyond medical pluralism in the Middle East, little has been written about such important topics as perceptions of pain and suffering, the body as the site of social inscription and control, the therapeutic encounter, including in clinical settings, strategies for coping with mental illness and disability, stigma and social labeling, the socialization and professionalization of healers, symbolic healing, the pharmaceuticalization and commodification of health, the household production of health, therapy management and health-seeking behavior, the reproduction of biomedical knowledge and praxis, and the technological imperative in health care. Obviously, this is not an exhaustive list; however, it does point to some important, unexamined issues.

Furthermore, although a great deal of recent scholarship has been devoted to Middle Eastern women, including to the understanding of contemporary Egyptian women's lives,[13] little if any attention has been devoted specifically to women's healing pilgrimages, although a few authors have touched on this subject in their examination of Muslim women's religious experience and everyday life (Betteridge 1992; Early 1993b; Mernissi 1977). Yet, as we shall see in the case vignettes to be presented in this book, infertile Egyptian women are peripatetic pilgrims, traveling not only to sacred sites, but to physicians, pharmacists, and healers in what they so poetically call their "search for children." As Morinis (1992:1) states: "Pilgrimage is born of desire and belief. The desire is for solution to problems of all kinds that arise within the human situation. The belief is that somewhere beyond the known world there exists a power than can make right the difficulties that appear so insoluble and intractable here and now. All one must do is journey."

In this book, we will meet many sojourners, women searching for a solution to their unacceptable childlessness in a world filled with fertile others. Whether or not they solve their problem (and, in this book, few do), many of these women manifest a heroic quality in their refusal to give up on their costly, time-consuming, often tortuous quests for conception; in their resilience following sickening therapeutic regimens; in their sacrificing of meaningful possessions, bodily integrity, and emotional well-being in their determination to be cured; and in their bravery in confronting and learning to cope with the problematic social world of discontented husbands, adversarial in-laws, suspicious neighbors, fraudulent healers, and supercilious physicians. That they survive multiple encounters of an overtly taxing nature is a testament not only to their suffering, but to their courage and to their unceasing hope.

The (Infertile) Anthropologist and the Egyptian Infertile

That this book is concerned with the conceptive quests of poor infertile Egyptian women is not simply fortuitous. As an American medical anthropologist, I first became interested in the problem of infertility while conducting fieldwork on blinding eye disease in an Egyptian Delta village in 1985–86. In the course of casual conversation, I noticed that asking women about their children was often disturbing to them. Women with children tended to dissimulate, either telling me that they had fewer children than they actually had, or that they wished they did not have so many children, or that they wished that I, too, would someday have many children. On the other hand, when I asked married women who had no children whether they had them or wanted to have them, the discomfort on their part was so obvious that I felt I had made a grave faux pas by even asking. The typical response was "*lissa*," which glosses as "still," "not yet," or "waiting." The obvious implication was that these married women without children were waiting for something that they wanted but still did not have.

It soon became apparent to me that *not* having children was nothing short of a cultural calamity for women in Egypt. I, as a 28-year-old woman with no husband and no children (and frankly over-the-hill by rural Egyptian standards), was perceived as an anomaly by some, especially given my tendency to wear pants, a distinctly male garment. Among other women, I was viewed as a threat, an unmarried women deemed potentially envious of them and their marital and reproductive success. In fact, in one household in which I spent a day conducting structured observations, little did I know that the many children on whom I was bestowing lavish compliments and attention were being systematically removed from the household, lest I cast the covetous evil eye on them.

In other words, during the initial stages of my first Egyptian fieldwork, I was extremely naive about the importance of children to Egyptians and the importance of being a married mother—a status that I could not claim and for which I was either pitied or feared. With additional, subtler inquiry, I soon learned that Egyptian women who are married but infertile face a rather unhappy fate, one that I resolved to study.

Two and a half years later, I returned to Alexandria, Egypt, to examine the impact of infertility on women's lives. Ironically, a week before my departure for Egypt, I had been given a presumptive diagnosis of endometriosis, a condition related to infertility. This, coupled with the fact that I had been married for nearly two years and had not yet produced any children, made me infertile in the eyes of my informants. In fact, within days of my arrival in Egypt, I began to recognize a series of five questions that I would be asked during virtually every encounter (including even the most casual encounters with taxi drivers and shopkeepers). The conversation proceeded as follows:

> "Are you married?"
> "Yes."

"Is your husband Egyptian or American?"
"American."
"Do you have any children?"
"No."
"Do you want children?"
"Yes."
"Then why don't you have any children?"
"It hasn't happened yet."

To my informants who asked me such questions, I explained that children are not as crucial to most American marriages and that some couples practice birth control throughout marriage so as to prevent conception altogether. However, I was quick to point out that I wanted children and that I hoped my purported endometriosis would not prevent me from having them. The disclosure of information on my part, which often occurred early on in my interactions with infertile women, served to break the ice and to encourage these women, who had often been extremely guarded in their relationships, to open up to me. Indeed, our joke with one another was "*fil hawā' sawa*," or, "in the air together," which is the Egyptian equivalent of the American expression, "We're all in the same boat."

Because of this relationship of camaraderie and because of my assurances of confidentiality, many women disclosed for the first time, sometimes accompanied by weeping, the problematic realities of their lives. For example, one woman sobbed as she described the deaths of all three of her sons, the fact that she could not get pregnant again, and her husband's current wish to remarry. Another woman burst into tears as she related the utter loneliness of being a childless woman confined to a small, dark, one-room apartment and sleeping alone at night while her husband traveled aboard a ship in the Mediterranean three weeks out of every month in order to support her infertility treatments. Several women who were in various stages of divorce because of infertility wept as they recounted the humiliations endured at the hands of their husbands and in-laws, who had initiated the divorce proceedings with insults and arguments.

I soon realized—and was often told as much by these women—that my private interviews and conversations with them were serving as therapeutic encounters. Although I could offer relatively little in the way of tangible aid (see Appendix 1), I was able to serve as a nonjudgmental, sympathetic listener for women who had had little opportunity to express their pent-up anxieties, grievances, and fears.

The fact that I dealt almost exclusively with these troubled women, as opposed to men, was both intentional and an artifact of the fieldwork process itself. On the one hand, I intended to produce a study that was gynocentric, given my feminist interests in women's issues in general and women's health issues in particular. In designing this research, I was extremely cognizant of the fact that in Egypt, infertility tends to be viewed as a woman's, rather than a man's or a couple's, problem. In fact, among poor women, infertility treatment is rarely undertaken by couples, given that, on the official social structural, ideological, and linguistic levels (Bourdieu 1977), "couples" do not exist in Egypt (see Inhorn n.d. for a fuller discussion of this theme). In the research setting, I soon discovered that husbands only occasionally accompany their wives for infertility treatment and usually only on days in which their semen is needed for analysis or artificial insemination. Furthermore, because most Egyptian men work during morning hospital or clinic hours, they are unable—or, in some cases, unwilling—to participate in their wives' infertility diagnosis and management.

The woman-centered focus of this book is also a reflection of the research process and my differential access to women and men. My study was based in a woman's hospital, the infertility clinic of the University of Alexandria's Shatby Hospital, and my informants, naturally, were women. During the fifteen-month research period, from October 1988 through December 1989, I conducted both participant observation and semistructured but highly open-ended interviews in this hospital with 190 women, 100 of whom were infertile and 90 of whom were fertile and served as a comparison group. These interviews, which were conducted in Egyptian colloquial Arabic in a private room, lasted anywhere from two to twelve hours, depending on the loquaciousness of the informant and the depth of her personal biography. Following the interviews, I visited many of these women (particularly the infertile women) in their homes and home communities, where I socialized and conducted informal interviews with them, their husbands, families, and neighbors in some cases; collected the life histories of a number of infertile women; was introduced to and subsequently interviewed several traditional healers; observed women undertaking ethnogynecological remedies; accompanied women on pilgrimages to holy sites; and generally observed and participated in the ebb and flow of daily life in Alexandria's poorer neighborhoods where these women lived. (See Appendixes 1 and 2 for a fuller discussion of the fieldwork process and informants participating in the study.)

Through this research process, I eventually met many husbands—some of whom were infertile themselves and some of whom were quite open with and friendly toward me. Yet, I would characterize my interactions with men in my informants' homes — as well as in my own, where my informants and their husbands sometimes visited me — as being limited to formal hospitality. My level of understanding of men's lives, including those of my informants' husbands, was exceedingly superficial compared to my eventual knowledge of women's lives, both infertile and fertile. Thus, it is extremely important to state at the outset that I came to know much more about Egyptian *husbands*, as seen through the eyes of Egyptian wives, than about Egyptian *men* in either the general or the specific sense. In other words, this is a book about Egyptian women and their therapeutic quests, and to a much lesser extent, about Egyptian men, but only *from the women's point of view.*

Theoretically, I was not opposed to including men in my study. Nor would it have been impossible, given that urban Egyptian society is, generally speaking, not rigidly sex segregated. However, my own status as an American woman posed some obstacles to cross-sex research. Just as male anthropologists before me have found it difficult to mix with women, I found it difficult as an American woman to interact with Egyptian men on anything but a formal and somewhat superficial level. Any attempts at more intimate interaction, including the process of confidential interviewing about infertility, might have been mistaken as meaning something else, given the general impression of most Egyptians that American women are promiscuous, like the ones they view on the nighttime soap operas (for example, "Dallas," "Dynasty," "Falcon Crest," "Knots Landing") that are imported from the United States. Given this widely held impression, I was extremely cautious in my behavior with women's husbands, and I spoke to them about infertility only when I felt it was appropriate or when they had specific medical questions they wished to ask me, which was sometimes the case.

Second, given that infertility is both an intimate and sensitive issue, I felt that most Egyptian men might be uncomfortable speaking with me about this subject, just as many infertile Egyptian women are uncomfortable speaking about their problems with men, including male physicians. Although women's husbands occasionally shared confidences with me regarding their infertility problems, infertility was a subject that was rarely raised in conversation with me by men and never in the presence of others. Women, on the other hand, were rarely reluctant to divulge the most intimate details of their lives, including issues of infertility and sexuality. That very little is actually known about sexuality in the Middle East has been attributed, in part, to Western researchers' own reluctance to probe in this area (Keddie 1979). However, I found that women were not only willing to discuss their private lives, but were quite curious about Americans' lives and practices, which I attempted to explain to them. I attribute this sharing of information in large part to the privacy in which discussions took place and to my repeated assurances of confidentiality.

Frankly, I am quite certain that the ideal anthropological study of infertility in Egypt would be one conducted by a male-female research team, particularly by a husband and wife, who could interview husbands and wives separately and privately. Not only is information on men's social and therapeutic responses to male infertility desperately needed for Egypt and elsewhere, but there is relatively little information on men's responses to their wives' infertility or, on a more general level, the meanings and practices of fatherhood cross-culturally (Lamb 1987). That this is a prime area for anthropological research seems abundantly apparent. Yet, I will also argue that the study of infertility described in this book could not have been conducted by a male researcher, who, I believe, would have been unable to elicit information of such an intimate nature from women informants.

Meeting such infertile women was greatly facilitated by the location of this study, which, as mentioned earlier, was based in the infertility clinic of the University of Alexandria's Shatby Hospital. As a large, public teaching hospital, Shatby caters primarily to lower-class women from the Alexandria vicinity, who use the facility for both primary and tertiary care. In addition to the large number of deliveries that occur at Shatby each day, the hospital provides contraceptive services, a walk-in outpatient clinic for minor gynecological complaints and prenatal care, inpatient services for gynecological surgeries and childbirth, and an outpatient infertility clinic. As a public teaching hospital, most services are offered at a nominal charge.

The women attending the outpatient infertility clinic at Shatby were largely representative of the patient population as a whole: namely, poor urban women from Alexandria and its provincial outskirts. Occasionally, patients traveled to Shatby from as far away as Cairo for infertility services that they could not obtain at a low cost in that city. Likewise, rural women were occasionally referred to Shatby for infertility treatment that they could not obtain elsewhere, and they, too, were included in this study. In the vast majority of cases, these women were economically disadvantaged, uneducated, and illiterate, as seen in Appendix 2.

Although conducting fieldwork at Shatby allowed me access to a large population of poor infertile women, working with this particular population of women presented some interesting limitations. For one, those women who became my informants were (1) all seeking treatment for infertility, and (2) seeking that treatment at a hospital. Obviously, not all Egyptian women seek biomedical treatment for infertility, although I would wager a guess that most do, given the infertility histories of nearly a third of the *fertile* women who participated in my study and who had once sought treatment for perceived conceptive problems. In addition, infertile Egyptian women who end up seeking treatment at a hospital may represent more difficult, intractable cases of infertility. Thus, these women may not be representative of the wider population of infertile women, who may become pregnant spontaneously or with minimal interventions by either ethnogynecologists or biogynecologists working outside hospital settings.

Furthermore, it is important to note that this study was based in Alexandria, which, as will be described in the following chapter, may differ in some ways from other Egyptian cities and, as a large metropolis, is certainly different from Egypt's vast rural areas. Nevertheless, many of the women in this study were not Alexandrian by birth, hailing originally from other regions of Egypt, including rural areas. Ethnically, they represented all four of the major groups in Egypt, as indigenously defined (that is, Lower Egyptian, Upper Egyptian, Nubian, Bedouin). Thus, in a sense, women of the entire nation of Egypt were included in this study, and, from the standpoint of infertility, their problems and responses were very similar, suggesting that the infertility quest shares common features among women from all parts of the country.

It is also important to mention, I believe, how the findings of this study might have differed had I been an Egyptian anthropologist (educated, middle- or upper-class, Arabic and English speaking) working with these women (illiterate, lower- or lower-middle-class, and Arabic speaking). I would argue that, despite my lack of complete fluency in Egyptian colloquial Arabic and my reliance at times during formal interviews on the help of a bilingual research assistant, being an American woman—and, hence, an entirely anomalous being—was a distinct advantage in carrying out this study in some senses. For one, most of these women had never before met an American—or any foreigner, for that matter—and were extremely excited about making my acquaintance and, in some cases, becoming my friend. Not only was I proudly introduced by my informants to their neighbors as an "American *duktūra*," but I was often asked for pictures of myself and for other items that I could autograph in both English and Arabic. I believe that my very "Americanness" helped me to secure the

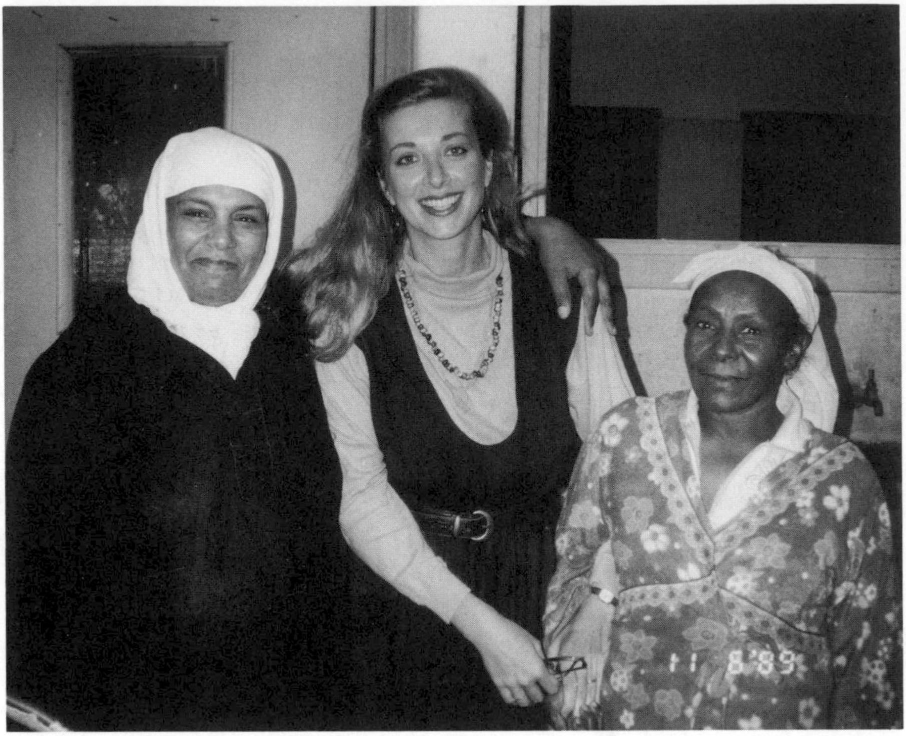

Photograph 1. The author with patients at Shatby Hospital. (Photograph by Margaret Hutchinson)

confidences of these women, since they knew that I would be returning to America, taking their secrets far away. Finally, and perhaps most important, my being American allowed me to overcome to some degree the class distinctions that sometimes radically separate Egyptians from each other. I was extremely conscious of attempting to overcome any power differentials between myself and the women with whom I was interacting, insisting that they dispense with the almost automatically ascribed *duktūra* title and call me by my first name, accepting invitations to their homes, inviting them to mine, and generally treating them with the respect and kindness that were sometimes lacking in their encounters with more educated, upper-class Egyptians, including physicians. Although the inherent asymmetries between "Self" and "Other" in the anthropological research encounter can never be overcome entirely, I attempted as much as possible to create a relatively egalitarian relationship between myself and my informants. I believe that, in most cases, women came to trust me and to view their interactions with me as cathartic experiences, as mentioned earlier.

Representing Women's Lives

In this book, I attempt to represent the lives of these infertile women as ones deeply engulfed in the care-seeking process. Because their "search for children" shares common features, I will concentrate on crosscutting themes. Nevertheless, these women's individual stories contain unique features and are usually poignant—some extremely so. In an attempt to represent both the commonalities and the special circumstances of their quests for therapy, I will draw upon individual case studies of women throughout this book and, on occasion, present fragments of women's therapeutic narratives in an attempt to give voice to their realities. Although I intend to make clear the profound difficulties of overcoming infertility for most of these women, I also intend to represent the dignity and resourcefulness with which they face the dilemmas of their infertile lives.

Furthermore, through case vignettes, I intend to focus on the lived experiences of infertile Egyptian women and the "local moral worlds" (Kleinman 1992) in which their quests for therapy take place. Because analysis of the experiential level has so often been overlooked in the literature on Middle Eastern women's lives—in favor of textual analysis, discourse analysis, symbolic analysis, and structural-functionalist analysis—certain subjects have been privileged at the expense of others. For example, in the Middle Eastern literature on women, concern with the discourse of "honor" and "shame" is widespread and, in my view, might have been usefully included as a fourth major theoretical metonym in Abu-Lughod's (1989) recent review of Middle Eastern anthropological theory (along with segmentation, the harem, and Islam).[14] Yet, the Egyptian women represented in my study were adamant that infertility has "nothing to do with honor and shame," given that infertility is nonvolitional and honor violations usually are. In other words, the preoccupation with certain subjects and discourses in the literature on Middle Eastern women has limited our understanding of other important issues, including problems of women's health that Middle Eastern women *themselves* perceive as morally problematic and even deeply threatening.

That infertility presents both moral dilemmas and serious disruptions in women's lives should become apparent in the chapters that follow. It is largely because of the *threatening* nature of infertility—to women's self-esteem and social status, to men's procreativity and lineage continuity, and to the reproduction of Egyptian society at large—that women who are infertile struggle so to overcome their childlessness. Their quest for conception—a quest that often involves pain, suffering, revulsion, violation, fear, despair, *and* inordinate hope and occasional joy—comprises the subject of this book.

2. Ancient Alexandria and Its Modern Poor

Afaf's Story

In the back alleys of Manshiyyah, the old market district of central Alexandria, there lives a young woman named Afaf, whose life is, and always has been, grim. From a poor family with too many mouths to feed, Afaf was "given away" at the age of three and a half to a wealthy Alexandrian family, with whom she was to spend more than twenty years as a domestic servant. In their spacious apartment in an upper-class neighborhood, Afaf was like a prisoner, who knew nothing of the world beyond the apartment walls. Kept inside, prevented from seeing her family, uneducated, unloved, and poorly paid, Afaf simply existed, washing the floors, wringing the laundry, and cooking the meals of her employers. When she reached her mid-twenties, her employers decided that they should not keep Afaf a spinster for life and so arranged a marriage for her with an employee of the husband's company. The groom, an exceptionally short, balding, chain-smoking, uneducated electrician, was totally unappealing to Afaf. However, as a domestic servant without active family ties, Afaf had virtually no say in the matter and felt compelled to accept the marriage arrangements—the only way out of her present degrading circumstances. Because Afaf's mistress continued to desire her services, the wedding was delayed for three years, during which time Afaf continued in the drudgery of domestic servitude. Yet, when the wedding day finally arrived, Afaf's spirits were low. Rashid, the little bald man with a nervous addiction to tobacco who was to become Afaf's husband, was a virtual stranger to her. Rashid and Afaf had never spoken at length, nor did Afaf feel attracted to him in any way. Because Rashid's monthly salary of thirty-five Egyptian pounds (equal to fourteen dollars) was extremely low, his savings over the years had enabled him to secure the most minimal of all apartments for himself and his new bride. On their wedding day, Rashid took Afaf from her employer's palatial apartment to her new home, a room about five-by-five meters in size in a dank, deteriorating building in the back streets of old Alexandria.

Since that day five years ago, Afaf has continued simply to "exist." Her days are spent alone in the cramped room—so small that the double bed occupies the bulk of the floor space. Afaf has learned how best to conserve square footage—for example, by hiding her antiquated, wringer-style washing machine under a small table with an obscuring tablecloth, by stuffing all of their possessions in the one wardrobe at the foot of the bed, and by using the refrigerator, the one "luxury" appliance, as a storage space as well. Because Afaf has no running water, she must fetch it each day from the building's communal tap, located near the communal squat toilet and shower in the first-floor interior atrium. The atrium, three floors in height, is dimly illuminated, and around it on each floor are the cramped rooms of other families living in similar conditions of dire poverty. Afaf mixes little with these neighbors, because, as an infertile woman, she is suspected of giving their children the "evil eye." Thus, Afaf's days are spent mostly alone in her room, with occasional forays out through the narrow, litter-strewn, mud alleys to the market or to the Islamic charitable clinics in her neighborhood where she often seeks free treatment for her infertility.

During only five years of an infertile marriage, Afaf has visited nearly twenty physicians, mostly at mosque-run Islamic clinics or public hospitals where treatment is largely free. Afaf believes in the ability of physicians to cure her of her infertility. "They examine you to see what's wrong," she says. "Doctors know what's inside of you, but these 'quacks' don't." The "quacks" to whom Afaf refers are ethnogynecologists, several of whom she has also consulted. For instance, shortly after her marriage, a *dāya*, or traditional midwife, made a house call to Afaf, examined her vaginally with her finger, and told Afaf that she had *dahr maftūḥ*, or an open back, which was causing her delayed conception. For two Egyptian pounds (eighty cents), the *dāya* provided Afaf with three *ṣūwaf*, or vaginal suppositories made of sheep's wool and a "smelly" substance. The *dāya* inserted one of these *ṣūwaf* deep inside Afaf's vagina to "close her back," and then told Afaf to insert and remove the remaining two over the next two days. However, Afaf "wasn't convinced" of the validity of the *dāya*'s recommendations and therefore failed to complete the cure.

However, as her infertility persisted, Afaf tried a number of other ethnogynecological therapies. On one occasion, she went to a special *'aṭṭār*, or herbalist, known for making *ṣūwaf* to "remove infections" and to "help with the things, the sisters, underground" (spirit-sisters believed to dwell beneath the surface of the earth and cause infertility). The herbalist made Afaf a series of seventeen *ṣūwaf* containing cloves, ground corn, wheat, barley, rose water, molasses, and "other things" with which Afaf was unfamiliar. The *ʿaṭṭār* told Afaf to dip one of these *ṣūwaf* in molasses and to wear it vaginally from morning until evening, beginning on the first day immediately following her menstrual period. She was to repeat this every other day until her next menstrual period arrived. However, Afaf's period came early, and seven unused *ṣūwaf* remained. Although the *ṣūwaf* did not cause Afaf to become pregnant, they "did some good" by removing all the water from her reproductive organs.

Eventually, Afaf did become pregnant, but she miscarried twice, both times early in the pregnancy. Following her miscarriages, her neighbor put an elastic band around her waist, upon which was a small lock to "close her back." Afaf was told to wear the lock and band until she became pregnant again and to continue to wear it throughout her pregnancy. On the day of delivery, the waistband could be unlocked. However, Afaf did not become pregnant again, so after two months, she removed the band.

After the failure of this method, her husband's sister brought her the *mushāharāt*, a collection of pebbles and clamshells from the sea. Afaf was told to immerse the *mushāharāt* in water during the time of the Friday noon prayer, and then to bathe herself with this water. She was to repeat this over three consecutive Fridays. According to Afaf, "They said at the time of my miscarriage, someone who shaved entered on me [in her room], or someone carrying raw meat or chicken—anything with blood." However, Afaf did not believe that she suffered from *kabsa*, or reproductive binding caused by such an entrance into her room. Rather, she attributed her infertility and miscarriages to her *dahr muftūḥ*, or open back, caused by her excessive childhood labor. Afaf recalled carrying something very heavy as a teenager and hearing her back crack. At that very moment, her menstrual period arrived several days early. Because she was forced as a servant to continue to carry heavy things, her back was never able to "close," and therefore she is unable today to become pregnant easily or to carry a pregnancy to term.

Although Rashid pressures Afaf to continue working as a day-laboring servant so as to alleviate somewhat their desperate financial situation, Afaf, tired of manual labor and annoyed that Rashid does not feel dishonored by the thought of his wife working, refuses his requests on account of her open back. When Afaf visits physicians, she always tells them about her open back, but the doctors never believe her, saying "this is empty talk." Instead, the doctors at Shatby, the public women's hospital where Afaf has decided to seek additional free treatment, have told her that her infertility is due to a postmiscarriage infection which has "blocked her ovaries." They have scheduled her for tubal surgery. Although Afaf will undergo the surgery reluctantly, she continues to believe that her miscarriages and subsequent infertility are caused by her open back. She also believes that Rashid, as the eldest son in a close-knit, pushy family, will repudiate her and take another wife if her surgery fails and she is unable to become pregnant. If this should come to pass, Afaf insists that she will never remarry, since she has "had enough of marriage to last a lifetime." Afaf does not really love Rashid, finds having sex with him to be deplorable, and fights with him almost continuously. Indeed, Afaf has never experienced love in her life. Yet, she continues to survive as one of the growing legions of urban poor Alexandrians.

In fact Afaf's present circumstances are not so unlike those of many other women in Alexandria, Egypt, whose lives are characterized by poverty, crowding, marital strife, uncertainty about the future, and perpetual distress. As the Alexandrian population continues to grow, with rural migrants to the city swelling the ranks of the urban poor, living space becomes less available, more expensive, and further afield from the city's core, and human relations in the urban environment become more and more attenuated. For many Alexandrians, the oft-cited expression *mafish khair* ("there is no goodness [anymore]"), is a reflection of their economic and social deprivation fostered by lack (and maldistribution) of basic economic resources, social isolation from extended-family networks, the stresses of male labor migration and asymmetrical gender relations, and the *anomie* of impoverished urban living, as described in Chapter 1.

Yet, when considering life as it is for millions of poor Alexandrians today, the question remains: Was life in Alexandria, Egypt, one of the most ancient metropolises in the world, always this way? To understand the changes that have affected this city—and the lives of the poor women who are its residents and the subjects of this book—it is necessary to consider briefly the cultural and political-economic history of the Mediterranean seaport that Alexandrians such as Afaf call home.[1]

Historic Alexandria

To begin, Alexandria was not part of Egypt's unique, pharaonic civilization dating to roughly 3000 B.C., but rather was founded much later, in 332 B.C., by twenty-five-year-old Alexander the Great, for whom Alexandria was named. Although Alexander is often thought of as being Greek in origin, he was actually the son of the Macedonian ruler, King Philip. Alexander continued his father's campaigns against the Greeks, overcoming them and making them vassals of his expanding empire. However, extremely appreciative of Greek culture and intellectual life—a love inculcated in part by his private teacher, Aristotle—Alexander ordered the building of Alexandria, the capital of his new Egyptian kingdom, according to Greek architectural plans. (Having given his orders, however, he never stayed long enough to see a single building rise.)

Upon the death of Alexander the Great in 323 B.C., one of his comrades, Ptolemy Soter, whom Alexander had placed in Egypt as satrap, came to rule the country, and it was during this Ptolemaic period, lasting from 323 to 51 B.C., that Alexandria became the seat of Egyptian culture and government, a cosmopolitan and religiously eclectic community, and a widely renowned center of learning. Under the first three Ptolemies, Alexandria was transformed into a magnificent Hellenistic city, complete with an immense lighthouse and a causeway connecting it to the shoreline, a great palace, a temple and royal tombs (including the Soma, the grand temple erected over the tomb of Alexander the Great), a theater, a racetrack, various gymnasiums and covered markets—all of it surrounded by a fortified wall.

According to one writer, "Alexandria was the New York of the ancient world; it was the first world city, enormously rich. . . . Like Manhattan, it was bordered by water and its streets were laid out in unvarying straight lines intersected by stately avenues. It, too, was the meeting and melting point of diverse races, languages, cultures, and religions, and was the city with the largest Jewish population in the world. . . . For more than three centuries, Alexandria was the most learned place on earth" (Elon 1988:44).

Indeed, the Mouseion, the great university of Alexandria, was the most stunning achievement of the early Ptolemies. The Mouseion housed lecture halls, laboratories, observatories, a park, a zoo, and, most important, a great library holding a purported 490,000 scrolls. According to Forster (1986: 20), "in some ways it resembled a modern university, but the scholars and scientists and literary men whom it supported were under no obligation to teach; they had only to pursue their studies to the greater glory of the Ptolemies."

During this period, science and mathematics advanced dramatically in Alexandria, and the city also became famous for its medical school, which was attended by a number of famous Greek physicians. Most important among them was Galen, the follower of Hippocrates and founder of a particularly influential brand of Hippocratic Greek medicine, which has come to be known as "Galenism," to be discussed in the following chapter.

Within three decades, however, Alexandria—and the last of the Ptolemies, Cleopatra—fell to the Romans. Octavian, later the Emperor Augustus, was installed in Egypt and adopted it as his personal property within the Roman Empire. Apparently, he so disliked Alexandria, which reminded him of the Greeks, that he founded another town to the east, turning Alexandria into a vast imperial granary. Following his death, however, Alexandria's situation improved, despite the fact that Christians, who had entered Alexandria and begun conversions in A.D. 45, suffered persecution and martyrdom during the Roman period (B.C. 30–A.D. 313). However, with the downfall of the Roman Empire, Christianity, which had continued its dispersion from Alexandria and had been made official in Egypt at the beginning of the fourth century, was made compulsory toward its close, and all things "pagan," including the great Alexandrian library and its holdings, were destroyed.

When the Muslims, under the Arab general Amr, invaded Christian Alexandria in A.D. 642, the city was still an architecturally magnificent Hellenistic capital, with most of its main buildings constructed from white marble. The Arabs did not destroy the city and its library, as is often suggested, but rather allowed many of these structures, as well as Alexandria's shoreline, waterways, and fortified walls, to fall into disrepair. For some time, the city was administered as a separate province. But, in the ninth century, Alexandria was administratively incorporated into the rest of Egypt, remaining the second most important city after Cairo, which became the new seat of Egyptian commerce and government.

Alexandria, now thoroughly Islamized, had a stable if uneventful history under the Arabs and Ottoman Turks. Under the Ottomans, a large foreign community received special protection and areas of the city reserved for their use, because they were important to Alexandria's maritime connections. However, at the turn of the eighteenth century (1798–1807), Alexandria experienced a series of foreign military invasions, including one by Napoleon, whose troops occupied the country from 1798–1801. The withdrawal of the French under British military pressure was followed by a period of anarchy, during which time a Turkish-speaking Ottoman officer of Albanian origin, Muhammad Ali, was able to jockey for power and seize control of Egypt as its governor.

Despite many disreputable features of his forty-three-year reign over

Egypt, Muhammad Ali realized the importance of maritime domination of the Mediterranean and proceeded to build an immense fleet, headquartered at Alexandria. It was thus Muhammad Ali who was responsible for rebuilding Alexandria as Egypt's major maritime port and cotton-exporting capital; for cutting the Mahmudiya Canal between Alexandria and the Nile and thus providing passage of Egyptian commodities to the Mediterranean and the European market; for converting Alexandria into the summer seat of government; and, as we shall see in the following chapter, for importing a system of European biomedicine into Alexandria and the rest of the country. Under Muhammad Ali and his imported European technical advisers, Alexandria once again became a thriving cosmopolitan city, eventually attracting both wealthy Egyptians and Europeans of predominantly Greek, Armenian, Italian, French, British, Spanish, and Maltese stock. These foreigners—many of whom like Muhammad Ali himself never bothered to learn Arabic—set up hotels and other businesses, influenced the transfer of their consuls general from the Levant ports to Alexandria, built palatial summer villas for themselves along the shores of the Mediterranean and the Mahmudiya Canal, and generally attempted to rebuild Alexandria along European lines.

The "Europeanization" of Alexandria continued under the British, who first bombed the city in 1882 and then came to control and reconstruct it, building a vast promenade along the seafront. In fact, the British, who began to arrive en masse in the 1890s, attempted to convert Alexandria into a British-style, seaside resort city—one which would become the eventual subject of wartime British writers, including E. M. Forster, who wrote Alexandria's history, and Lawrence Durrell, who wrote *The Alexandria Quartet*, a series of four novels set in the city.

But Durrell's Alexandria—enormously rich, romantic, and peopled only with wealthy, non-Muslim Egyptians and Europeans, including the mystical Greek poet, Cavafy—was an Orientalist fantasy. In reality, the ratio of Alexandrian Egyptians to Europeans, even during the foreign communities' acme, was always more than four to one, and the indigenous population did not necessarily fare so well economically under the British, who were not compelled to leave the country completely until the signing of the Anglo-Egyptian treaty in 1954.

Today, most of Alexandria's foreign communities, including its large Greek population, have left, some voluntarily and others by expulsion under Nasser. For example, English and French residents were expelled in 1956–57 following the Suez war and their property was confiscated. Within a few years, most of the Greeks and Italians were compelled to leave, along with Alexandria's ancient Jewish community, which once numbered more than twenty thousand. It is estimated that today there are fewer than ten thousand *khawagāt*, or foreigners, left in the city of an estimated five million.

Modern Alexandria

Today's Alexandria—once the ancient jewel of the Hellenic world—is a thoroughly Egyptian city, with relatively little other than a few deteriorating monuments and statues to remind its inhabitants of its two-thousand-year history. The western harbor of Alexandria, once one of the busiest seaports of the Mediterranean, is relatively inactive. And since the 1952 revolution, the Egyptian population of the city has soared—both through in-migration and natural increase—necessitating numerous hasty construction projects with none of the aesthetic appeal of the city's once glorious architecture. Furthermore, during the summer months, Alexandria's population overflows with affluent Cairenes, who venture to Alexandria as summer renters and tourists in order to escape Cairo's scorching summer heat and dry winds. However, because of Alexandria's recent, rapid industrialization, air quality—once considered superior to that of dusty, landlocked Cairo—has declined considerably in the past decade, adding asthma to rheumatism as major health complaints of the city's inhabitants.

Yet, despite Alexandria's "general air of exhaustion" (Elon 1988), Alexandrians are proud of their city's unique heritage and of their own identity as *Iskandarīyyīn*, or "the people of Alexandria"—whether or not their ties to the city have generational depth. To the residents of the city, Alexandria still has much to recommend it. Its Mediterranean climate is ideal—neither too hot in the sunny, breeze-cooled summers, nor too cold in the mild, rainy winters—and even the poor are able to take advantage of pleasant summer outings via public transportation to any one of Alexandria's many public beaches. Perhaps more important, the city is still less than half the size of Cairo; this means that it is less congested, less expensive to live in, and represents greater potential in terms of housing and employment, especially in the city's new industrial zones. And even the poor are able to afford occasional meals of delicious Mediterranean fish, brought in off wooden fishing dinghys and sold fresh at stands in the Bahriyyah section of Alexandria's western harbor.

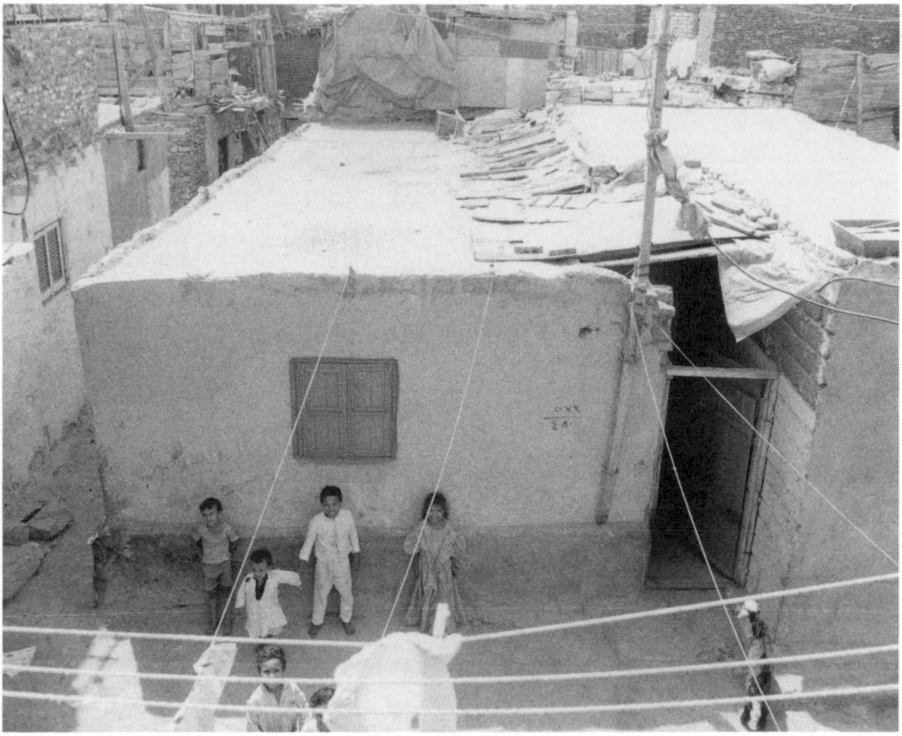

Photograph 2. A poor neighborhood in Alexandria's western harbor district. (Photograph by Mia Fuller)

Furthermore, for many Muslims, Alexandria represents an attractive spiritual community, home to a growing Islamic movement. Beginning primarily among the university-educated, the Islamic revival in Alexandria has spread to the masses, including growing numbers of poor men and women. During the past decade, more and more Alexandrian women have donned Islamic garb, including various forms of veiling, and many men have grown untrimmed, "Sunni" beards, which, along with the calloused "prayer spots" on their foreheads, mark them as devout Muslims.

Yet, when all is said and done, it is simple pleasures—and less Alexandria's attractions per se—that make life among the urban poor worth living. Among life's joys are the visits from relatives who have been missed; the sharing of a freshly prepared meal; the festivities accompanying Ramadan and the other religious holidays; the laughter and commentary shared with others over the evening television soap operas; the purchase of material for a new dress or *gallābīya*; the celebration of a neighbor's wedding; the trip to a special mosque on a saint's day; the sharing of sweet tea and gossip with friends on a cold winter morning; the success of a child in school; the letters from a son or husband at work in the Gulf; the words of tenderness uttered during a private moment with a loved one; the birth of a desired child.

These are what fuel life among the urban poor, what make life tolerable in the face of sometimes insoluble economic hardship and uncertainty. However, for poor infertile women like Afaf, who have yet to experience the joy of an infant's soft skin or sweet breath, the anguish of infertility often overshadows life's other happinesses and obliterates the potential for relationships marked by love, sharing, and commitment. This is why thousands of poor infertile Alexandrian women such as Afaf continue to "search for children," a search that holds the promise of reducing this unmitigated suffering.

3. Past and Present in Theories of Procreation

Nashwa's Story

Like Hind and Afaf, Nashwa, a young Alexandrian woman hailing originally from a village in Upper Egypt, has "suffered a lot," both in childhood and now in an infertile womanhood in which her marriage and very future are at stake. As the eldest daughter of a poor family with eight children, Nashwa was forced to assume all of the domestic responsibilities when her mother died. Not only did she take care of the house and her younger siblings, but she fed and watered the family cattle and fetched her family's drinking water from a well far away. With all of this strenuous work, Nashwa's body seemed to waste away, and people in the village began to notice her weight loss and apparent exhaustion. Thus, when Nashwa's father took a young bride, the village women hoped that Nashwa would be relieved somewhat of her chores. Instead, Nashwa's stepmother developed an instant aversion to Nashwa and was able to turn Nashwa's father against her (which Nashwa attributes, in part, to her own close resemblance to her dead mother, a resemblance that served as a reminder to her father of his mistreatment of his first wife). Furthermore, Nashwa's stepmother kept Nashwa in servitude, while she, herself, assumed none of the domestic responsibilities. To add insult to injury, Nashwa's stepmother went on to have two children, whom she gave to Nashwa to raise.

When Nashwa herself reached marriageable age, two suitors came to ask for Nashwa's hand, but her father turned them away, saying "she is no good." Nashwa was exceedingly demoralized. How was she ever going to marry, to escape this misery, if every suitor was chased away by her hateful father? However, when a young man named Fathi and his mother came from Alexandria to look for a bride in Nashwa's village, Nashwa's luck changed. A neighbor woman, taking pity on Nashwa, told them, "Come to see [so-and-so]'s daughter. She's skinny not because she's weak. She's so tired because her stepmother is torturing her, and she has the whole house to take care of. She is suffering." Fathi's mother replied, "I don't care what she looks like. I just want to know her." With her neighbors serving as intermediaries, the marriage contract was written for Nashwa and Fathi, who were distant relatives from the same patrilineal *'a'ila* (extended family). Within days, a large wedding feast was held in the village. According to Nashwa, this day "made up for a lot. I was happy because I was out of tragedy, and he was good, and his family was good." Fathi and his mother took Nashwa and her few items of clothing with them to Alexandria, where Fathi's family lived together in one building. Both Fathi and his parents were very kind to Nashwa and hoped to fatten her up so that she would become healthy and fertile. However, Nashwa remained thin, sickly, and barren. When children were not forthcoming, Fathi's parents asked Nashwa, "Would you like to go for medical care? It's up to you. If you want to go, we'll give you the money. We'll take care of you. Since your mother is dead, it would be a shame for us not to."

Thus began Nashwa's pilgrimage for pregnancy—a pilgrimage that has taken her to nearly twenty-five biogynecologists, three female ethnogynecologists, and several mosques, morgues, slaughterhouses, and cemeteries where she has enacted healing rituals and prayed for a child. The list of ethnogynecological remedies Nashwa has tried—"all against her own will"—is impressive. These include: stepping over gold, a slaughtered cow, clamshells, and a bead necklace; entering and exiting from a cemetery where she peered into a skeleton-filled tomb; bathing herself with the loofah sponge used to cleanse a dead body; circumambulating the cadavers in a darkened hospital morgue; undergoing cupping on both her back and abdomen; wearing vaginal suppositories of animal blood and herbs; visiting and vowing at the mosque-tomb of Shaikh Abū 'l-'Abbās al-Mursī; and making prayer-requests to nine dead *shuyūkh* all named Muhammad. Nashwa herself does not believe in these *wasfāt baladī*, or folk cures. But, as she explains, "there are people who told me it worked for them. I don't really believe it, because God created medicine and treatments and so I believe that if I'll ever be cured, it's by this, and not traditional remedies. My husband also believes in what doctors say, but he tells me, 'Maybe, just in case. If it worked for someone else, why not you?' Mostly, I did these things for my mother-in-law, because she's nice to me. But it's all nonsense."

Coincident with her ethnogynecological therapy, Nashwa has also undergone numerous biogynecological tests and treatments, many of which have made her "fed up." These include two pelvic X rays, one brain X ray (to rule out a pituitary tumor), two hormonal assays, one endometrial biopsy, several postcoital tests, several cervical mucus analyses, two diagnostic laparoscopies, three D & Cs, three tubal insufflations, fourteen sittings of shortwave (infrared) therapy, and nine years' worth of almost continuous drug therapy. Finally, three years ago, after receiving conflicting reports from numerous physicians, Nashwa was diagnosed with tuberculosis, which had spread to her pelvis, making her infertile. Although a pharmacist, taking pity on her, supplied Nashwa with the expensive, injectable, antitubercular drugs, the first treatment regimen did not work, and she has been forced to repeat her antitubercular treatment several times—to no avail.

Meanwhile, because of all of her exposure to both ethno- and biogynecologists, Nashwa has picked up considerable information about the body, its reproductive parts and processes, and the way in which conception takes place. She explains that

> after sex, if the thing [the semen] that the man puts in [the woman] remains inside, it means that the ovaries have caught it. If it comes down again, it's not caught. After the period, the ovaries come down to catch the man's thing, and they come up again after ten days. The ovaries are the tubes, so it's the tubes that catch the thing. The man has something that comes down, and she does, too. But his is more important, because this is what forms the child. *He* has the children. She, too, has something; if he has and she doesn't, she doesn't get pregnant. If she gets pregnant, her menstrual period doesn't come. When the child is born, he gets measles because he is formed from the blood of the period and after he's born it comes out on him in red spots. The menstrual blood is *part* of his formation. But it's bad blood from the ovaries. It's a mistake for a man to have sex with a menstruating woman because it brings diseases to the man.

As for why she is infertile, Nashwa now realizes that her pelvic tuberculosis is an "infection that is preventing my tubes from catching my husband's thing." The doctor who is currently managing Nashwa's case has told her that if the infection is not cleared, she will never be able to get pregnant. Nashwa's husband, Fathi, realizing the severity of his wife's illness, has become demoralized over the future of his marriage to Nashwa and the likelihood of having children by her. According to Nashwa, Fathi has developed a psychological "complex," has become religious, growing a beard, and spends most of his time at a mosque praying. Nashwa is certain that Fathi would be more motivated to work if he had children to support, but instead he relies on his sympathetic parents, who provide them with money for food. Meanwhile, many people, including Nashwa's own contemptuous father, have encouraged Fathi to remarry. Nashwa is deeply concerned about this and would undertake *any* treatment just to avoid a divorce and the unimaginable misery of having to return to her stepmother and father. At this point, Nashwa believes Fathi still feels sorry for her, which is the only reason he has stayed with her for so long. She is certain he will remarry if no children are forthcoming; in fact, he mentioned it recently, and they fought, but Fathi told Nashwa afterward, "I'm only joking. It's only talk. Nothing like this will happen." Nashwa, however, doubts that Fathi is being frank. She knows that he is under pressure from his extended family and friends to remarry for children. If he does, she will ask to be divorced rather than to remain in a polygynous marriage. But, insisting that she will never return to her daughter-hating father and stepmother, Nashwa, with her chronic tuberculosis and lack of employment skills, says she will "go far away and knock on any door."

The History of Medicine and Procreative Theory in Egypt

Little does Nashwa realize that, in her quest for conception, she has encountered therapies and theories of procreation dating back literally thousands of years. In fact, in order to understand Egypt's medical present, including the syncretic amalgam of beliefs and practices which characterizes patients' therapeutic narratives, it is necessary to gaze into Egypt's medical past—a past in which the city of Alexandria played a prominent role.

As we will see in this chapter, within a five-thousand-year medical history in which four, major literate medical systems achieved ascendancy, we find clues to the theories of procreation held by poor urban Egyptians today. Most important, the widespread belief in what Delaney (1986; 1987; 1991) has called "monogenesis"—the notion that only men contribute substantively to the creation of the fetus—hails from pre-Islamic times in Egypt, deriving considerable support from both pharaonic traditions and the teachings of Aristotle, the Greek philosopher-physician whose influence in Egypt and the rest of the Arab scientific world was profound.

However, contemporary theories of procreation, as well as beliefs about men's and women's reproductive bodies, have also been significantly influenced by the most recent medical system to be introduced into this region, that of "modern" biomedicine, which has achieved rapid, historical ascendancy in the urban Egyptian landscape. Not only have many poor Egyptians come to accept what Martin (1991) calls biomedicine's "romance of the egg and the sperm," but because of the "machine metaphor" of the body so prominent in biomedicine (Kirmayer 1988; Martin 1987; Osherson and Amarasingham 1981; Renaud 1978), most poor urban Egyptians now view the body mechanistically, which has profoundly affected their understanding of the reproductive process and its failure. As we shall see, while men's bodies are seen as productive machines, ones that produce fetus-laden "worms" through the process of spermatogenesis, women's reproductive bodies are viewed largely as unproductive storage containers, with movable parts that break down from time to time. Thus, women are usually deemed responsible for infertility because of faulty reproductive equipment, a view that has further marginalized women in the reproductive process and profoundly affected the nature of the "search for children" undertaken by the infertile.

In other words, to understand contemporary conceptions of procreation, procreative failure, and ways of overcoming this failure among the Egyptian urban poor, it is necessary to understand the historically situated, cultural construction of reproductive knowledge in Egypt and the ways in which such knowledge has been transmuted and translated into quotidian discourse over time.

Fortunately, from an historiographic standpoint, the Middle East is one of the few regions of the world in which written materials concerning health-related ideologies, practices, and professional standards are available and date back thousands of years. Many of these records provide an exquisitely detailed account of the medical systems and accompanying ideologies that gained hegemony in this region throughout the millennia, as well as the cultural and socioeconomic milieus in which they existed (Gran 1979; Millar and Lane 1988). Within the Middle Eastern region, perhaps nowhere is a richer, more complete, and ancient medical corpus available than for the contemporary nation-state of Egypt. Medical historians of the Middle East, including, among others, Bürgel (1976), Dols (1984), Gallagher (1990), Gran (1979), Kuhnke (1990), Leake (1952), Musallam (1983), Sandwith (1905), Sonbol (1991), and Ullman (1978), have examined the medical history of Egypt and have documented the historical presence of four major literature medical systems in the country.

Pharaonic Medicine

The earliest recorded medical practice in Egypt occurred during the pharaonic period. Between 1900 and 1200 B.C., eight medical papyri were written (Leake 1952). Four of these documents—the Kahun (1990 B.C.), the Ebers (1550 B.C.), the Erman (1550 B.C.), and the Berlin (1350 B.C.) papyri—were specifically concerned with "female conditions" and matters of pregnancy. The Kahun papyrus in particular was devoted largely to the diseases of women and animals and explained "female diseases" on the basis of uterine conditions, or "wanderings." Included in this document, as well as in the later Berlin papyrus, were a number of recipes for determining whether a woman was infertile, and both this papyrus and the later Ebers papyrus suggested treatments for promoting pregnancy. However, the Erman papyrus is particularly noteworthy, in that its focus on childbirth and infancy reflected ancient Egyptian attitudes toward motherhood and the importance of children. For example, included in it were various magical incantations designed to provide protection during childbirth and infancy, thereby ensuring survival of the newborn.

As Leake (1952) has concluded, these eight medical papyri from the pharaonic period show us that ancient Egyptian practitioners: (1) were relatively keen and accurate observers; (2) possessed a systematic method of examination; (3) were exploring principles of diagnosis; (4) had an idea of the significance of prognosis and thus were aware of the natural course of untreated disease; and (5) had accumulated a large body of tested agents and methods for the treatment and management of disease. Furthermore, as Leake notes, there is little evidence in these papyri of excessive "supernaturalism," indicating that these ancient medical practitioners were, for the most part, empiricists.

The empirical tradition extended to the preparation of herbal remedies, which were used extensively by pharaonic medical practitioners and constituted perhaps the major component of their materia medica. According to Manniche (1989), the pharaonic medical texts relied chiefly on the rich choice of plants that were available in Egypt or were cultivated in medicinal "physics gardens." As a result of this herbal knowledge, the pharaonic medical papyri provided an extensive pharmacopoeia, detailing remedies to be applied externally as poultices, unguents, and fumigants, or internally as inhalants, potables, suppositories, and vaporized sitz baths. As we shall see in Chapter 6, most of the important herbal substances used today in the ethnogynecological treatment of infertility, as well as their methods of application, can be traced to this "ancient Egyptian herbal" (Manniche 1989).

In addition, contemporary monogenetic procreative beliefs received their first expression during the pharaonic period in myths of creation that were also recorded in papyri. In these creation myths, male gods—

including Amun, Atum, Ptah, and Khnum—gave birth to, *inter alia*, their spouses, their children, other humans, animals, cities, sanctuaries, shrines, perpetual offerings, earth, and the planets themselves. For example, Atum, the sun god of Heliopolis, exemplified "the procreative act of the Monad," which, according to Hart (1990:12–13), was "a male principle in solitary splendour." Extracts from the Bremner-Rhind papyrus record Atum's initial procreative act as follows:

> All manifestations came into being after I developed . . . no sky existed no earth existed . . . I created on my own every being . . . my fist became my spouse . . . I copulated with my hand . . . I sneezed out Shu . . . I spat out Tefnut. . . . Next Shu and Tefnut produced Geb and Nut. . . . Geb and Nut then gave birth to Osiris . . . Seth, Isis and Nephthys . . . ultimately they produced the population of this land. (Hart 1990:13)

As Weigle (1989) concludes, it is clear from even the most superficial reading of pharaonic mythology that men had appropriated for themselves sole creative and procreative power and represented this power in parthenogenetic cosmogonies about masturbation and anthropogenies about the sperm's creative supremacy. Ergo, "Atum's act of masturbation . . . not only shows that the male factor in generation was already understood: it indicates that the male factor was regarded as decisive" (Brandon cited in Weigle 1989).

Yūnānī Medicine

Following the demise of the pharaonic dynasties of the Nile Valley by the third century B.C. and Alexander the Great's conquest across the Mediterranean, Greek physicans gained access to Egyptian intellectual circles, where, at the famous Alexandrian medical school founded by the Ptolemies, they introduced the second literate—and by far the most historically influential—medical system, known as *Yūnānī*, or Greek, medicine (Sandwith 1905; Adamson 1973; Longrigg 1981; Millar and Lane 1988).

Yūnānī medicine was based largely on the teachings of Hippocrates, the son of a midwife who is best known for the famous physicians' oath that bears his name (Sandwith 1905). Hippocrates was a proponent of the so-called humoral theory of pathology. According to the tenets of the Hippocratic humoral pathology, the physiological functions of the body were regulated by four basic humors: blood, phlegm, yellow bile, and black bile (Dash 1978; Dols 1984). These humors represented the primary qualities of the four basic elements: that is, air corresponded to blood which is hot and wet; water to phlegm which is cold and wet; fire to yellow bile which is hot and dry; and earth to black bile which is cold and dry. The equilibrium of the four humors created bodily well-being, which, in Greek medicine, was termed "eukrasia," or "symmetria" (Dols 1984). Therefore, any disturbance in their relative preponderance was thought to cause disease and even death, and the goal of the physician and his treatments was to restore the delicate balance of the four humors through a system of therapeutic opposition, or "contraria contrariis," in which hot substances were used to treat cold diseases, wet and cold substances to treat dry and hot conditions, and the like.

As with the early pharaonic practitioners, Hippocrates was also extremely interested in matters of fertility and infertility. For example, Hippocrates proposed the following test of fertility, which is very similar to a contemporary ethnogynecological treatment used by the Egyptian infertile: "If a woman does not conceive, and wishes to ascertain whether she can conceive, having wrapped her in blankets, fumigate below with oil of roses, and if it appear in the nostrils and mouth, know that of herself she is not unfruitful" (Aiman 1984).

Hippocrates also proposed a theory of conception that lasted in the Muslim world for centuries. In order to account for the resemblance of children to their parents, Hippocrates proposed that both males and females contributed similar reproductive material, namely, semen, to the fetus (Musallam 1983). Male and female semens, which were formed during sexual excitation and which were made up of particles from all parts of the body, were defined as similar in that both were equally capable of passing inheritance to offspring. Hippocrates' theory of two semens and its explanation of duogenetic inheritance was similar to that proposed in the nineteenth century by Darwin, a theory that was then given the name "pangenesis."

Aristotle, who followed Hippocrates and who was the teacher of Alexander the Great, was also interested, as a philosopher-physician, in reproductive physiology and the nature of conception. Although Aristotle's theory of transmission of resemblance was similar to Hippocratic pangenetic theory, it diverged considerably from it in its dualistic, biologically deterministic, misogynistic statement of male and female roles in this process (Berman 1989; Weigle 1989)—a formulation that Musallam (1983: 44) calls "the most radical statement of the difference between male and female in the history of biology, the strongest statement on record for the biological inferiority of women."

According to Aristotle's conception theory—which, as we shall see, persists in popular notions of monogenesis held by Egyptians today—semen was the "ultimate residue" of the body's nourishment in its final form. Blood was transformed into semen only in males, because of their adequate vital heat. Females, on the other hand, were not "hot" enough, according to Aristotle, who stated:

> (1) The male and the female are distinguished by a certain ability and inability. Male is that which is able to concoct, to cause to take shape, and to discharge, semen possessing the "principle" of the "form"; and by "principle" I do not mean that sort of principle out of which, as out of matter, an offspring is formed belonging to the same kind as its parent, but I mean the *proximate motive principle*, whether it is able to act thus in itself or in something else. Female is that which receives the semen, but is unable to cause semen to take shape or to discharge it. And (2) all concoction works by means of heat. Assuming the truth of these two statements, it follows of necessity that (3) male animals are hotter than female ones, since it is on account of coldness and inability that the female is more abundant in blood in certain regions of the body. (Aristotle in Weigle 1989:76)

Thus, according to Aristotle, menstrual blood was the analogous substance in females to the male's semen (Anees 1989; Musallam 1983); but, as "passive matter," it served only as the basis of the physical body of the fetus and the nutritive element for the growing embryo, whereas semen provided the "form," the "principle of movement," and was the source of the soul, or the "essence" of a body. This semen-originated soul guided and determined embryological development, which occurred in a series of chronological stages known as "epigenesis." Meanwhile, surplus blood from the female body that could not be transformed into fetal nutritive matter was expelled as menstruation (Anees 1989).

Despite the profound influence of Aristotle's masculinist theory on ancient Greek and Egyptian thought, it was Hippocrates' *duogenetic* theory of procreation that came to be promoted by Galen, a Greek who lived from A.D. 130 to 200 and who studied medicine at the medical school in Alexandria from A.D. 147 to 158 (Sandwith 1905; Aiman 1984).[1] As a prolific scholar and writer, Galen was the leading proponent and formalizer of Hippocratic medicine, and as a student of anatomy through dissection, he was the first to declare physiology to be its basis (Sandwith 1905).

Of all the Greek physicians, Galen was the most influential in the ancient Middle East, and his teachings, which have been termed "Galenism" (Temkin in Dols 1984), dominated the medical thinking of Arab physicians throughout the Middle East for nearly thirteen centuries (Ullman 1978). Unlike Hippocrates' works, nearly all of Galen's works had been translated into Arabic by the second half of the ninth century (Ullman 1978), in part by the prodigious Arab translator, Ḥunayn ibn Isḥāq, who lived from A.D. 808 to 873 (Dols 1984). Because of this translation effort, Galen and his teachings came to rule over medieval medicine, inspiring the "Arabic" or "Islamic" medicine of the Middle Eastern region in all of its essential points (Dols 1984; Ullman 1978). This included the acceptance by Islamic medical practitioners of (1) Galen's comprehensive theory of humoral pathology, including the six "non-naturals" (surrounding air, motion and rest of the body, sleep and wakefulness, food, excretion or retention of superfluities, and the passions of the soul) thought to affect humoral balance; (2) the system of therapeutic opposition in which drugs of four degrees of potency were administered as correctives to humoral imbalance; (3) the physiological theories of metabolism, digestion, and circulation suggested by Galen, as well as the teleological thinking that sought to recognize and explain the function of each organ; (4) the idea of the miasmatic corruption of the air by noxious vapors as the cause of epidemic disease; and (5) the rationalism and nonmoralizing, noncondemnatory interpretation of disease which characterized Galen's work (Dols 1984; Ullman 1978).

Furthermore, Galen essentially revived Hippocrates' duogenetic conception theory and energetically criticized Aristotle's rejection of that theory (Musallam 1983). Like Hippocrates, Galen argued that both male semen *and* female semen contribute to the fetus, and although he adopted the Aristotelian theory of semen formation, he insisted that male semen, too, contributes to the formation of the *body* of the fetus and not just to the soul.

As Musallam (1983) explains, the new evidence that Galen used to support this theory was the discovery that both sexes have left and right reproductive "parts"—namely, the ovaries in the female and the testes in the male—where, according to Galen, semen collects and is finally concocted. Galen also believed that each woman has a bicornuate uterus, and he attributed all gynecological disorders to malpositions of this uterus (Speert 1958; Aiman 1984). Furthermore, menstruation was viewed by Galen as a means of disposing of "surplus" blood, blood that is used by a woman's body during pregnancy to nourish the fetus (Good 1980).

In effect, Galen became the "great champion of Hippocrates against Aristotle" (Musallam 1983:46), and the Arab physicians who came to practice *Yūnānī* medicine were confronted by two sides of a scientific debate regarding human generation. On the one side were the Muslim philosophers, primarily Ibn Sina (Avicenna) and Ibn Rushd (Averroës), who were among the major Aristotelians. In his volume *Hayawan* (literally, *Animals*), Ibn Sina, the most important physician of the Middle Ages and the major scientific and philosophical authority for the premodern Europeans, attempted to merge the Hippocratic-Galenic and Aristotelian schools of thought by accepting unconditionally the argument of Hippocrates and Galen that females produce semen and that semen rather than menstrual blood represents the most important female contribution to conception, yet still assigning the female semen the exact role that Aristotle had assigned to menstrual blood, namely, the substance forming the bodily "matter" of the fetus and not its soul-guided "principle of movement" (Musallam 1983). "It is clear," Ibn Sina wrote, "that the seed of women is fit to be matter, but not fit to be the principle of movement. The seed of men is the principle of movement" (Ibn Sina in Ahmed 1989:49). On the other hand, Ibn Rushd, who was even more of an Aristotelian purist but who was ultimately less influential than Ibn Sina, argued that women did not contribute any semen at all, even of an inferior variety (Ahmed 1989).

On the other side of the debate were the great Muslim jurists, primarily al-Ghazali and Ibn Qayyim, who pointed to Islamic religious texts in support of Hippocratic-Galenic duogenetic theory (Ahmed 1989; Musallam 1983). Because of the seeming correspondence between the Islamic scriptures and Hippocratic-Galenic medical writings, the Muslim jurists sided with Hippocrates and Galen and rejected Aristotle's theory of procreation completely, which had important consequences for Islamic legislation regarding the sexes and provided the theoretical underpinning for the consensus among Muslim jurists from the tenth to nineteenth centuries that contraception was permissible in Islam. For example, Ibn Qayyim was able to convince the Muslim majority of his day that the fetus was formed of both male and female semens following their union. Furthermore, although subject to opposition, Ibn Qayyim argued that the contributions of the two semens were *equal* in value and quality—"as clear a statement of the biological equality of male and female as Aristotle's was of their biological inequality" (Musallam 1983:52).[2]

According to Musallam, "the most formidable opposition came from the Islamic religious sources where, to put it mildly, all the cards were stacked against Aristotle; for the statements about parental contribution to generation in the *hadith* paralleled the Hippocratic writings, and the view of foetal development in the Quran agreed in detail with Galen's scientific writings" (1983:49).

As suggested in this statement, the primary religious sources to which the medieval Muslim jurists referred for supportive evidence were the Qur'an which, to Muslims, is the word of God as spoken to the Prophet Muhammad by the angel Gabriel, and the sayings and deeds of the Prophet Muhammad as recorded in the Hadith. Passages in the Hadith were particularly explicit about the female contribution to conception through female "semen," the role of which was deemed by the Prophet to be equal to that of male semen. As Ahmed (1989) argues, the reason for the Prophet's egalitarian notions of conception may, in fact, be due to the profound influence of women in the Prophet's life and, hence, in the Hadith material. As she notes:

> Furthermore, the authors of many of the Hadith, in the sense of the person who was its original source, were often actually women, although the texts of the Hadith literature were physically written down by men. The Prophet's wife Aisha alone, for example, according to one estimate, was the author—or source—of one sixth of the entire Hadith corpus. . . . Thus . . . women's perspective is present in the texts—in a way that it is not in, say, Aristotle's texts. And it may be that it is this fact about the Arabic source texts that accounts for the difference between the specifically Arab theory of human biology with its notion of the equal contribution of both sexes—and the quite distinct masculinist Greek and Hebraic views. (Ahmed 1989:50–51)

It is important to note, however, that although the procreative debate may have been won on scriptural grounds by pro-Galenic duogenecists in Muslim theological circles, the influence of these jurists over the masses, including the Arab physicians who tended to those masses, may have been less convincing. As Gran (1979) has shown for Egypt, from the time of the rise of Islam in the seventh century until the mid-nineteenth century, there were three "main phases" in medical philosophy, at least one of which was dominated by Aristotelian-inspired "Avicennianism" rather than by Galenically inspired *Yūnānī* medicine. In fact, Gran decries the "scholarly fixation on the *Yūnānī* tradition," which, according to him, does "serious injustice both to the past of Arab medical history and to the present" (Gran 1979:339). Rather, Gran argues that throughout Egyptian medical history and up until the present historical moment, medical systems have achieved shifting hegemony, leading to an extremely pluralistic medical climate. Furthermore, within this pluralistic setting, Avicennianism—which promoted Aristotelian monogenetic procreation theory—dominated for at least six hundred years and was present along with Galenism for at least three hundred others. Thus, although Galen's influence on the Egyptian medical landscape was profound (Dols 1984; Ullman 1978), the influence of Ibn Sina, Aristotle's major defender, should not be forgotten and may explain the continuing authority of monogenetic procreative beliefs among the urban poor of Egypt today.

Prophetic Medicine

During the same period in which Hellenistically inspired Islamic medicine enjoyed ascendancy in Egypt, another literate medical tradition, known as "prophetic medicine," was being widely practiced in Egypt and elsewhere in the Arab world (Dols 1984; Gran 1979; Ullman 1978). Prophetic medicine differed from the Islamic medicine just described, because the former constituted a quasi-medical "religious medicine," based exclusively (at least putatively) on passages in the Islamic scriptures (Dols 1984). After the Prophet's death in A.D. 632, Muslim believers such as Al-Suyuti in his *Tibb-ul-Nabbi*, or *Medicine of the Prophet*, collected everything the Prophet was reported to have said about, for example, hygiene, alcohol consumption, circumcision, menstruation, breastfeeding, sanitation, and diseases and then institutionalized these sayings into a form of medical practice (Gran 1979).

According to medical historians, however, prophetic medicine was actually a syncretic blend of biblical "Jewish medicine," as contained in the book of Leviticus; Persian medicine, as taught in the famous medical school of Gondēshāpūr, which was attended by several of the Prophet's relatives; nomadic Bedouin medicine, as practiced in Arabia (particularly in Medina and Mecca) during the Prophet's lifetime; and Hippocratic-Galenic *Yūnānī* medicine. Furthermore, as Ullman (1978) has argued, many of the Hadiths on which prophetic medicine was supposedly based were actually inauthentic, prescribing pre-Islamic folk practices that were then reinterpreted using concepts from *Yūnānī* medicine.

Nevertheless, prophetic medicine acquired greater and greater significance during later Islamic history and, in some cases, came to counter and supersede *Yūnānī* medicine, which was suspected as being a science of heathen origin. Prophetic medicine was also popular with the people, for it incorporated traditional concepts and practices from Arab folk medicine, such as the use of magical incantations and spells, the writing of *ḥugub*, or religious sayings in curative amulets, belief in the evil eye, and the practice of cupping[3]—all of which, as we shall see, are widely practiced in Egypt today.

In addition, by the sixteenth century, cults of popular Islamic mystics, known as *Ṣūfīs* or marabouts, began to proliferate in Egypt, although the presence of these cults dates back to the tenth century. As Gran (1979) points out, the *Ṣūfī* cults and their shrines flourished in Egypt because they were able to cater to the spiritual, psychological, and political needs of the lower classes, as well as to their medical complaints. Furthermore, these cults offered medical specialization; for example, some dealt specifically with the ailments of women, whose social condition began to deteriorate with the penetration of Western market conditions in Egypt, while others specialized in psychiatric problems, which were usually attributed to spirit possession.

Despite its association with Islam, *Ṣūfī* medicine (or "maraboutic medicine," as this form of practice is sometimes called in North Africa) was not entirely synonymous with prophetic medicine (Gran 1979). Whereas prophetic medical practitioners claimed to draw upon the exacting, literate tradition of the Islamic scriptures, *Ṣūfī* medicine did not derive from a book tradition, nor was it uniformly practiced. Rather, it attempted to be holistic, and, as such, it drew upon all of the medical systems described so far. Thus, it was truly syncretic and has remained so until present times, as we shall see in Chapters 4 and 7.

European Biomedicine

Just at the time when *Ṣūfī* medicine was flourishing in Egypt, Europe was on the verge of the Enlightenment, a time of rapid scientific expansion and discovery in which Galen's humorally based medical system, unchallenged for more than a millenium, was largely overturned. This was, in fact, the period in which "biomedicine"—the term used in this book to connote biologically based "Western" medicine[4]—experienced its inchoate stages of development. During the pre-Enlightenment period, studies of human anatomy and physiology had been revived, leading to the publication in 1543 of a biomedically accurate atlas of human anatomy by Vesalius, which included a representation of the female pelvic organs (Aiman 1984). In addition, during this period, William Harvey expressed the opinion that all creatures originate from eggs, and, about twenty years later, in 1672, Rejnier de Graaf published a book on the female reproductive organs, in which he described the female ovaries with their egg-containing follicles (Zander

1988). Only five years later, with the invention of the microscope, sperm were first identified (Zander 1988).

These scientific discoveries, and especially the invention of the microscope, yielded some curious results in terms of theories of procreation. Namely, during the seventeenth and early eighteenth centuries, scientists began expounding "preformation" models, theories of conception in which the human being was already preformed, either in the ovum or the sperm (Child 1922; Jordan 1987; Musallam 1983). The "ovulists"—those who favored the ovum as the site of the preformed fetus, even though the ovum itself was not seen until 1827 by Karl Ernst von Baer—went so far as to refer to the semen as "mere manure for the ovum" (Jordan 1987). Alexander Hamilton, one such ovulist, declared in 1781 that the child existed in the ovaries and was only excited into life by the "seminal worms" (Jordan 1987). On the other side of the debate were the "animalculists"—or those who argued that tiny microscopic beings called "homunculi," or little men, existed in the spermatozoa, which, under the primitive microscope, were found to be tiny, swimming creatures complete with heads and limbs (Jordan 1987; Musallam 1983). As in Aristotle's formulation, the animalculists either denied the existence of the ovum altogether, or argued that it only existed as nourishment for the tiny beings carried in the semen.

How the animalculists' preformation views reached Egypt, given the demise of this model in eighteenth-century Europe and the ascendancy of the duogenetic model of equally contributing ova and sperm, will probably never be known. But, given the history of Egyptian monogenesis described so far, it is not surprising that masculinist preformation beliefs eventually took hold, probably with the introduction of European-based biomedicine. (As we shall see, they have continued in Egypt ever since, but are gradually being superseded by the biomedically based duogenetic model.)

Given the birth of biomedicine in Enlightenment Europe, it is not surprising that the history of biomedicine in Egypt is largely tied to the history of European colonialism and military expansion in that country. The first introduction of biomedicine occurred at the turn of the nineteenth century, when the French and later British armies mounted expeditions in Egypt. Because their troops were ravaged by diseases unknown to the Europeans, including blinding eye diseases, the French and British military commanders were forced to import physicians from their home countries, some of whom influenced Egyptian medical practice for years to come (Millar and Lane 1988).

However, it was Muhammad Ali, the ex-Ottoman Albanian who seized control of Egypt in 1805, who was most responsible for the introduction and initial development of biomedicine in Egypt. In 1827, Muhammad Ali founded the first Western-style medical school in the Middle East—Qasr al-Aini in Cairo—which was intended in part to train Egyptian physicians to care for Egypt's conscript army (Kuhnke 1990; Sonbol 1991). However, Muhammad Ali's interest in bringing European biomedicine to Egypt extended beyond his military ambitions. As Sonbol notes:

> [Muhammad Ali's] medical reforms were meant to revive medical learning so that Egypt would be provided with the services it had been accustomed to at times of security and prosperity. Being a man of the nineteenth century, however, he was concerned with introducing the most up-to-date facilities and knowledge, and that meant borrowing the form of medicine practiced in Western Europe. Consequently his medical projects, which involved establishing a medical school, a school of maternity, and a school of veterinary science as well as hospitals and clinics, adopted modern medical science and made use of Western medical personnel. . . . Perhaps for this reason, Muhammad Ali's reforms enjoyed a good measure of success, unlike the abrupt changes that took place during the British takeover of Egypt's medical institutions and services in 1892. (1991:12–13)

The differences between Muhammad Ali's pro-Egyptian medical reforms of the mid-1800s and the anti-Egyptian stance of the colonial British medical reformers of the late 1800s were striking. For example, with the help of the French physician, Antoine-Barthélemy Clot (better known as Clot Bey), who was the major implementer of Muhammad Ali's medical reforms, Muhammad Ali was able to initiate truly innovative changes in Egyptian medical education and practice. In addition to the impressive medical infrastructure he created in both urban and rural areas, Muhammad Ali encouraged (1) the training of women physicians, or *ḥakīmāt*, to cater to the maternal and child health needs of the Egyptian populace; (2) the training of traditional barber-surgeons, or *ḥallāqīn aṣ-ṣiḥḥa*, as ancillary medical personnel and vaccinators in the vast Egyptian countryside; (3) the study of human anatomy based on autopsies, which won the support of the skeptical Muslim clergy; (4) the translation of vast numbers of European medical texts into Arabic and, thus, the creation of an Arabic medical terminology; (5) the government's payment of all expenses for medical students and government-sponsored training missions of Egyptian medical students to Europe; (6) the establishment of standards and penalties for medical malpractice; and (7) the emergence of an authentic, indigenous medical profession that did not bar potential practitioners on the basis of creed or class (Sonbol 1991). Furthermore, spurred by two great epidemics—cholera in 1831 and plague in 1835—Muhammad Ali commissioned an international Quarantine Board, the first in history, which provided the basis for a rudimentary public health service (Kuhnke 1990).

With the British occupation of Egypt in 1882, virtually all of Muhammad Ali's most important reforms were reversed (Sonbol 1991). The Qasr al-Aini medical school was completely taken over by the British, who severely restricted the enrollment of Egyptian medical students and based their admissions on upper-class status and ability to pay. With too few physicians to meet the needs of the Egyptian populace, the British encouraged the importation of foreign doctors, many of whom had been found guilty of malpractice and other misdemeanors and thus were forbidden to practice medicine in their own countries. Furthermore, professionalism and specialization among Egypt's own medical practitioners was discouraged by the British, who effectively turned medicine into a trade for profit, practiced for gain by those who could afford to pay for a medical education and set themselves up as private practitioners, primarily in urban areas, which were considered superior. In addition, medical education would no longer be conducted in the Arabic language under the British, and this further restricted entry to the medical profession to students with sufficient linguistic ability to learn and pass exams in a second language. The traditional barber-surgeons, whose access to English language training was obviously limited, were no longer educated as ancillary medical personnel. Likewise, the female physician program designed to meet the needs of Egypt's women was discontinued, and the title *ḥakīma* gave way to *dāya* (midwife). Furthermore, few Egyptians were treated at the government hospitals set up by Muhammad Ali, because, under the British, patients were required to pay. Thus, the British failed to meet the medical needs of Egypt's large urban and rural underclass, which was forced to rely exclusively on home remedies and the treatment of traditional healers.

As we shall see in Chapters 8 and 9, the deleterious ramifications of British imperial rule are still remarkably evident in Egyptian biomedicine today, exactly a century later. As it now stands, Egyptian biomedicine is blatantly elitist, urban-biased, technologically oriented, and excessively entrepreneurial, and it is characterized by inadequate medical education with resultant scientific traditionalism, lack of subspecialization, and frequent iatrogenesis (without an accompanying system of malpractice). Furthermore, boundaries are effectively maintained between physicians and patients through the continuing use of English as the language of medical discourse—a discourse that is rarely shared with poor patients. As Sonbol sees the contemporary situation:

> British rule had long-term adverse effects on Egypt by making it dependent on foreign assistance and by pursuing policies that increased the gap between the westernized wealthy and the traditional poor. . . . Today Egypt's doctors continue to be the recipients, rather than the initiators, of medical discoveries. They still travel to Western universities to sharpen their knowledge of medicine, and they depend on importing foreign technology and medical instruments to be used in their practices. . . . Furthermore, notwithstanding the fact that today Egypt has thirteen universities and graduates thousands of doctors each year, there is still a long way to go in the type of services provided. Hospitals exist in large numbers, but only a few provide high-quality service, and those cater to the very rich.
>
> British colonial rule played a direct role in bringing this situation about . . . as a result of British policy Egypt would be kept constantly a few steps behind the West in technological and scientific advancements; it would grow in its dependence on Western knowhow; and, most seriously, it would be molded into a two-class society in accordance not only with wealth, which was not new for Egypt, but with culture, outlook, and expectations. (Sonbol 1991:134–35,139)

Despite its many inadequacies, which have been documented by a number of investigators in addition to Sonbol,[5] biomedicine now provides the system of care preferred by most Egyptians, who have been convinced of its "modernity," its "high technology," and hence its superior efficacy. Furthermore, biomedical hegemony in Egypt has profoundly affected popular ideologies regarding the nature of the human body, its structures, and its physiological processes. Nevertheless, biomedical hegemony in Egypt is far from complete, in the realm of both ideology and praxis. In terms of praxis, biomedicine has clearly not usurped the authority of the practitioners of many other forms of medicine in Egypt—forms based largely on the aforementioned historical traditions. But, as will be clear later on, most biomedical practitioners know and care little about their ethnomedical competitors, and they have only the foggiest notions of what these ethnomedical practitioners offer to their patients. In their disregard for ethnomedicine of all kinds, Egyptian biomedical practitioners tend to disregard patients' ethnomedical beliefs, rarely inquiring about them or attempting to replace these beliefs through education from a biomedical perspective. Thus, Egyptian patients tend to learn about biomedicine largely on their own, absorbing bits and pieces of information during their encounters with biomedicine in various settings throughout their lifetimes. As a result, beliefs tend to become amalgamated, with biomedical notions absorbed only when they make sense within larger, preexisting belief systems. This ideological syncretism is perhaps nowhere clearer than in contemporary theories of procreation among the Egyptian urban poor, theories that can be seen to contain disparate elements from the historical medical traditions discussed so far.

Contemporary Theories of Procreation

The degree to which biomedical ideologies have or have not permeated Egyptian ways of thinking can be seen in the realm of procreative theory, or how Egyptians conceive of the "coming into being" of human life (Delaney 1991). Despite its historical exposition of monogenetic preformation models, biomedicine, grounded as it is in Western biology, is now quite emphatically duogenetic in its theoretical position. It is argued in Western biology, the underpinning of biomedicine, that men and women contribute equally to the hereditary substance of the fetus, which is formed through the union of a woman's ovum and a man's spermatozoon. In the West, we take such a theory for granted, for it seems to us to be self-evident. But, bearing in mind the historical recency and potential cultural specificity of such a model, the question must be asked: Is this duogenetic theory of procreation universal? Do all peoples conceive of conception in this way?

In fact, anthropological evidence gathered from around the world shows that not all people theorize conception in a duogenetic framework—that is, as an act entailing an egalitarian, substantive contribution from both a male and a female partner (Delaney 1991; Jordan 1987; Valsiner 1989). This is certainly true of the Middle East, where ethnographers from Iran (Good 1980) to Morocco (Crapanzano 1973; Greenwood 1981) have pointed to procreative models in which men are seen as contributing more to conception than women. For example, while working in rural Turkey, Delaney discovered that it is men who are seen as "planting seeds"—who carry the substance of life in their sperm—while women are imagined as "fertile fields," in which these seeds are nurtured. Thus, in rural Turkey, children are seen as the product of men—not women—making procreation an inherently male act with numerous important implications for gender relations and village social life.

Like Turkish villagers, many poor urban Egyptians also hold a monogenetic theory of procreation—a theory that, I argue, underlies patriarchal gender relations in Egypt and the particular backlash suffered by infertile women who fail to facilitate the virile, procreative act (Inhorn n.d.).[6] However, as nonagrarian peoples who have been deeply affected by the congestion of urban living and the hegemony of biomedicine, most poor urban Egyptians view procreation not as the planting of seeds in fertile fields, as Delaney found among the rural Turks, but rather as the passage of microscopic, seminal "worms" into women's waiting "womb houses," which carry the fetuses that men create. In other words, the metaphorical language of procreation in urban Egypt has been transformed. Moreover, the biomedicalization of thought is apparent in the belief among a growing number of poor urban Egyptians that women, too, contribute substantively to the creation of fetuses—sometimes in ways and means equal to those of men.

What exactly are the procreative beliefs of poor urban Egyptians? To begin, it is widely believed that sexual intercourse is a necessary, although not sufficient, prerequisite to pregnancy. Intercourse is not sufficient because not every act of intercourse results in pregnancy, as is apparent in the case of the infertile. During intercourse, a man "brings" (that is, ejaculates) a substance that causes pregnancy.[7] This substance is called various names by Egyptian women, including "fluid," "seminal fluid," "the fluid of children," "discharge," "running water," "milk," and "a drop." *Sā'il*, the Arabic term for fluid or liquid, is used most commonly, although *nutfa*, the term used in the Islamic scriptures to describe the male contribution to conception (which is translated with some indeterminacy as "seed" [Ibrahim 1976], "semen" [Musallam 1983], or "sperm" [Cowan 1976]), is occasionally employed. The Arabic term for "seed," *bizra*, is sometimes used by Egyptian women to designate the male contribution to conception, and hence women are like the "soil," or *arḍ*. However, in the overall scheme of things, the "seed-field" metaphor found by Delaney in the rural Turkish setting and by Boddy (1989) among the rural northern Sudanese is less frequently employed in the urban Egyptian landscape.

Rather, the vast majority of poor urban Egyptian women believe in the transmission of "sperm" in men's "fluid"—a notion that has definitely been disseminated through biomedical channels in urban areas. Egyptian physicians use an Arabic approximation for the English biomedical term "sperm"; in speaking to their patients, they call sperm *ḥayawānāt il-minawī*, literally, "spermatic animals," a term that is subsequently used by many patients. That sperm are living creatures—"animals," in fact—has not been lost on the Egyptian collective imagination. Since "spermatic animals" are creatures so small that they can only be seen through the physician's microscope (as in semen analysis), then they must resemble *dīdān*, literally, "worms," which are animals known to be microscopic in size. As one woman put it: "The man has fluid with worms, like bilharzia exactly. They see them in the microscope." Thus, with the widespread knowledge of both semen analysis and bilharzia (a parasitic blood fluke infection endemic in the countryside) in Egypt, the vast majority of poor urban Egyptians now equate sperm with worms—an idea that has definitely outstripped the language of seeds in the urban Egyptian setting. (Yet, it is worth noting that both "worms" and "seeds" are associated with "soil," the nurturant earthly substance of insemination.)

Men's worms, furthermore, are deemed quite remarkable, for, in the monogenetic view espoused by many poor urban Egyptians, they are seen as containing preformed children, or, as Egyptians are apt to put it, "the worms carry the kids." Thus, it is *men* who through spermatogenesis—conceptualized by some as occurring in a nerve in the male back or in the spine itself—actually *produce* preformed offspring, which are carried by their wriggling "worms of kids" to women's wombs.

Because men carry preformed fetuses in their sperm, it is they who determine the sex of the child, according to those who adopt this preformation model.[8] But, such preformation adherents point to a cruel irony: When no sons are forthcoming in a marriage, the woman, and *not* the man, is usually blamed for the failure, just as she is blamed for other reproductive failures for which the man may, in fact, be responsible. Thus, as Morsy (1980b) has noted, gender asymmetries in Egypt find their justification in theories of procreation that are "victim-blaming," placing women outside the realm of procreation, yet faulting them for procreative failure.

Yet, as we shall see here, it would be a mistake to assume that the monogenetic theory of procreation, which sees men as worm-bringing life-givers, is monopolistic in urban Egypt. Rather, in this markedly pluralistic environment, three primary versions of the procreative story can be found and are characterized by a significant degree of overlap and fluidity. Although two of these variant theories contain distinctly duogenetic features, all three of them are often construed so as to place women in a marginalized procreative position, often secreting bodily substances inferior to those of men. For heuristic purposes, I shall call these three theories "women as fetal catchers and carriers," "women as suppliers of menstrual blood," and "women as egg producers."

Women as Fetal Catchers and Carriers

The most emphatically monogenetic of the three theories is also the one most widely held: namely, the belief that women serve as fetal "catchers and carriers," with no role in conception and a minimal role in nurturing the fetus. In this view, a woman's major role lies in the mechanical functioning of her reproductive organs, primarily her uterus and, to a lesser extent, her ovaries. The role of the woman's ovary, or *mibyaḍ*, is to "catch" the fetal-carrying worms upon their entrance into the womb. Ovaries are typically viewed as "coming down" to (or into) the uterus to perform this function, that is, they are "wandering" or movable organs as the pharaonic physicians once suggested. The uterus—called the *raḥim* in biomedical parlance and the *bait il-wilid*, or "house of the child," by most poor urban Egyptians—is viewed as the initial receptacle for the man's fetal-containing worms and the nine-month gestational home of the developing fetus, or *ganaina*, that is liberated from one of those worms. Thus, it is commonly thought that the ovaries "catch" and the uterus "carries," although these functions are occasionally reversed by women. In this view, then, these mostly mechanical functions constitute a woman's primary role in the reproductive—as opposed to procreative—process, and the uterus, the "house of the child," is less a home than a nine-month storage space.

Women express this view of their limited role in conception in a variety of ways. As one woman stated, "Here in Egypt, we say the woman is just a container. It is something from God, but she is only a container. It is God who determines the sex of the child through what the man gives. The child is in the man. She has no role. She only carries the pregnancy. God blows the soul into the uterus, as much as I believe in God."

Another woman explained, "Of course, they must have sex to get pregnant. From where would she get the children? It's the fluid of the man that makes the woman pregnant. God made it like this so that men can have children. Of course, the woman is more important in pregnancy, because as soon as she's pregnant, the man's out of it. But she's the one who carries and gets tired. She has nothing, but she carries his fluid. The children are in the fluid, so that's why the sex of the child is from the man."

Another woman expressed the view that

> the man is the important one. Since I went to all these doctors, I know from them that the man is the important thing. He is the main thing in determining pregnancy. He has the kids in the sperm. If there is no fetus in his sperm and he's weak, she can't get pregnant. The woman, her role is to carry the child. The fluid [of the man] carries the baby, and she provides a place for it to grow.

> Her ovaries also have to function for her to get pregnant. If they don't, she can't get pregnant because her ovaries are weak; that's why she can't get pregnant and carry the baby.

It is important to note that the roles of women's other reproductive "parts"—especially the *anābīb*, or fallopian tubes—are left unclear in this scheme. Although most urban Egyptian women acknowledge the existence of tubes, they are unsure of their function or location in relation to the ovaries and uterus—a connection of parts that very few women can easily identify. Likewise, women are well aware of their cervices, or the *ʿunq ir-raḥim*, "the neck of the uterus," which they physically manipulate while manually douching on a daily basis; however, they are also uncertain about the role of the cervix in reproduction.

In addition, women believe that once the man's fetus begins to grow in their "womb houses," its weight is carried mainly in their lower backs—or, as they put it, "the child is carried in the back." This is why lower backache occurs so frequently during pregnancy, and this is also why an "open back," which prevents carriage of the child, is deemed a major cause of both infertility and miscarriage.

Women as Suppliers of Menstrual Blood

A less common but potentially more empowering view of the role of women in the reproductive process conceptualizes them as the crucial suppliers of menstrual blood. According to this view, which, as we have seen, is historically rooted in both Aristotelian and Galenic theories of conception and gestation, menstrual blood is the component that women contribute to the reproductive process, either as (1) the product of conception, which helps to form the child by mixing with the man's worms (a modified Aristotelian view); (2) the product that nourishes the fetus during its nine-month developmental period (part of the duogenetic Galenic view); or (3) the product that forms "cushions," or "mattresses," for the fetus in its uterine "home."

Of these three possibilities, the modified Aristotelian "menstrual mixture" theory, involving a mixture variously described as "blood and worms," "blood and fluid," "blood and seeds," or "blood and milk," is most common. Like Aristotle, who saw menstrual blood as a "passive material" leading to the physical body of the fetus and semen as an "essential material" leading to the soul of the fetus, contemporary Egyptian women who hold this view generally see blood as a lesser substance in this formative mixture. Indeed, a woman's blood may only help to form the child's body *after* the preformed fetus, carried in the man's sperm, has been picked up by a woman's ovaries and settled in its uterine home, where, as one woman put it, "the menstrual period and the child get mixed together."

Speaking about the role of menstrual blood in fetal formation, one woman explained, "The baby is actually *from* the man, but what *forms* the boy or girl is their mixing together." Or, as another woman added, "The child comes from the worm, but [the woman] has a great role in *forming* the child as it grows; he gets the benefit of the food she eats and some of her blood."

However, because menstrual blood is deemed insalubriously polluting, many Egyptian women who hold this view are also troubled by what they perceive to be the contribution of a dangerous, defiling substance to the development of a healthy child. As one woman put it, "If the menstrual blood is bad, then why does it form the child?"

Like Turkish (Delaney 1988, 1991), Iranian (Good 1980), and Sudanese (Constantinides 1985) women, most Egyptian women hold that "dirty," "rotten" menstrual blood can be *very bad*—even "poisonous"—when it comes in contact with men, other women, or, as suggested here, fetuses. The strength of this menstrual-pollution theory, which is historically rooted in both Greek Galenic and Islamic notions of women's bodies (Bouhdiba 1985), is most apparent in Egypt in widespread sexual abstinence during the menses.[9]

However, most poor urban Egyptian women, while viewing themselves as regularly defiled, are uncertain about why they menstruate and from where this blood originates. The most common belief is that once proposed by Galen: menstruation is the means of disposing, or cleansing the body, of "extra blood," either from the entire body, the brain, or the woman's reproductive organs, especially the uterus. Thus, if excess blood—polluted or not—is employed during pregnancy to form, feed, or cushion (depending on one's viewpoint) the fetus, then the empirically verifiable relationship between menstruation and pregnancy makes a great deal of sense. If a woman is pregnant, she does not menstruate; if she menstruates, she is not pregnant; and if she is unable to menstruate, she is unable to become pregnant, because "How would the child form without blood?"[10]

Thus, the "women as suppliers of menstrual blood" theory actually incorporates three variant formulations regarding the nature of menstrual blood and its role in the related processes of conception and gestation. At least one of these variants—the menstrual mixture one—is potentially duogenetic in its formulation, given that women are sometimes thought to contribute substantively and *equally* to the formation of the fetus. Yet, that men and women do *not* contribute equally to this mixture is the view most commonly espoused, as is the disturbing notion that women's contribution to fetal formation is, in fact, polluting to the fetuses that men are largely responsible for creating. Thus, here we see that even when assigned a procreative role, women continue to be marginalized as procreators, contributing less than their male counterparts, as Aristotle once argued, and even tainting the union with their blood.

Women as Egg Producers

Of all of the theories of procreation found among the urban Egyptian poor, the one that appears to be increasing in acceptance—even supplanting in some cases the other two theories—is the duogenetic "sperm-ovum union" theory promoted by biomedicine. Now held by most educated and semi-educated women, this theory is also beginning to take hold among uneducated women who have had significant exposure to the biomedical system or to popular health messages in the media.

In this duogenetic view, both men and women have a "fluid" or "discharge" that serves as a medium for the conceptive products: *ḥayawānāt il-minawī*, or "spermatic animals," among men and *buwaiḍāt*, or "eggs," among women.[11] These spermatic animals and eggs are believed to meet in the woman's ovaries, "tubes" (fallopian tubes), or uterus and merge there to create a fetus. From this perspective, then, sperm alone are not sufficient to produce the fetus; eggs are also necessary.

This expanding discourse of procreative eggs in Egypt receives varying expression, depending largely on educational background. Educated women, whose first exposure to human reproductive biology usually comes in junior high school, are often able to recite the egg-sperm theory in some detail.

For example, a woman who had completed junior high school, was an avid reader of popular health literature, and had spent considerable time in doctors' offices, explained, "After sex, the egg from the ovaries comes down the tubes, and sometimes the sperm fertilizes the egg in the tube and it stays for one week. Then it comes down to the uterus. The best time for fertilization to occur is thirteen to fifteen days after the beginning of the period. It's better to have a lot of sex—for example, once a day—during this period."

Another woman, college-educated and currently working as an agricultural inspector, stated, "Of course, the egg meets the sperm in the fallopian tubes and this starts the phases of pregnancy. After the egg is fertilized, it travels to the uterus, and the fetus forms over nine months. Fertilization occurs on day fourteen of the period. The egg is ready to be released from the ovaries, and if fertilization happens, the period doesn't come." When asked, she added, "Of course, it's fifty-fifty—the sperm and the egg."

Less educated women often conceive of eggs as being contained in a woman's body "like chickens" or "a bunch of grapes." As one woman explained, "The woman has a predetermined number of something like eggs inside her, and this is the number of children she gets. It's not necessary that all live; some live and some die." Or, as another woman put it, "She has a bunch of eggs like a chicken, and when this is finished, she can't have any more children. The woman has eggs in a bunch, and they're just as important [as a man's sperm]." Or, as one woman said, "A woman has a bunch of children, like grapes, which decides how many children she's going to have, and some [women] don't have any."

The idea that eggs might contain preformed children, just like men's sperm, is not widely held but is occasionally articulated by poor urban women. For example, commenting on the possible etiology of her own infertility, one woman remarked, "Women have children in them or have no children in them. If a woman has no period at all, she has no children at all. Maybe I ran out of my children."

However, much more common is the view—pervasive even among some educated women—that, in the union of egg and sperm, women's eggs are less important, either contributing "less than half," or, in the view of some, contributing little at all to conception. In other words, despite the duogenetic philosophy of modern Western biology, which is firmly upheld in official Egyptian biomedical and educational circles, *unofficial* versions of the egg-sperm story popular among the masses are, in fact, markedly less duogenetic. This is why women who demonstrate knowledge of eggs often situate this knowledge within other, more monogenetically inspired, procreative discourses, leading to artfully blended, conceptually consistent theories in which fetus-laden worms, polluting menstrual blood, eggs, seeds, milk, and other reproductive secretions may *all* play an important role. The degree of conceptual indeterminacy and fluidity between the three theoretical variants so neatly separated above is often remarkable. Take, for example, the syncretic procreative explanations offered by these women:

> The ovaries are on the sides of the uterus, and they make the woman get her enjoyment. And they help excrete the eggs, which mix with the man's eggs. The man has something like the egg, the thing which forms the fetus. His is more important, of course, than the woman's. I heard this. These things come out from a nerve of the man's back, and this is what forms the fetus. So, its the seminal fluid, together with the egg from the woman, plus her blood—this makes the child.

When asked about the blood, she added, "It's the blood of the period. That's why it doesn't come out during pregnancy. The blood of the period is rotten blood that we let out every month. It comes out when the egg is broken; this is what causes the blood to come. So, when a woman is pregnant, this egg is used in forming the fetus, so it's not broken and no blood comes down."

Another woman stated,

> After sex, something white comes from the man, like milk. The milk is the thing forming the child, like the seed. Of course, this is why he's more important [in conception], because he has the seed. This milk enters the woman's inside and if she has no problems, she can catch it right away and start her pregnancy from the first time she has sex. She just catches it and carries it. But she also has something—I heard like eggs—which waits inside. When she becomes pregnant, her period doesn't come because the blood forms the child. As soon as the man's milk is caught, the blood starts collecting and forming a child.

She added, "Because I have a problem, I don't catch the milk, and it goes out again."

Another woman explained, "She receives something from the man—worms—and these start forming the child. She has worms, too, and they meet in the house of the child [uterus]. If hers are good and his are good, pregnancy happens, and if they're no good, it doesn't happen. His are more important, of course, because she gets the pregnancy *from him*, not vice versa. Her major role is to carry. He has the seed, and she's the field." When asked about menstrual blood, she added, "She doesn't have her period when she's pregnant, because the blood forms the child."

Thus, in the theories of procreation held by poor urban Egyptian women today, we see a multiplicity of beliefs—sometimes neatly bounded, sometimes creatively merged—reflecting the pluralistic medical history of this region and the relatively recent, but influential legacy of Western biomedical ways of thinking. Yet, amid newer notions of eggs and sperm, the age-old monogenetic theory of procreation — in which men bring and women receive life — still prevails among this population, receiving symbolic confirmation in religious beliefs about the life-giving powers of a male God, who, as we shall see in Chapter 7, is the *ultimate* creator.

The Assignment of Procreative Blame

But the question remains: If men make babies, then are men also responsible for failures in the procreative realm?[12] Ironically, in the monogenetic system described above, it is *women* who are most often deemed responsible for reproductive failure, of thwarting the creation of life. Just as men are seen as giving life, women are seen as taking life away, by virtue of wombs that fail to facilitate the most important act of male creation.

To wit, in the masculinist preformation model described above, men cannot be blamed for failures of procreation, unless, because of impotence or premature ejaculation, they are unable to pass their worm-enveloped children into women's wombs. In other words, barring male sexual inadequacy, men cannot fail reproductively so long as their bodies are the least bit spermatogenic. On the contrary, women's bodies may be plagued by numerous problems that bar the facilitation of male procreation or result in an unsuitable gestational "home" for the child that a man "brings" in his ejaculate. This is why every act of sexual intercourse does not result in pregnancy. This is also why women are seen as suffering from a whole host of infertility conditions, both ethno- and biogynecological in nature. As we shall see in Part 2 of this book, in the Egyptian ethnogynecological explanatory system, women's bodies are viewed as quite susceptible to numerous natural and supernatural afflictions. Men, on the other hand, are seen as being relatively immune to infertility-producing bodily pathology. Although they may suffer impotence through acts of sorcery or a shock to the body that renders them nonspermatogenic, such conditions are deemed relatively rare when compared to the host of corporeal maladies thought to incapacitate a woman's fecundity.

Such differential assignment of bodily blame has also been perpetuated by the biomedical system in Egypt. As we shall see in Part 3 of this book, biomedicine has identified numerous etiological factors in infertility — problems such as blocked tubes, weak ovaries, uterine tumors, ovarian cysts, and cervical erosions. Amazingly, these are problems that many Egyptian women — fertile and infertile, educated and uneducated — can cite, describe, and analyze, often in great detail. Thus, biomedicine has expanded substantially the realm of known female bodily pathology, thereby perpetuating the notion among Egyptians that women's bodies are *extremely* vulnerable to a host of infertility-producing setbacks.

Yet, on the more positive side, biomedicine in Egypt has certainly shifted the blame for infertility toward the male. With the widespread advent of semen analysis in Egypt over the past two decades, virtually every Egyptian has heard of the problem of "weak worms," and most have come to accept the idea that men, too, may be infertile because of worms that are slow, sluggish, dead, or even absent altogether. In fact, "worm" pathology — to be discussed further in Chapter 8 — is a popular and even titillating topic of conversation among poor urban Egyptians.

Yet, it is extremely important to note here that accepting male infertility in theory is not the same as accepting it in practice. Although Egyptians are willing to discuss the possibility of weak worms when a couple is childless, they tend to be less willing to accept male infertility as the absolute cause of any given case. In other words, even when men are acknowledged as having "worm problems," their problems are seen as correctable through "strengthening" medications that are thought to enliven dramatically even the most moribund of worms. Women, on the other hand, are usually blamed for having more severe, intractable infertility problems and are usually suspected of having such problems even in cases of proven male infertility. In the realm of infertility in Egypt, the persistence of women-blaming cannot be overstated. Purportedly infertile women who have been given a clean bill of health by numerous physicians continue to be condemned as infertile by family members, neighbors, and even husbands and continue to search for therapies under the assumption that there *must* be something wrong with them. In fact, the internalization of blame on the part of Egyptian women is often quite remarkable and is what motivates, in part, women's relentless quests for therapy.

It is this quest for therapy — ethnogynecological, biogynecological, or combining features of both — to which we now turn.

Part 2

Ethnogynecology

4. Healers, Herbalists, and Holy Ones

Siham's Story

Like every little girl in her poor Alexandrian neighborhood, Siham's hopes for the future included marrying a handsome husband and becoming a mother of many children. But, little did Siham realize that, as an adult, her "destiny" would also include delivering the children of other women and helping the childless overcome their plight.

Siham's introduction to ethnogynecology came when, as a new bride, she moved into her husband's family's home in an old neighborhood near the port of Alexandria. The multiple-story structure was known in the neighborhood as *bait id-dāyāt*, or "house of the midwives," for all of the women of Siham's husband's family, including his grandmother, great aunt, mother, and married sisters, were practicing midwives. Indeed, Siham's mother-in-law was an "educated" *dāya*, one who practiced midwifery "by certificate."

At first, Siham had no interest in the deliveries which occurred in the family's compound and to which her female in-laws were constantly called. But, when she came to work as an all-purpose aide in a gynecologist's private clinic, Siham, an uneducated but intellectually gifted woman, began observing the doctor and learning to "circumcise and deliver and do abortions and everything." Siham worked in the doctor's clinic for eight years, during which time her knowledge of biogynecology grew tremendously. However, when her mother-in-law died, Siham decided to quit her job and take over the family midwifery business. In addition to doing deliveries, she introduced into her practice the circumcision of girls; the induction of abortions for unmarried women who had been "tricked" by men; and the performance of *wasfāt baladī*, or folk remedies, for infertile women.

Today, Siham, who is in her mid- to late forties, has a thriving ethnogynecological practice, because, as she admits, she "knows everything" about ethnogynecology and much about biogynecology as well. She is called upon to deliver two or three infants a day, although she is unable to assist all of the women who request her midwifery services. Furthermore, she sees at least two infertile women a day, because she has developed a reputation in her neighborhood and beyond as a highly skilled infertility specialist. Siham says she helps as many of these infertile women as possible because she feels sorry for them. "They're upset because they can't get pregnant, and, psychologically, they're bad," she explains. She also notes, "Some come to me before they go to doctors, because they don't like doctors. And some come to me after they've seen doctors, because they get bored from their treatments. Some are young, fifteen to sixteen years old, and some are thirty-five."

When an infertile woman comes requesting Siham's services, Siham asks the woman to lie down, and she puts her finger in the woman's vagina to "see if the uterus is tight or the uterus is up or buried. If I find the uterus in the middle and open, this is good. But if it's on the side and became reversed because of humidity, that's wrong. It doesn't catch [the sperm]. It needs electrocautery and dilatation and curettage [i.e., biogynecological therapies]." She adds, "The most important thing is the uterus and the ovaries. If the ovaries are active and working and the uterus is in the right position and wide enough to catch, nothing can possibly happen."

If Siham finds that a woman's uterus is not in the right position and that all the fluid (semen) flows out immediately after sex, she attempts to "put it right." She asks the woman to get on her knees with her face down near the floor, and she manually raises the uterus "from behind" (anally). Afterward, she instructs the woman to lie on her back after sex until the morning to "keep the liquid inside."

If Siham finds that a woman's uterus is positioned correctly but she still suffers from infertility, Siham offers a wide variety of treatments, depending on what she suspects to be the probable cause. If she thinks the woman may suffer from utero-ovarian *ruṭūba*, or humidity, she asks the woman to return the following day for *ṣūwaf*, or vaginal suppositories, which she prepares for the patient overnight. In order to make *ṣūwaf*, Siham obtains "a medicine from the *'aṭṭār*" (herbalist)—usually a combination of *ḥulba* (fenugreek), *shīḥ* (wormwood), and a medicine called *abū kabīr*, or "old father," consisting of tiny seeds to be heated on a fire and ground to a smooth consistency. Once Siham has purchased all of these ingredients, she first picks through and washes the *ḥulba*, then sends it out to a nearby mill to be ground. Then she peels and grills several onions and mashes them in "something very clean." Next, she combines all of the ingredients and grinds them together. Taking small handfuls of the mixture, she kneads in some black glycerin and molasses, forming the mixture into a small lump. Then she places this lump in a piece of clean white gauze, and ties off the ends with a piece of thread to be used for removal (much like a tampon). Each *ṣūfa*, or vaginal suppository, is smaller than a teabag and is to be worn by the infertile woman for one day. In the evening, the *ṣūfa* is removed, and in the morning, a new *ṣūfa* is inserted for a period of three days immediately following the menses. According to Siham, "all the discharge and water comes down, and she's *very* dry underneath. The woman is very comfortable and feels good."

If, however, a woman is infertile and has a period that "comes too heavily," she is probably suffering from *dahr maftūḥ*, or an open back, which prevents her from becoming pregnant. For *dahr maftūḥ*, Siham performs *kasr*, or cupping, which serves to "hold the back." First, she asks the woman to remove her upper clothing and to lie on her stomach. Then, she takes a piece of gauze, fills it with salt, and ties it with a thread like a teabag. Dipping the tied-off end in oil, she flattens the gauze, lights it, and then places it on the woman's back. Immediately, she sets a small glass jar over the ignited gauze, thereby extinguishing the flame and preventing the gauze from burning the woman's skin. The resultant suction effect "sucks the flesh" for a period lasting five minutes. Siham then removes the jar and repeats the cupping six more times from top to bottom on both sides of the back. Although she knows that other *dāyāt* perform *kasr* on women's ovaries (that is, the abdomen), she believes this is a "mistake," a practice that "spoils the ovaries." Rather, by performing *kasr* on the back alone, Siham knows that she "closes the back" and prevents the infertile woman's period from coming (in other words, she causes her to become pregnant).

If, however, a woman has already had at least one child but suffers from an infertility-producing open back, Siham "locks" the woman's back, after providing *ṣūwaf* and performing *kasr* over two consecutive Fridays. On the third Friday of the therapeutic regimen, Siham takes one meter of rubber band, places a small lock on this band, and ties it around the woman's waist exactly at the time of the Friday noon prayer. She then fastens the lock, thereby closing the woman's back and allowing her to become pregnant and "carry" the pregnancy to full term.

Siham also treats women who are infertile from *khaḍḍa*, or a shock or fright that prevents them from becoming pregnant. This is because Siham owns the special *ṭast it-tarʿba*, or "pan of shock," a flat, copper pan from Saudi Arabia that is used to treat anyone who is sick or infertile from fright. When an infertile woman has been shocked, Siham provides her with the *ṭast it-tar'ba* and tells her to soak both dates and *ḥulba* in the pan overnight. The *ṭast it-tar'ba* is to be covered and left outside "in the open air." The next morning, the infertile woman must drink the contents of the pan, and, according to Siham, "the shock goes."

In addition to treating these relatively simple problems, Siham specializes in "unbinding" women who have been rendered infertile by way of *kabsa*, or an unexpected entrance of a ritually polluted person into the woman's room, an entrance which results in the "binding" of the woman's reproductive organs. According to Siham, a woman becomes *makbūsa*, or bound by *kabsa*, if she is a new bride and, during the lunar month following her wedding, someone "enters on her"—either a woman who has just delivered a child, a woman who has just miscarried, a girl who has just been circumcised, a man who has just shaved, or a woman who is wearing *dhahab bundu'i*, or twenty-four-karat gold in the shape of nuts. Likewise, women who have just miscarried or have just delivered a child can experience *kabsa* from such entrances and become infertile.

If Siham believes that a woman has suffered *kabsa*, she tries one or more of four remedies. First, she may tell the woman to go to a cemetery near Pompey's Pillar (a historic Alexandrian landmark)—or any cemetery for that matter—and to enter the cemetery through one door and leave it by another. While inside the cemetery, she mustn't speak to anyone, but, if a gravedigger can be found, she must ask him to dig up a bone or a skull and show it to her, thereby shocking her and unbinding *kabsa*.

If the woman is reluctant to go to the cemetery, Siham tries *kabsa* remedies at home. If she happens to be delivering a baby on a Friday morning before the Islamic noon prayer, Siham may summon the infertile woman to come to the site of the delivery, so that she can cause "pregnancy under the delivering one." Namely, she asks the infertile woman to sit underneath the delivering woman or to lie beside her. When the infant has emerged and the placenta is expelled, Siham takes small pieces of both the umbilicus and placenta and places them immediately inside the infertile woman's vagina, "while the blood is still hot." According to Siham, this unbinds the effects of *kabsa*, because the infertile woman's "uterus gets jealous, and she gets pregnant right away."

If the infertile woman cannot be summoned during the delivery itself, Siham may retain the bloody placenta and, when the infertile woman arrives, she may ask her to sit on the placenta or step over it seven times. Likewise, Siham keeps a miscarried fetus in a jar in her home and she may ask an infertile woman to step over it seven times or to place it in water and then to bathe with this water at the time of the Friday noon prayer. In every case, these *kabsa* rituals are to be repeated over three consecutive Fridays at the time of the Islamic noon prayer.

Siham also knows that some infertile women are *marbūṭīn*, or "tied" by *ʿamal*, an act of sorcery. Although she specializes in reproductive unbinding, Siham is by no means a sorceress. If she suspects a woman is *marbūṭa*, she advises her to go to "one who knows how to untie it." According to Siham, these are mostly "black people" from *Ṣaʿīd* (Upper Egypt) or Sudan, who know how to find an *ʿamal* which has been buried in a cemetery or inside the thick, fatty tail of a sheep.

Likewise, Siham knows that some infertile women must be seen by physicians. She explains, "There are injections and lots of things from the pharmacy. Now, medicine is not like before. It is more enlightened." But she adds,

> With doctors, you pay a lot and buy medicines and pay for operations. And some people are very poor, and they're scared of doctors. That's why they go to *wasfāt baladī*. [Doctors'] treatments are surgical operations, like *nafq* [tubal insufflation] and *kaḥt* [curettage] and *kawī* [cervical electrocautery]. They just do *nafq* and such things to get money. Believe me, I'm frank. They get five hundred or six hundred [Egyptian] pounds [$200–240]. The doctor I worked with did that, and the cure is from God. If some women go on with doctors' treatments, they can get pregnant, and if a woman is comfortable and relaxed and her nerves are okay, she can get pregnant. There are lots of treatments from doctors, and there are some very good doctors. And there are doctors who only want money and don't help you. They ask for more and more money and nothing happens. And there are some who are simple; they give you a simple treatment, and you get pregnant.

According to Siham, she sends her infertile patients to doctors only when all of her *wasfāt baladī* fail to cause pregnancy. However, she concludes that, "thanks to God," her success rate is 60 percent.

Ethnogynecology

Siham is one of thousands of ethnogynecologists practicing in urban Egypt. Although their numbers are unknown and their activities have been largely unaccounted for, Egyptian ethnogynecologists — both young and old, male and female—are prominently involved in the diagnosis and treatment of the infertile, who seek them out with perhaps greater frequency than they seek out the services of physicians.

Despite the increasing authority and influence of biomedicine in Egypt, what should not be underestimated is the extent to which most infertile Egyptian women hold beliefs about infertility causation that can be termed ethnogynecological in nature—causes of infertility for which only *wasfāt baladī*, or folk remedies, are considered to be effective. The vast armamentarium of ethnogynecological beliefs and practices relating to infertility alone is so rich and elaborate in Egypt that long-term fascination with and concern over the problem of infertility can only be assumed.

Siham, a female ethnogynecologist who specializes in the treatment of infertility, is in some ways representative of her fellow Egyptian ethnogynecologists. For one, she is a woman, as are most ethnogynecologists. Because those who seek treatment for infertility tend to be women, ethnogynecologists who "lay on hands" tend to be women as well, and, in most cases, they are senior, postmenopausal women, who have accumulated knowledge about infertility over time, eventually beginning to practice. In addition, Siham is, first and foremost, a *dāya*, or "ethno-obstetrician," who sees delivering infants as her major calling. However, many Egyptian *dāyāt* like Siham begin specializing in ethnogynecology as well, and this often includes the treatment of infertility and miscarriage, in addition to the performance of female circumcisions and traditional abortions in some cases.

Although Siham is representative of her fellow ethnogynecologists because she is a female *dāya*, she is also different from her compatriots in some ways. For one, she has firsthand experience in the biogynecological world, a world that she has come to understand perhaps better than most ethnogynecologists. Although Siham has never been certified in one of the biogynecological *dāya* training programs once attended by her mother-in-law, most of her noninfertility-related training came from observing the practices of her biogynecologist employer, a male physician who performed deliveries, female circumcisions, abortions, and infertility "operations." In fact, with the exception of her infertility therapies, Siham bases her practice on biogynecological methods. But, in cases of infertility, she sees what she has to offer patients as being quite different from the biogynecological procedures that physicians perform "for money." In fact, Siham believes that the most common causes of infertility—causes that she knows biogynecologists refuse to recognize—are probably responsible for the vast majority of infertility cases, responding only to the kinds of therapies that she and other ethnogynecologists can provide.

Thus, Siham, an ethnogynecologist who is somewhat atypical in bridging medical worlds, sees herself and her fellow Egyptian ethnogynecologists as performing an invaluable service. Not only are their infertility treatments more affordable to poor patients than those of biogynecologists, but their services are essential for the many causes of infertility denied by biogynecology. Given this scenario, it is not surprising to Siham that most poor urban Egyptian women begin their search for children in the ethnogynecological world.

But how does one typify the Egyptian ethnogynecological world—a world that has been largely overlooked by scholars and dismissed by the orthodox forces of Egyptian medical practice? To understand Egyptian ethnogynecology, it is necessary first to contextualize this area of specialized knowledge and praxis in terms of the much broader scope of contemporary Egyptian ethnomedicine.

Historical Continuities and Discontinuities

At the present historical moment, it is most accurate to characterize Egyptian ethnomedicine as consisting of a syncretic, unsystematic, loosely woven fabric of beliefs and practices gleaned in large part from the four major discursive traditions of medical practice described in Chapter 3. None of these traditions has disappeared completely in Egypt, despite the potent forces of both Islam and Western biomedicine as agents of social transformation. The documented history of medical pluralism in Egypt attests to the cultural embeddedness and continuity of these historically antecedent medical traditions dating to pharaonic times (Gran 1979; Sonbol 1991).

Yet, even though the medical past is embedded in the present, it is important to understand that contemporary medical pluralism in Egypt is not reducible to antecedent literate traditions (Morsy 1993), given that these medical traditions no longer exist in any recognizable, systematic form. It would be a mistake to emphasize the historical continuities and the contemporary survival of ancient medical traditions while ignoring the historical ruptures and discontinuities of continuously "shifting medical pluralism" in Egypt (Gran 1979). For, as we shall see, discontinuities between what once was and what is practiced today are abundantly apparent in contemporary Egyptian ethnomedicine. To take but one example, certain ethnomedical beliefs and practices common in Egypt today appear to be vestiges of Egypt's Galenic-Islamic medical past. Yet, Galenic humoral theory, so important in Egypt's history, is no longer articulated in any comprehensive fashion by patients or healers, nor can *Yūnānī* practitioners—those who base their practice exclusively on this literate tradition—be found in Egypt. In fact, despite the impressive histories of the great medical traditions traced in Chapter 3, unified schools of ethnomedicine rooted in these traditions are entirely absent in Egypt, as are practitioners formally trained in such schools or informed by textual guides. Rather, most ethnomedical practitioners receive training and ultimately operate independently, lacking professional associates and associations. Furthermore, like Siham, most offer services that can only be described as markedly heterogeneous and syncretic in nature, and they do not view themselves as adherents to any of the historic medical philosophies. Moreover, because they do not zealously follow particular literate traditions, most ethnomedical practitioners do not actively compete with one another or with biomedical physicians; some ethnogynecological specialists, for example, are cooperative, providing each other with ingredients and patient referrals. Furthermore, most see their services as *complementing* those of physicians, and they may actively refer patients to doctors when they believe their remedies will fail to provide relief.

Curative Eclecticism

That the majority of the Egyptian populace accepts the expertise of ethnomedical healers and the validity of their healing practices—which often counterpose the formally legitimated, purportedly authoritative, but nonetheless problematic tenets of biomedicine as it is practiced in Egypt today—is evident in both the serial and simultaneous use of ethnomedical and biomedical therapies on the part of many patients. Early (1993a, 1993b) has characterized the Egyptian tendency toward holistic health-seeking as curative "eclecticism" and has viewed it as a strategy for maximization of therapeutic benefits.

Perhaps nowhere is such curative eclecticism more evident than in infertile women's quests for therapy—quests that typically resemble therapeutic pastiches of ethnomedical and biomedical curative attempts. For example, Ragah, an infertile woman plagued by multiple medical problems, was deeply involved with biogynecological therapies, including a six-month regimen of artificial insemination with her husband's sperm (AIH). Yet, during the course of her AIH therapy, Ragah placed a small, clove-imbued lemon in her vagina, following the suggestion of a healer who told her that her uterus might be "disgusted," preventing pregnancy. After leaving the lemon in place for several hours so as to allow the refreshing fumes of clove and lemon to waft into her uterus, Ragah was unable to remove the lemon suppository on her own. Her trip to a competing hospital's emergency room was engendered by her embarrassment at having to explain to her probably incredulous physician why she had attempted such a cure in the midst of her ongoing, carefully monitored AIH therapy. Yet, for Ragah, active belief in and utilization of biomedicine did not preclude equally active belief in and utilization of alternative forms of care. Although Ragah could not articulate the exact meaning or desired therapeutic outcome of a lemon-clove suppository, she surmised that the effects of such natural substances, used medicinally since ancient times and placed nontraumatically in her vagina, might be just as beneficial to her reproductive organs as the painful, transcervical "injection" of her husband's medicated, incubated, and centrifuged ejaculate into the inner recesses of her womb.

Like Ragah, most poor urban women accept the validity of ethnomedical beliefs and practices, despite their lack of understanding of the historic origins and medical meanings of these beliefs and practices and regardless of their degree of belief in or understanding of biomedical notions of causation and cure. To wit, ethnomedical and biomedical beliefs and practices are seen as being of different logical orders; thus, most women do not experience cognitive dissonance or cultural conflict over the acceptance of ideas from presumably competing medical philosophies. Rather, many Egyptian women believe wholeheartedly in the nature of *both* bio- and ethnoetiologies, and thus they are willing to undertake remedies for a variety of potential conditions.

When remedies fail to cure, as they often do, most women do not question the treatment rationale, the potential efficacy of the cure, or the healer who administered it; rather, they explain the treatment failure by considering the likelihood of etiological causes of a different logical order. In most cases, women who have tried ethnomedical remedies seek explanations on the biomedical level, attributing their problem to a "medical cause" that could not have been overcome by *wasfāt baladī* alone. Such is typically the case when an ethnogynecological cure fails to produce a pregnancy; instead of condemning the cure, the woman who undertook it may realize, upon a posteriori reflection and contextualization, that she was not suffering from the ethnogynecological condition after all and must seek help for a medical problem that only a physician can cure. Or, as is often the case, an ethnogynecological treatment failure may be attributed to God—namely, his decision to postpone the woman's conception for reasons that only he can know. Thus, Egyptian women, who tend toward retrospective reflection and intellectualization of their therapeutic experiences, also tend to be tolerant, even forgiving, of ethnomedical failures, turning to "God and his medicine" as an explanatory paradigm when the ethnomedical model fails to satisfy.

As we shall see in the following chapters, for the Egyptian infertile, their quest for therapy typically includes appeals to *all* levels—ethnomedical, biomedical, and the divine. Even women who contend that ethnomedical beliefs are superstitious or religiously heretical may be swayed to try ethnomedical therapies out of concession to influential family members or out of resignation when biomedicine fails to provide an answer. In most cases, however, infertile women employ these therapies along with biomedical ones—often simultaneously—to increase the likelihood that all etiological possibilities are being considered and therapeutically countered. Failures on one level are met with attempts on another level, leading to a "search for children" that is complex, syncretic, creative, and ambitious, although often consuming, enervating, impoverishing, and ultimately unsuccessful for many.

Biomedical Dismissal

Although poor urban Egyptians tend to be open-minded, therapeutic holists, the physicians they encounter tend to be narrow-minded, biomedical purists, who dismiss ethnomedical beliefs and practices out of hand as "harmful superstition" or who contend that ethnomedicine has "died out" in Egypt altogether. This contemporary biomedical dismissal of ethnomedicine—in terms of both its significance and prevalence in the country—is not new. Rather, medical historians have documented the derisive attitudes of physicians, particularly imported European ones, toward Egyptian "traditional medicine" since the founding of European biomedicine in Egypt in the early 1800s (Gallagher 1990; Kuhnke 1990; Sonbol 1991).

That early European denigration of Egyptian ethnomedicine was to influence *Egyptian* biomedical practitioners is not surprising, given the influence of the British in convincing Egyptian medical students of the superiority of a nonindigenous medical model. In the late 1800s, for example, Dr. ʿAbd al-Raḥmān Efendī Ismāʿīl, an Egyptian graduate of the British-run Qasr al-Aini medical school, wrote a book entitled *Tibb al-Rukka*, or "The Medicine of the Old Women." Although the book today provides a fascinating account of Egyptian ethnomedical beliefs and practices at the *fin de siècle*, the author *intended* for his book to be an attack on the quackery of

Egypt's traditional medical practitioners, primarily "old women." His invective includes the following derogatory passages:

> I am referring to a low trade and mean occupation, which charlatans engage in as a means of obtaining spoil and as a source of plunder. Indeed, we ought rather to designate them as public robbers because they go around the countryside sometimes in company, sometimes alone, so that no village is free from their mischief, nor does any land escape from their guile. Some of them disguise themselves in the garb of pious derwishes and of learned *ulemas* [i.e., religious scholars]. Others make the speaking in a foreign language the snare by which they appropriate much of the property of those whose strength has been reduced by diseases, and who are ignorant even to-day of the methods of physicians and of the water-holes of healing. (Ismā'īl cited in Walker 1934:15)

The author continues, "Now that we have demonstrated by actual instances the influence of imagination, there only remains for us to set down here, in order, all the falsehoods and absurdities in which the 'old women' trade; for anyone who buys from them comes away fleeced . . . these stupidities as a whole are named the *Science of the Rukka*, or of the 'old wives'" (Ismā'īl cited in Walker 1934:17).

Contemporary biomedical practitioners in Egypt seem to lack such overt antipathy toward their ethnomedical counterparts. But this is due to the fact that most Egyptian physicians, especially those practicing in urban areas, have no idea of the extent to which ethnomedicine and ethnomedical practitioners continue to influence the actions of their patients. For example, urban biogynecologists tend to be wholly unfamiliar with (1) ethnogynecological practices, including the variety of types of practitioners, (2) ethnogynecological beliefs relating to infertility causation, (3) the significant degree to which poor urban Egyptian women participate in the ethnogynecological world, and (4) the magnitude of Egyptian women's beliefs in ethnogynecological causation and the efficacy of ethnodiagnosis and therapy.

Most biogynecologists admit that they possess no knowledge of ethnogynecological beliefs and practices, given their lack of interest and resultant failure to inquire about such things from their patients. However, others are adamant that such beliefs and practices have disappeared altogether in the urban areas of Egypt and are maintained at a low level, if at all, by "ignorant" people living in the countryside of the Nile Delta or in Upper Egypt. Furthermore, those who dismiss the significance of ethnomedicine contend that only desperation would drive a woman to believe in and undertake ethnogynecological practices and only after prior biomedical treatment had failed to provide a cure for her infertility.

On the other hand, not all physicians are so sanguine about the moribundity of ethnomedicine. Because of their exposure to patients' "extra-biomedical" beliefs, some biomedical practitioners (but the minority to be sure) have come to consider these beliefs widespread, although misguided. As one biogynecologist practicing in a provincial Nile Delta city explained, "They come and ask me what they can do about these [ethnomedical] causes. I cut it short with them; I don't like them to tell me. I tell them, 'Don't believe these things. We've got medical causes, and we're going to treat you, and you'll be pregnant.' I convince them that it is rubbish."

However, a university-based biogynecologist, whose own mother had once treated him with *wasfāt baladī*, was more philosophical about the motivation of patients who seek ethnomedical explanations and therapies. As he stated: "Yes, of course, at all levels of social class, they use these [traditional remedies]. If our president's wife didn't find a solution with doctors, she may ask a *dāya*. And I think there is something inside the female that causes her to do this. I think everywhere in the world if you don't get your problem solved by a specialist, you may ask anywhere else for help."

Interestingly, *dāyāt* such as Siham tend to share this biogynecologist's outlook. According to *dāyāt* and other ethnogynecologists, most of their infertile patients do not restrict their searches to either physicians or traditional healers, but rather utilize both in the hope of achieving pregnancy. In fact, like Siham, most urban *dāyāt* say they *encourage* their patients to visit physicians when ethnogynecological treatments fail to cause pregnancy. Physicians, they acknowledge, are best at handling the "big problems" of infertility, whereas *dāyāt* are equipped to deal with less complex, "little problems." Furthermore, most *dāyāt*, like Egyptian women in general, are well aware of a range of possible biomedical causes of infertility, which they can explain at length and which do not conflict with their alternative views of infertility causation.

Thus, whereas ethnogynecologists share an interest in and acceptance of the biomedical causes of infertility, believing such causes to be legitimate and treatable only by physicians, biogynecologists show little or no interest in the subject of ethnomedical causation, deeming such beliefs to be nonsensical, superstitious, and irrelevant in the modern world. Not only do they grossly underestimate the degree to which these beliefs are still present and acted upon by their patients, but some of them also scorn the promoters of such beliefs, particularly *dāyāt*, as ignorant, illegitimate, and potentially dangerous to patients. (It is important to note, however, that *dāyāt* are viewed as competing with them for obstetric clientele.)

Yet, the actual pervasiveness of ethnogynecology in urban Egypt is, in part, a reflection of the contemporary character of Egyptian biomedicine and its tendency to repel patients who might otherwise avail themselves of biomedicine exclusively. Put another way, biomedicine itself serves as a force for therapeutic diversification, given characteristics of biomedical practice that cause many patients to reject it. As we shall see, these include, *inter alia*, economic and social class barriers to access and utilization of biomedical services; asymmetrical power relations between biomedical practitioners and patients and the willingness of physicians to increase social distance through interactions with their patients that are patently authoritarian, paternalistic, and undermining of patients' self-esteem; promotion by physicians of purportedly therapeutic, invasive procedures that are biomedically unfounded, often iatrogenic, and are perceived by patients as profit-making ventures for physicians; and the resultant inability of many patients to find solutions within the biomedical system. Given the frequent outcome of "no results" following biogynecological treatment, infertile Egyptian women may turn to ethnogynecological therapies in what for many is a desperate quest for a cure. For some infertile Egyptian women, ethnogynecological remedies might be less appealing were biomedicine to offer more certain solutions. However, given Egyptian biomedicine's structural inadequacies and its inherent difficulty with infertility as a diagnostic and therapeutic problem, ethnogynecological therapies are compelling, especially for women who uphold the ethnomedical notions of infertility causation to be described in the following chapters. Furthermore, because biomedical practitioners often fail to offer adequate explanations to their patients, many Egyptian women, out of desperation for understanding, are willing to consider and accept a wide range of nonbiomedical etiological possibilities. As Egyptian women are apt to put it, "When one is sinking, one will hang on even to a straw."

Religious Opposition

Opposition to ethnomedicine does not come from biomedical quarters alone. Increasingly, Islamic religious leaders and groups in Egypt are spreading the word that *wasfāt baladī*—especially those that involve unorthodox religious elements—are "against the religion." Whereas biomedicine is viewed for the most part in Egypt as being *ḥalāl*, or compatible with

Islamic doctrine,[1] many ethnomedical practices are considered *ḥarām*, or forbidden, by religiously literate Muslims and conservative Islamists (popularly known as Islamic "fundamentalists"), who see these practices as being "against God," "a mistake in the religion," or "like believing in something besides God." This religious argument is becoming increasingly apparent as a result of the contemporary Islamic revival in Egypt, which, as noted earlier, has gained momentum among the urban underclass during the past decade.

Interestingly, contemporary Islamists tend to condone most biomedical therapies as the creation of God—as being "God's medicine." Yet, it is truly ironic that only modern, Western-based biomedicine is deemed religiously acceptable, given the rich history of *Yūnānī*-inspired Islamic and prophetic medicine in Egypt. As we shall see, many of the contemporary ethnomedical practices found in Egypt derive from these earlier, religiously acceptable medical traditions, which are now viewed as unorthodox by Islamist elements in Egyptian society. Certainly, this opposition to ethnomedicine attests to the powerful hegemony of European-inspired biomedicine in Egypt, the ideologies of which have permeated the thinking of the religious elite. For example, in her article, "Islamic Clinics in Egypt: The Cultural Elaboration of Biomedical Hegemony," Morsy (1988) argues that the medicine being practiced in charitable, mosque-run "Islamic clinics" throughout Egypt is not Islamic at all, but rather the standard brand of Egyptian biomedicine transplanted to a so-called Islamic setting. Thus, Islamic clinics are not counterhegemonic to Western imperialist biomedicine in Egypt, but rather serve as a force for its globalization and entrenchment.

Unlike biomedicine, ethnomedicine has been increasingly discredited as superstition, given its origins in the pre-Islamic *jāhilīya*, or "age of ignorance," and its practice by quasi-religious *shuyūkh* who blaspheme Islamic orthodoxy through practices involving animism and sorcery, among other things. Even pilgrimages to the mosque-tombs of dead religious *shuyūkh*, pilgrimages which are religiously inspired, are viewed as heretical by orthodox Muslims in Egypt. According to them, praying to human *shuyūkh* is like "giving God a partner"—a partner who is "just as human as we are." Thus, spiritual pilgrimages, like other components of the ethnomedical "search for children," are seen by increasing numbers of urbanites as being religiously heretical.

Yet, despite this increasing religious opposition, ethnomedicine continues to be vigorously practiced in both urban and rural areas and is often overtly syncretic, combining at once the natural and the supernatural, the profane and the sacred. As we shall see, practices that can be traced to pre-Islamic times, as well as practices that have arisen since then but are clearly unorthodox in terms of Islam, are often undertaken in conformity with Islamic ritual—primarily their performance in concordance with the Islamic prayer cycle. Although this convergence of "folk" with religious practices is extremely troubling to orthodox Muslims, such forms of so-called popular Islam continue to be extremely common in Egypt, particularly among the religiously illiterate, urban and rural Muslim poor, who comprise the majority of the country's populace. Thus, it is important to bear in mind that many of the ethnogynecological practices to be described in the following chapters are representations of the less orthodox elements of "Islam in praxis" (Early 1993a), elements that are found throughout Egypt and the rest of the Middle East.

Popular Rejection

Because both biomedicine and Islam, and the popular media through which they are promoted, are powerful institutions in Egyptian society, growing numbers of Egyptians, including women of the urban and rural lower classes, are beginning to reject ethnomedicine[2]—sometimes based on religious arguments, sometimes based on the scientific rationales of biomedicine, and, in most cases, based on both, given that biomedical science and religion in Egypt tend to reinforce one another. Although still in the minority, poor urban women (and more often than not their husbands) who reject ethnomedical interpretations and remedies usually do so by claiming complete faith in "God and doctors" or "science and medicine" to offer effective cures. For these women, ethnomedicine is no longer convincing and is often deprecated as "quackery," "nonsense," "ignorance," "stupidity," "silliness," "superstition," "empty words," "fairy tales," and "based on coincidence."

As one skeptic explained, "I don't believe in *wasfāt baladī*, although lots of people do. I think medicine is up to date now, and it's better to go after it instead of starting to do things at home. If you start doing *wasfāt baladī*, you won't stop."

Another commented, "Forget about *wasfāt baladī*, because these hurt a person. Doctors are much better. Maybe she'll do something wrong [with traditional remedies], and she'll feel sorry for her whole life. It's better to get information from the doctor. He knows the difference between one thing and another."

Another woman, who was infertile but literate and able to read the

Qur'an, said, "I don't believe in these things. I believe in God only. Many people told me to go to the cemetery, to get gold and bathe with it, to do *ṣūwaf*, to use a lock for my open back. But I only trust the doctor because he's educated. Anything from those 'retarded' people [i.e., ethnogynecologists] I don't believe. I know all this is nonsense. I can only ask God for help. I read the Qur'an, and I know this is *dagl* [quackery]. It's ignorance."

Another infertile woman, who had been coerced by neighbors to undertake two traditional remedies, explained,

> I didn't believe in it, but I just did two things because my neighbors told me to do them, and I had nothing to lose. Later, they told me they didn't work because I didn't believe in them. I believe it's empty words. Everything is from God, and God made medicine, so if I'm sick, I should get examined and treated [i.e., by a doctor]. My husband doesn't believe in *wasfāt baladī* either. He told me, "This is nonsense, and it was ignorant of you to do them."

The experience of this final commentator is not unusual. Ethnomedical disbelievers say they are often coerced into undergoing ethnomedical therapies at some point in their lives by overzealous friends, neighbors, and relatives, particularly older women in their own and especially their husbands' families. For many, the pressure becomes unbearable, and they end up undertaking ethnomedical remedies—sometimes in great numbers—just to "keep others quiet."

As one infertile woman explained, "Whatever anyone tells me, I do. Otherwise they say, 'Why aren't you pregnant? Are you searching?' The whole building gives me advice, because here we don't have anyone who leaves the other alone."

Another infertile woman, whose neighbor was "dragging" her into both biomedical and ethnomedical treatment, lamented, "I don't believe—not even in *munaggimīn* or *dāyāt*. But I'm afraid people would blame me if I don't try. My friend is just *forcing* me. She's a neighbor who's good with me. All the other neighbors are saying, 'Where are you going?' I tell them, 'For exams.' They say, 'All day every day for exams?' I'm tired of all this."

Another infertile woman, whose husband didn't agree with the ethnomedical remedies advised by his family to his wife, explained, "During my fourteen years, I've been doing *everything*. My in-laws give me *lots* of advice. I did *many* things. When they say, 'There's a doctor,' I go to the doctor. 'There's a *dāya*,' I go. 'A *shaikh*,' I go. 'A *munaggim*,' I go. 'A mosque,' I visit. Also, when I'm fed up with injections, operations, and so on, and see it's no use, I try other things [i.e., *wasfāt baladī*]."

Like this woman, some poor urban Egyptian women who are skeptical about ethnomedicine may try *wasfāt baladī* when biomedicine appears to offer little hope for curing their infertility. Most rationalize the experience by saying "*maybe* it can get me pregnant . . . just to see if it helps." Furthermore, many infertile women report being exposed to bountiful rumors of women who have become pregnant following these treatments; so, they try them—"just to give some hope."

For the vast majority of poor urban Egyptian women, however, ethnomedical remedies pose no crises of conviction. Their belief in the potential efficacy of ethnomedicine to cure them of their afflictions is wholehearted, and they visit ethnomedical specialists with faith in their knowledge and expertise. In this regard, poor urban infertile women who accept the conditions of ethnomedicine are particularly fortunate, because, as we shall see, several different types of ethnogynecological specialists hope to avail the infertile of their services.

Ethnogynecologists

Ethnogynecology, practiced primarily by Egypt's numerous *dāyāt*, is a particularly active area of ethnomedicine, given Egypt's high total fertility rate of 4.8 births per woman (Egypt National Population Council 1989), the maternal health problems that accompany such high fertility, the concern with fecundity among childless women, and the various barriers, both social and economic, that prevent Egyptian women from seeking biomedical care (Carney 1984; Institute of Medicine 1979; Lane and Millar 1987; Morsy 1980a, 1980b, 1993). In Egypt, the vast majority of poor rural and urban women consult an ethnogynecologist, usually a *dāya*, at least once in their lifetimes and usually much more often. However, as we shall see, ethnomedical specialists other than *dāyāt* also treat women's reproductive health problems, although their contributions to Egyptian ethnogynecology have received relatively little scholarly attention.

Furthermore, it is important to note that these various ethnogynecologists often serve as the primary proponents and perpetuators of ethnomedical beliefs relating to infertility causation. Unlike biomedical practitioners, who tend to retain etiological information for a variety of reasons to be explored in Chapter 8, ethnogynecologists tend to disclose causal and sometimes therapeutic information to their patients, although often without dogmatic verification. Because this information is not considered sacred by healers, it is disseminated widely throughout the Egyptian populace, especially among the rural and urban poor. As a result, most poor urban Egyptian women, even those who have never experienced infertility problems, are familiar with the more commonly held ethnomedical beliefs regarding infertility causation, even though their understandings and interpretations of these causes may vary. Those who tend to have acquired the most ethnogynecological knowledge, however, are usually older women, who may eventually accrue enough expertise in this area to begin to serve as lay healers, dispensing advice and remedies to younger women of reproductive age. Furthermore, many young infertile women begin their therapeutic searches at home, because their mothers, mothers-in-law, and older female relatives and neighbors may be able to provide them with much needed advice on, and even administration of, appropriate ethnogynecological therapies. In other words, because of the rather casual spread of information from ethnogynecological healers to their patients, knowledge of ethnogynecological beliefs and practices is widespread, especially among women, who may learn to heal other women without ever claiming an official healer's status.[3]

The vast majority of infertility problems, however, are viewed as requiring specialized expertise, be it biomedical or ethnomedical. In Egypt, infertile women have a large number of ethnogynecologists from which to choose, given the presence of five major types of healers who specialize in ethnogynecological problems as shown in Table 1.

Sittāt Kabira

In urban areas of Egypt such as Alexandria, it is possible for women to visit healers who specialize only in the treatment of infertility. These healers are typically postmenopausal women, or *sittāt kabira* (literally, "elderly women"), who distinguish themselves from *dāyāt* because they do not perform deliveries or other roles normally associated with traditional midwifery. Rather, these women, who have no special title other than "elderly women," perform various cures for infertility and especially those cures requiring ritual healing objects. Most commonly, these women are owners of the *ṭast it-tar'ba* (the pan of shock) and/or the *mushāharāt* (the various items necessary to unbind the effects of *kabsa*). Because these objects are difficult to obtain, originating as they most often do in Saudi Arabia, women who own them may begin to specialize in the treatments associated with them and become recognized for this specialized knowledge.

In Alexandria, the most famous *sitt kabīra* was an elderly woman

TABLE 1. The Roles of Ethnogynecological Specialists in Egypt.

TYPE OF SPECIALIST	ETHNOMEDICAL CAUSES OF INFERTILITY TREATED	TYPE OF TREATMENTS PRESCRIBED
Sittāt kabira (elderly women)	*Ruṭūba* (humidity)	Cupping
	Kabsa (polluting entrance)	*Kabsa* preventives, rituals
	Khaḍḍa (shock)	Pan of shock
Dāyāt (midwives)	*Ruṭūba*	Suppositories, cupping, vapor sitz baths
	Dahr maftūḥ (open back)	Cupping, cauterization, locking, twining
	Khaḍḍa	Pan of shock
	Kabsa	*Kabsa* preventives, rituals
	Vaginal tightness	Vaginal stick
	Uterine malposition	Anal correction
	Other	Herbal potables
ʿAṭṭārīn (herbalists)	*Ruṭūba*	Suppositories, vapor sitz baths, ointments
	Kabsa	Suppositories
	Ukht taḥt il-arḍ (spirit-sister under the ground)	Suppositories
	Female infertility (general)	Herbal potables
	Male infertility (general)	Herbal edibles
Munaggimīn (spiritist healers)	*Kabsa*	Divination, *kabsa* rituals
	ʿAmal (sorcery)	Sorcery divination/nullification
	Ukht taḥt il-arḍ	Spirit invocation/appeasement rituals
	Ḥasad (evil eye)	Protective amulets
	Miscellaneous	Diagnostic clairvoyance, quasi-biomedical healing, prayer, amulets, *zār* spirit placation ceremonies, semen suppositories, "artificial insemination" by intercourse
Shuyūkh bil-baraka (blessed *shaikhs*)	God's will	Divine intercession, amulets, prayers

Photograph 3. A Bedouin *sitt kabīra*. (Photograph by Mia Fuller)

named Sitt Naima, who was said to have specialized for many years in the performance of *kabsa* healing rituals. Over time, she gained wide recognition and notoriety throughout Alexandria and other parts of Egypt for her ability to unbind *kabsa* effects in infertile women. Infertile women were usually taken by their mothers or mothers-in-law to the home of Sitt Naima, located near the famous mosque of Abū 'l-'Abbās al-Mursī in the ancient Manshiyyah section of Alexandria. There, they participated in *kabsa* rituals either alone or with a small number of other infertile women, who were enjoined by Sitt Naima to circumambulate her well seven times, throwing in pieces of bread, sugar, and candles as they went. However, by

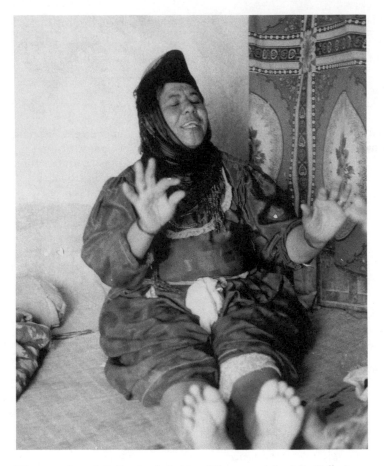

the late 1980s, Sitt Naima was no longer performing *kabsa* remedies, either because she had died, as some said, or because she was forced by religious or governmental authorities to cease her healing activities, as others claimed. As a result, infertile women who went searching for Sitt Naima during the late 1980s did so in vain, much to their disappointment.

Dāyāt

Throughout the centuries, Egypt has been home to thousands of *dāyāt*, or traditional midwives such as Siham, who have delivered the infants and cared for the health of Egypt's less privileged women (Kuhnke 1990). In Egypt today, it is estimated that approximately ten thousand *dāyāt* are active practitioners of midwifery, conducting between 80 and 90 percent of all deliveries among the rural and urban poor (Assaad and El Katsha 1981; El Malatawy 1985).

Although formal, six- to twelve-month practical obstetrics training of traditional midwives started as early as the 1940s in Egypt, the Egyptian Ministry of Health changed its policy in 1969, discontinuing all *dāya* training; revoking all previously issued licenses; warning women by radio against the use of "ignorant, unskilled, and often dangerous" *dāyāt*; and encouraging women to deliver with governmentally trained *ḥakīmāt*, or nurse-midwives, stationed at maternal and child health clinics and rural health units throughout the country (Pillsbury 1978; Khattab 1983; Sukkary 1981). Because of this governmental effort to essentially wipe out the position of the *dāya* (Pillsbury 1978), *dāyāt*, who most often learned their skills from older female relatives,[4] were forced underground, continuing their practices illicitly without the benefits of supervision, training, or hygienic supplies. Not until the 1980s, when the Ministry of Health realized that its program of modernization had failed to bring about intended changes in the state of Egyptian obstetrics, did it reinstitute limited *dāya* training programs in primarily rural governorates (Hong 1987).

Yet, despite recent attempts by the Egyptian government and international health organizations such as WHO and UNICEF to regulate and professionalize the *obstetric* practice of *dāyāt* (Assaad and El Katsha 1981; Bentley 1989; Hafez 1989; Hong 1987; Ismail 1989; UNICEF 1985), little attention has been paid within the international health and scholarly communities to the *gynecological* services performed by *dāyāt* on thousands of infertile Egyptian women.[5] This neglect is serious when one considers that *dāyāt* are Egypt's truest ethnogynecologists, performing the greatest variety of the most commonly employed ethnogynecological cures for infertility.

In fact, it would not be overstating the case to suggest that *dāyāt* are perhaps *the* major force in the attempted treatment of infertility problems in Egypt, gaining wide recognition for their infertility services and silently but effectively competing with unwitting Egyptian gynecologists for infertile patients.

However, to impute competitive motives to Egyptian *dāyāt* is unfair, given that the majority of them do not claim to treat the kinds of problems, such as "blocked tubes" and "weak ovaries," that only physicians are able to handle. Because *dāyāt* restrict themselves to the treatment of "little problems," they generally charge their patients relatively small fees for their services—usually half a pound to five pounds (twenty cents to two dollars) and rarely more than ten pounds (four dollars).[6] Some *dāyāt*, on the other hand, refuse payment, knowing that if the patient becomes pregnant, a gift will be forthcoming.

In treating their infertile patients, *dāyāt* often forgo diagnosis altogether, proceeding instead to empiric trials of the various infertility treatments they offer. However, some *dāyāt* like Siham perform diagnostic examinations, usually consisting of using the index finger to manually examine the patient's vagina or externally examining the patient's ovaries, breasts, and sometimes back by palpating them or by inserting a finger in her navel. Rarely, *dāyāt* become more sophisticated in their diagnostic procedures; for example, one Alexandrian *dāya*, who acts "too much like a *duktūra*," according to some women, asks her infertile patients to bring a sample of their husbands' semen in a glass jar, so that she may pronounce whether or not the "worms are swimming."

Generally speaking, however, *dāyāt* are best known for treating the "little problems" of infertility, including *ruṭūba* (humidity), *dahr maftūḥ* (open back), and *khaḍḍa* (shock), all of which will be described in detail in Chapter 6. Some *dāyāt* also own the *mushāharāt* objects necessary for *kabsa* healing rituals or specialize in advice on other ways of unbinding this state. Rarely, *dāyāt* perform purported anatomical corrections, such as "widening" the vagina or returning retroverted uteri to their correct position. *Dāyāt* do *not*, however, deal with the socially induced causes of infertility involving sorcery or spirits. As they are the first to admit, these problems are best left to the *munaggimīn*, or spiritist healers, whose services will be described shortly.

Because of their reported success in curing infertile women, many *dāyāt* are renowned in their communities as infertility specialists. Infertile women who seek the services of such *dāyāt* are often compelled to do so

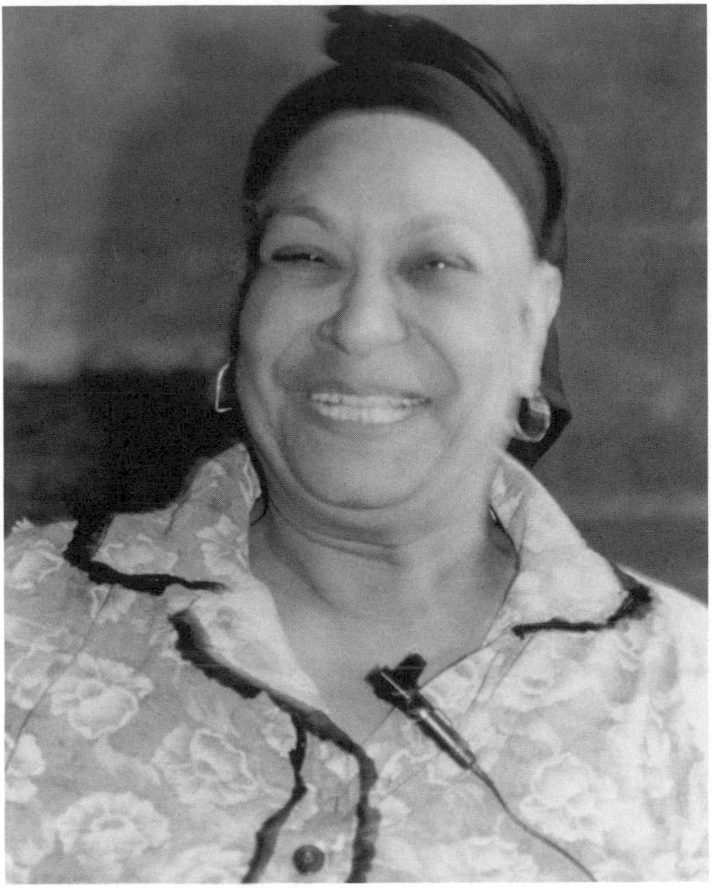

Photograph 4. An urban *dāya.* (Photograph by Marcia Inhorn)

because of their acquaintance with other women who have "gone and become pregnant." Even when the cures of *dāyāt* fail, many infertile women contend that they would have become pregnant had they not had some other intervening medical condition. In other words, faith in *dāyāt* is generally high among the infertile, and the reputations of these healers are constructed through curative success.

'Aṭṭārīn

To perform their cures, *dāyāt* work closely with *'aṭṭārīn*, or herbalists, who usually supply them with the botanical and mineral substances necessary for various infertility remedies. Like their predecessors in the pharaonic and *Yūnānī* eras (Dols 1984; Kuhnke 1990; Manniche 1989), many *'aṭṭārīn* are highly skilled ethnobotanists, with knowledge about the geographical origins, pharmaceutical properties, and medicinal uses of a wide range of plant substances. In fact, some *'aṭṭārīn* advertise their expertise in treating common maladies by way of signs hung in their small shops or marketplace stalls. Most *'aṭṭārīn*, it should be noted, are first and foremost commercial merchants, selling herbs and spices for household cooking use and offering ethnomedical advice only as a sideline.

Although most *'aṭṭārīn* are male, and the profession is transmitted hereditarily in some cases through the male line, *'aṭṭārīn* are quite knowledgeable about "female complaints," given the propensity of Egyptian women to employ herbal remedies for various common gynecological problems, including vaginal bleeding, severe labor pains, and menstrual cramps. In the case of infertility, *'aṭṭārīn* are specialists in uterine *ruṭūba*, or humidity, which is thought to be especially amenable to various herbal substances, administered by vapor sitz baths or vaginal suppositories. (Indeed, many *'aṭṭārīn* are famous for their *ruṭūba*-draining vaginal suppositories.) Although most *'aṭṭārīn* are strictly "naturalists" (Pillsbury 1978), some also dabble in the occult; namely, through manipulating the symbolic properties of the colorful, pleasing herbs and minerals placed in vaginal suppositories, some *'aṭṭārīn* believe they are able to placate the angered spirit-sisters who occasionally cause infertility.

Although *'aṭṭārīn* are the ones who dispense the necessary herbs and minerals, *dāyāt* are usually the ones who purchase these substances from *'aṭṭārīn*, thus serving as intermediaries between them and their infertile patients. However, in some cases, infertile women are asked by *dāyāt* to buy specific ingredients directly from *'aṭṭārīn*, who may dispense their own advice and remedies directly to patients. Because of their extensive pharmacopoeia, *'aṭṭārīn* often have specific ideas about the best treatments for *ruṭūba*, as well as detailed information about herbal cures for male infertility and impotence problems. Thus, in and of themselves, many *'aṭṭārīn* are skilled infertility specialists, although they usually provide their consultation services only to *dāyāt*, who pass this wisdom on to their patients in the form of ready-made treatments.

Munaggimīn

By far the most controversial class of urban Egyptian ethnogynecologists is *munaggimīn*,[7] or spiritist healers, who are known for specializing in diagnostic clairvoyance and the treatment of the more difficult, socially mediated causes of infertility, including angered spirits and the sorcery acts of enemies. Despite cautionary mention of them in the Qur'an, the practices of contemporary *munaggimīn* are clearly rooted in Egypt's prophetic medical tradition, and many *munaggimīn* draw upon "the power of the Book"—namely, the Qur'an—to help them diagnose and cure patients. Because of their professed religiosity, *munaggimīn* are often addressed and referred to by their religious title *shaikh(a)*. However, many Egyptians say that *munaggimīn* do not deserve such a title of respect, given that they do not truly "know God," and they refer to them pejoratively instead as mere *saḥḥārīn* (sorcerers or magicians) or *daggālīn* (quacks or charlatans).

Given the suspicion surrounding *munaggimīn*, it is perhaps surprising that they can be found to practice widely in both rural and urban poor areas of Egypt and can claim their fair share of infertile patients. Furthermore, to describe *munaggimīn* as spiritist healers alone is to diminish their role, because both male and female *munaggimīn* provide a considerable variety of services, for which they often receive significant payments (£E 10–250 or $4–100) and which appear to be gender-based to some degree.

Female *munaggimīn* are often sought out for their ability to tell fortunes, particularly in matters of concern to women, such as marriage and reproduction. Many female *munaggimīn* are, in fact, famed clairvoyants with large female followings and are able to divine whether a particular infertile woman is suffering from a biogynecological problem, such as "weak ovaries," for which she should seek a physician's treatment, or an ethnogynecological problem such as *kabsa*. The latter information is particularly useful for women who must decide whether to undergo *kabsa* unbinding, which is sometimes provided by female *munaggimīn* for their patients. Furthermore, some female *munaggimīn* cure other "natural" causes of infertility, including uterine *ruṭūba* (by way of vaginal suppositories and herbal potables) and open backs (through cupping and "sewing" of the flesh with an upholstery needle).

Unlike male *munaggimīn*, female *munaggimīn* generally do not traffic in malevolent sorcery—in either its creation or its dissolution. However, they may be deeply involved in the spirit world, either as "possessed" individuals, who use their spirits to diagnose and treat other spirit-troubled women, or as skillful agents of spirit invocation, who make the wishes of others' spirits known. For the infertile, female *munaggimīn* communicate with the *akhawāt taḥt il-arḍ*, or "spirit-sisters under the ground," who trouble their earthly sisters by making them infertile. However, because these spirit-sisters do not actually possess, or "wear" their earthly sisters, the female *munaggimīn* who treat the infertile for spirit troubles rarely ask them to participate in the communal *zār*, the spirit placation ceremony attended by the possessed, but instead perform private rituals to be described in Chapter 6.

Similarly, male *munaggimīn*, who are widely known in Egypt for their organization of *zār* healing rituals, do not ordinarily recommend the *zār* for their infertile patients. Instead, like female *munaggimīn*, they perform a number of alternative diagnostic and treatment services, which in some cases duplicate and expand upon those offered by their female counterparts.

For one, male *munaggimīn* are often renowned clairvoyants, who "open the Book" (that is, the Qur'an or some other presumed religious text) to discern and reveal the patient's future. Whereas many female *munaggimīn* restrict their divinations to simple diagnoses of women's conditions, male *munaggimīn* are often bold prognosticators, who predict whether a woman will have a child and even how soon in the future this will occur. Speaking of her own visit to a *munaggim*, one infertile woman explained, "On a piece of paper, he wrote my name and my mother's name. Then he put that paper in the Qur'an and waited for maybe five minutes. Then he opened the Book and started telling me things. Some pages of the Book, he knows the number of the pages, and he talks about them and tells me if I will get pregnant or not. He told me that I will have children, but when he doesn't know. When is up to God."

Furthermore, it is the content of these remarkable divinations—remarkable in that they often involve uncanny revelation by the *munaggim* of patients' most personal matters—that often convinces patients to undergo the expensive and unusual infertility "cures" sometimes suggested by the *munaggim*. As curers, male *munaggimīn* offer a variety of services, to be described in detail in Chapter 6. Most frequently, they write protective and therapeutic *ḥugub*, or amulets, which are said to contain passages from the Qur'an and which are to be worn or held against the body, burned with incense, or placed in water for drinking or bathing. Like female *munaggimīn*, some male *munaggimīn* may use their ability to communicate with the spirit world to suggest ways angered subterranean spirits can be appeased, thereby reversing a patient's infertility. Rarely, male *munaggimīn* use their divinational diagnostic powers to undertake quasi-medical healing. For example, some *munaggimīn* are reputed to be "*shaikh*-doctors," because they claim to "diagnose and treat any medical problem." For the infertile, they often dispense "prescriptions" consisting of unidentified injections and bottled "medicines." In most cases, however, the treatments prescribed by *munaggimīn* are herbal substances, administered as suppositories, additions to bathwater, or mixtures to be imbibed by both husband and wife. Occasionally, such *shaikh*-doctors become extremely sophisticated, performing physical examinations of patients, "analyzing" husbands' semen, examining patients' X rays, pronouncing "medical" diagnoses, and prescribing medications from the pharmacy.

According to a Christian woman who received treatment from one such Muslim *shaikh*-doctor over a period of seven months,

> Someone told me to go, because they said, "If you go to him, you'll get pregnant right away. He treats all kinds of medical problems." During a period when I wasn't going to doctors, I decided to go. My husband didn't accept my going there, but I convinced him, "Let me try." When the *shaikh* saw me, he told me, "Your treatment doesn't need doctors. In my hands, you'll get pregnant. But you should pay me seventy pounds [twenty-eight dollars] for a four-month treatment." It was my misfortune that I believed him. Each month for four months, I went. It cost me fifteen pounds [six dollars] each time and sometimes I had to sleep there because it was very far, in a village near Damanhur. He insisted I shouldn't go to a doctor. Instead, I must wash myself and come the first day of my period. He prescribed things for me, but, after four months, there was no result. So I stopped for two months, then I went back to him again for three months. At the end, I found it was useless, and he was taking advantage of me. But, at that time, it was a big fuss. And even doctors' wives used to go to that *shaikh* to get pregnant. But I didn't see [a successful result] with my own eyes; I heard only.

Although the thought of *munaggimīn* posing as doctors is troubling to some, male *munaggimīn* have gained their most unfavorable reputation from their ability to ensorcell innocent victims, causing, among other things, male impotency, and their reported impregnation of innocent infertile women through the provision of semen-imbued suppositories or through the rape of women whom they have "tricked" or made unconscious. In fact, stories of male *munaggimīn* impregnating hundreds of "infertile" Egyptian women with their own sperm abound in the media, in popular discourse, and in scholarly discourse as well (El Saadawi 1980; Morsy 1993). The frequency with which unscrupulous *munaggimīn* provide their own brand of "artificial insemination by donor" to women whose husbands may actually be infertile is probably much less than these stories suggest. For example, although many women in this study had heard of such practices on the part of male *munaggimīn*, only one woman had ever encountered a suspicious situation of this sort. Namely, a Sudanese *munag-*

gim who was visiting her neighborhood said that he could cure her of her infertility. He went to another room of her house, returning with a pan containing thirty cotton suppositories, which he told her to wear vaginally over a period of several days. She consulted with her husband and agreed to throw the suppositories away, fearing they might contain the *munaggim*'s semen. As she explained, "We may be *fallāḥīn*, but we're careful."

Although such occurrences are probably exceedingly rare, the Egyptian media run stories from time to time of male *munaggimīn* who are caught by the police and confess to having impregnated hundreds of women. In one such widely publicized 1989 incident, a husband had accompanied his wife to the *munaggim*'s home, and, when she failed to emerge from a "private" session with the "*shaikh*," her husband broke down the door to find his inebriated, sleeping wife on the floor of the darkened room and the naked *munaggim* on top of her—"doing his work." The husband grabbed the *munaggim*, dragged his naked body outside, screamed for other witnesses to come, and had the *munaggim* hauled off by the police. Upon his arrest, the *munaggim* confessed to having had sex with and impregnating hundreds of women, who were the helpless victims of their husbands' unacknowledged infertility.

Because of such reports, *munaggimīn* have a poor reputation as a class of healers, and Egyptian men are often quite reluctant to allow their wives to visit male *munaggimīn* alone or at all. In general, *munaggimīn* are regarded with a great deal of suspicion by most poor urban Egyptians, although they may actively employ their services, especially when they believe they have been ensorcelled. Many Egyptians doubt the characters of *munaggimīn*, because of their willingness to perform harmful sorcery and other "cures" that are immoral, their inauthentic claims to religiosity and consequent performance of quasi-religious divinational and healing practices which are condemned in the Islamic scriptures, and their avarice. Furthermore, because the questions *munaggimīn* ask patients are often indicative of prior knowledge of the individual, many Egyptians are suspicious of *munaggimīn*'s strategies of divination, believing that their knowledge must be based on illusive practices and trickery. Thus, *munaggimīn* are often accused of being bad men, quacks, charlatans, tricksters, liars, opportunists, and thieves, who take advantage of gullible, helpless Egyptians and cheat them of large amounts of money. Even those individuals who complete a *munaggim*'s suggested remedies are often unconvinced of their efficacy and may comment that the *munaggim* "stole my money for nothing."

As one woman who had once resorted to a *munaggim* explained,

> There are two kinds of *shuyūkh.* One is in a mosque. He's a *mufti* [cleric]. He only prays and reads Qur'an; he is wise. The other is a *saḥḥār* [magician]. This is a bad word, so we wouldn't call him that. So, instead, we call him "the *shaikh.*" He's not exactly a good man. He takes money for what he does, and he is *not* religiously educated. These people clean themselves before prayer with milk, not water; this is religiously incorrect. And they actually trick people. For example, they send two or three people to you in the street and they ask, "What do you complain of? There is a good man you should see." And they would know your complaint and one would go back to the *shaikh* and inform him. So when the lady comes, he would tell her, "You have this and that." So, the *shaikh* becomes famous, but the man is actually a thief. This is all nonsense.

It is interesting to note that this ambivalence toward a class of ethnogynecological healers appears to be restricted to *munaggimīn* alone.[8] *Dāyāt*, *ʿaṭṭārīn*, and *shuyūkh bil-baraka*, to be discussed next, are generally viewed as being honest and beneficent healers, who may, in fact, view *munaggimīn* with equivalent skepticism.

Shuyūkh Bil-Baraka

When speaking of healing *shuyūkh*, it is extremely important to differentiate *munaggimīn* from the other variety of *shuyūkh*: namely, religious *Ṣūfī*, or maraboutic, healers known by urban Egyptians as *shuyūkh bil-baraka*, or "blessed *shaikhs*." *Shuyūkh bil-baraka* are typically (but not necessarily) founders or followers of *Ṣūfī* orders, whose history in Egypt dates to the tenth century and whose members have been involved in healing since at least the sixteenth century (Gran 1979). Today, there are sixty-eight recognized *Ṣūfī* orders in Egypt, claiming to encompass up to 10 percent of the total population (Biegman 1990). The Egyptian government not only fully recognizes the existence and organization of such orders, but sees *Ṣūfī*s as allies in its fight against Islamic extremist groups that oppose both the government and all religious practices regarded as "novelties," including the veneration of saints, the celebration of saints' birthdays, and the various practices of sufism in general (Biegman 1990).

Among the practices regarded as heretical by Islamists is *Ṣūfī* healing, performed by *shuyūkh bil-baraka*, both dead and alive. The most famous *Ṣūfī* healers in Egypt are, in fact, dead *shuyūkh*—often founders of *Ṣūfī* orders who are buried in mosque-tomb complexes that have become major pilgrimage centers. Infertile women and others with serious health and personal problems often visit these "saints' shrines" (as they are often referred to in the scholarly literature) in order to receive some of the dead saint's *baraka*, or divine blessing, to make personal appeals for well-being and vows of repayment, to increase the likelihood that one's prayers for well-being are answered by God, and to pray for miracles (such as conception among the infertile) that the saints are thought to perform on pilgrims' behalf. According to infertile women, the power and intercessional abilities of these *shuyūkh bil-baraka* are "very strong," and women who visit them have been known to become pregnant "as soon as they arrive home to their husbands."

At these pilgrimage centers and at smaller mosques and shrines throughout Egypt, infertile women also visit living *shuyūkh bil-baraka*, who tend to congregate at mosques, especially at the time of saints' birthday celebrations, or *mawālid*. There, these living *shuyūkh bil-baraka*, some of whom are descendants of the saint and others who are simply followers of his *Ṣūfī* order, bestow their own inherited or acquired *baraka* on pilgrims through laying on of hands, reading the Qur'an and writing *ḥugub* with religious inscriptions, and praying over the afflicted. It is important to point out that these living *shuyūkh bil-baraka* are quite different from *munaggimīn*, who also write *ḥugub* and sometimes use the Qur'an; for, according to poor urban women who are familiar with both, the former "know God and do not do sorcery" like the latter.

Yet, as suggested above, these Qur'anically educated *shuyūkh bil-baraka*, who epitomize religiosity and God's favor in the eyes of most poor urban Egyptians, may nevertheless be frowned upon by the religiously literate and Islamist groups in Egypt, who are highly critical of the assumed role of these individuals as intermediaries between God and other human beings. This view is beginning to infiltrate poor urban areas, where skepticism about the role of *shuyūkh bil-baraka* in divine intercession is beginning to grow.

As one infertile woman explained, "Some people think they can get *baraka* from *shuyūkh*, and when their prayers are answered, they think it's those people who helped them. But it's all from God, and it's *ḥarām* not to treat these people as human beings. These *shuyūkh* are just as human as we are." Or, as one Muslim "fundamentalist" woman stated succinctly, "If you go to a *shaikh*, it's like giving God a partner."

The role of these *shuyūkh* in healing, the nature of their *baraka* and intercessional abilities, and the activities of poor infertile Egyptian women who visit them will be described in further detail in Chapter 7.

5. *Kabsa* and Threatened Fertility

Amina's Story

On her wedding day, Amina, a plump, freckle-faced farm girl from the provincial Delta town of Kafr al-Dawwar, never imagined that her marriage to Ali would be plagued by continuing childlessness. Ali, a strikingly handsome young man from the rural outskirts of Alexandria, had seen Amina while visiting his uncle in Kafr al-Dawwar and, finding her beautiful, he told his uncle, "I want to marry this one." Thus, marriage to Ali was Amina's "destiny." Following their wedding, Ali moved Amina to his father's extended-family household, because, as the eldest son, he was expected to set the example for his two younger brothers. However, soon after the wedding, Amina's in-laws, and particularly her mother-in-law, began "noticing" that Amina was not becoming pregnant. With each passing month, she would remind Amina of the need for "children, children." As Amina explains, "From the day of marriage, she wanted me to have children. After five months, she started telling me to search, to do the *mushāharāt.*"

Amina's search for children began at the home of a *dāya*, who told Amina that she was *makbūsa*, or suffering from the effects of infertility-producing *kabsa*. The *dāya* told Amina that *kabsa* had occurred during the first lunar month following Amina's wedding, when someone with *kabsa*-inducing potential had "entered upon" Amina in her bridal suite. According to the *dāya*, the person who entered upon Amina causing *kabsa* could have been any one of a number of individuals. For example, the person could have been Ali himself after he had just shaved. Or it could have been someone carrying meat or a black eggplant. Or it could have been a child, either a boy or girl, who had just been circumcised. Or it could have been a woman who was menstruating, had just weaned her child, or had just been married. Or the "person" could have been a cat—or any "nonspeaking animal"—that had just delivered a litter.

Amina considered carefully whether any such entrances might have occurred while she was still a new bride, and she remembered that a woman named Hasna, who had just had her daughter circumcised, had come to visit her, perhaps contaminated by her daughter's circumcision blood. Following her visit to Amina, Hasna, too, had been unable to become pregnant. When Amina told this to the *dāya*, the *dāya* suggested that Amina and Hasna had caused *kabsa* to each other, by virtue of the fact that they were both contaminated with genital blood (from the defloration and circumcision, respectively). Thus, she advised Amina to find Hasna and take her to a cemetery, where the two of them were to enter the cemetery through one door and exit by another. In front of the exiting door, they were to urinate on the ground together, to fashion the dampened ground into two mud dolls, and then to place these mud dolls in water and to bathe with this water. This was to be repeated on three consecutive Fridays during the Islamic noon prayer.

Amina convinced Hasna to perform the *kabsa* healing ritual with her, and, lo and behold, they both became "unbound" and pregnant immediately. Hasna went on to have a son, but Amina miscarried within the first trimester.

Thus, when no additional pregnancies were forthcoming, Amina returned to the *dāya*, who told Amina that a second *kabsa* might have occurred during the lunar month following Amina's miscarriage. Because Amina was uncertain about who might have entered her room during that month, she was advised by the *dāya* to undertake a number of different *kabsa* healing rituals.

First, the *dāya* provided Amina with a miscarried fetus and told Amina to place the fetus in water and then to bathe with this water during the time of the noon prayer over three consecutive Fridays. Although repulsed by the thought of bathing with the miscarried fetus, Amina undertook the ritual, which, unfortunately, failed to make her pregnant. Thus, the *dāya*, while delivering another woman's baby, called Amina to the delivery site and made her sit down on the bloody placenta. She also told Amina to go to any barbershop and to ask the barber for his tool kit (razor, comb, and scissors). She told Amina to place the barber's tools in water and to bathe herself with this water during the time of the noon prayer over three consecutive Fridays.

Amina did as she was told, and she also began performing the *kabsa* healing rituals suggested to her by friends and neighbors. For example, her husband's sister, to whom Amina was close, borrowed a *mushāharāt* necklace, consisting of beads, the figure of a person, a doll, and a horse. Like the *dāya*, she told Amina to place the necklace in water during the Friday noon prayer and to bathe with this water over three consecutive Fridays. Amina was also advised by women in the neighborhood to make some therapeutic "visits": one to a slaughterhouse, where she was to step over a slaughtered animal's blood seven times and then to smear her feet in this blood, and one to an eggplant field, where she was to walk across the field, stopping to eat some raw eggplant. Another woman told Amina to take a black eggplant, core it, and then to wear this core "inside" like a vaginal suppository. (Unfortunately, the eggplant burned badly, and Amina removed it and douched after only fifteen minutes.)

Furthermore, Amina visited a *munaggima* known for her clairvoyant powers. The *munaggima* told Amina that a newly delivered cat had entered her room during the lunar month following her wedding and had caused *kabsa*. Ideally, to unbind the effects of this *kabsa*, the placenta of another newly delivered cat must be found and worn as a vaginal suppository. However, given the difficulty of obtaining a feline placenta (cats are known to eat them hastily), the *munaggima* told Amina to find a newly delivered she-goat and to sit on its placenta.

Amina undertook all of these *kabsa* healing rituals and tried other sorts of remedies as well. For example, assuming that she might have uterine *ruṭūba*, she grilled an onion, put it in gauze, and wore it overnight in her vagina to release the discharge and humidity from her uterus. In addition, following her miscarriage, two separate *dāyāt* attempted to remove her uterine humidity and close her open back by undertaking *kasr*, or cupping, and *kawī*, a sort of branding of Amina's lower back with a lit corncob. Furthermore, one of these *dāyāt* provided Amina with *ṣūwaf*, vaginal suppositories consisting of *ḥulba*, *shīḥ*, and molasses. The other told her to go to a cemetery and to look at a dead child in its tomb in order to get shocked.

Amina also made four *ziyārāt*, or pilgrimages, to the mosque-tombs of famous *shuyūkh bil-baraka* in Tanta, Dasuq, Alexandria, and Cairo. After praying "regularly" in the mosques, Amina prayed for a child, asking "Oh God, give me children, let me stay in good health, and lengthen the lives of my mom and dad." After placing her prayer-requests, she circumambulated the tombs of the dead *shuyūkh*, in order to obtain their sacred *baraka*, or divine blessing.

Amina also consulted three additional *munaggimīn*, one man and two women. The male *munaggim* gave Amina a piece of paper with English writing on it and told her to put the paper in water and to bathe with this water during the noon prayer over three consecutive Fridays. Afterward, she was to throw the piece of paper in an intersection. He also told her to buy yellow lentils and to sprinkle them around the house so as to "unlock all the things in the house going against me." However, the *munaggim*, to whom Amina paid ten Egyptian pounds (four dollars), "tricked" her, because his therapy was "useless."

During that same year, Amina went to see a female *munaggima*, called "the *shaikha*," who was known in her neighborhood for treating women's problems. The *shaikha* told Amina to go to the neighborhood cemetery, to take a brick, and to place this brick in water and then bathe with this water during the noon prayer over three consecutive Fridays. Afterward, she was to return the brick to the cemetery, because "if I leave it at home, it may cause disturbances and noises." Furthermore, when a "fortune-teller *shaikha*" happened to walk through Amina's neighborhood, peddling her clairvoyant services, Amina decided to visit her. The *shaikha* told Amina that she had *jinn*, or spirits, "on her" and that these spirits wanted Amina to give them a white headscarf, a bar of scented soap, and a bar of unscented washing soap. The *shaikha* also pulled out the *mushāharāt*, consisting of a replica of a human face, a doll, a horse, a seashell, and a barber's tools. She put the *mushāharāt* in some water and then threw some of this water suddenly into Amina's face, in order to both shock her and to unbind the effects of *kabsa*. She then told Amina to drink some of this water and to bathe with the rest of it during the noon prayer over three consecutive Fridays. Afterward, Amina was to throw the remainder of this water into the street in front of her house. Finally, the *shaikha* asked Amina when her period was due. After Amina calculated the date, the *shaikha* predicted, "God willing, you're not going to see it [the period]."

However, despite such predictions and innumerable exhausting, time-consuming, and costly remedies, Amina is still not pregnant—five years after her wedding to Ali. Although the two doctors Amina has visited have both told her that she needs "an operation"—namely, a diagnostic laparoscopy at Alexandria's Shatby Hospital—Amina continues to believe that she is *makbūsa*, a condition which has plagued her throughout her infertile marriage and for which, as of yet, she has failed to find the appropriate cure.

Kabsa and the Ritual Process

Many other Egyptian women like Amina believe that they are *makbūsīn*, or suffering from infertility-producing *kabsa*. *Kabsa*—also known by the synonymous term *mushāhara*[1]—is, by literal definition, a "raid" or a "surprise attack." However, among contemporary Egyptian women, *kabsa* has taken on a much different meaning. In Egypt today, *kabsa* represents the unwitting and unexpected entrance of a symbolically polluted individual into the room occupied by a sacredly vulnerable female ritual initiate, whose bodily "boundaries" (and, more specifically, her reproductively significant genitalia) have been recently violated through circumcision, defloration, or childbirth. As the result of the symbolic "penetration" of these boundaries by a polluting substance, the polluter who has mistakenly "entered" upon the vulnerable, "open" female causes the latter to enter a state of liminal suspension called *makbūsa* (also known as *mitshāhara*)—more exactly, a binding of her reproductive capacities, rendering her infertile or incapable of providing the breast milk necessary to sustain the life of her newborn child. In other words, *kabsa* threatens the reproductive bodies of individual Egyptian women and, by extension, the social reproduction of the Egyptian body politic.

The threat of *kabsa* to society lies in the fact that it is not uncommon; indeed, it is thought to affect large numbers of Egyptian, Nubian, and Sudanese women, all peoples of the Lower Nile.[2] In Lower Egypt, *kabsa* is widely viewed by poor urban women (often of rural backgrounds) as *the* major ethnogynecological cause of female infertility, among women who have never conceived as well as those who have. Because infertility-producing binding is the primary outcome of *kabsa* and because infertility is a severely stigmatizing condition in Egypt (Inhorn n.d.), *kabsa* is greatly feared by Egyptian women.

To make sense of the disparate beliefs, practices, and meanings surrounding *kabsa* in Lower Egypt, it is necessary to examine *kabsa* in terms of theories of ritual and rites of passage in particular. From the perspective of the ritual process, *kabsa* can be understood as a socially threatening disruption to normal female reproductive rites of passage, the three stages of which were first described by Van Gennep (1960) and later explicated by Turner (1964, 1969, 1974). More specifically, *kabsa* constitutes polluting boundary violation into the two inner sanctums—room and womb—of sacredly vulnerable female ritual initiates who have been separated (stage one) from the "normal" female world in order to undergo solitary rites of reproductive transition, or limen (stage two). Such violation produces an abnormally extended stage of transition, in which childlessness is the hallmark of liminality. Hence, rites of incorporation (stage three) involving birth celebrations are waylaid, and alternative, compensatory rites of incorporation are necessary to "undo" the extended state of liminality. These rites involve complex, depolluting rituals of consubstantiality, designed to bring liminal personae into contact with that substance which is thought to have penetrated their room / wombs, thereby binding their reproductive bodies. If successful, such rituals allow ritual initiates to complete the normal rite of transition, ending in the birth of a healthy, living child.

Thus, through ritual analysis, it is possible to make meaningful the conditions under which *kabsa*, as reproductive ritual disruption, is produced and how it is manifest among female Egyptian ritual initiates. In addition, "cures" for *kabsa* can be seen less as cures than as healing rituals of depollution necessary to release ritual initiates from a suspended state of limen via an alternative rite of incorporation. Through ritual analysis, it is also possible to explore the symbolism of the ritual paraphernalia used in *kabsa* healing and to highlight the syncretic incorporation of what is presumably a pre-Islamic rite into the formal, Islamic ritual cycle. Indeed, *kabsa*, as a ritual complex, is intricately tied to the corpus of Islamic purity and pollution beliefs, which is why *kabsa* represents such potent danger to Muslim believers and to the Muslim body politic at large.

It is also important to focus on the highly gendered nature of *kabsa* and its accompanying ritual complex. Given that *kabsa* is experienced and, hence, understood almost exclusively by women, it involves (at least in Lower Egypt) reincorporative rituals over which women exert virtual control. Thus, despite the persistent patriarchy existing within Egyptian society at large (Inhorn n.d.), *kabsa* healing rituals are gynocentric, involving the active help *of women by women*, in their roles as ritual facilitators, officiants, and coparticipants.[3] Furthermore, because women undertake *kabsa* rituals beyond the official gaze of men—at sacred times and in sacred spaces where men neither congregate nor would expect women to heal each other—these rituals effectively subvert male authority, constituting an example of subaltern women's everyday resistance (Hammami and Rieker 1988).

Although poor urban Egyptian women neither construct an overarching analytical "*kabsa* model," nor explain their disparate notions of *kabsa* causation and cure in terms of ritual and resistance, examining *kabsa* etically within a dynamic theory of ritual offers perhaps greater understanding of this symbolically rich complex than that rendered through other interpretive and explanatory paradigms, including theories of culture-bound syndromes (Early 1993a), imitative magic (Morsy 1980a), taboo (Kennedy 1978a), and symbolic ambivalence in the context of spirit possession (Boddy 1989).

Indeed, for nearly a century, scholars of Egypt (and northern Sudan) have encountered the exotic beliefs and practices relating to *kabsa* and have puzzled over their meaning and significance. In one of the earliest accounts, the Egyptian physician ʿAbd al-Raḥmān Efendī Ismāʿīl—whose 1892–94 text *Tibb al-Rukka*, or "The Medicine of the Old Women," is a mordant condemnation of Egyptian ethnomedicine—relates considerable descriptive information on *kabsa*, including its association with death, eggplants, breast milk, and mysterious beaded necklaces, concluding that "the harm of these is limited to their delaying the patient from calling in a doctor" (Ismāʿīl in Walker 1934:23).

Since Ismāʿīl's early vilifying summary, numerous scholars have offered more neutral descriptions of *kabsa*, although their accounts tend to be brief and partial in terms of important detail.[4] Only Kennedy's (1978a) work on *kabsa* among the Egyptian Nubians and Boddy's (1989) among the rural northern Sudanese move substantially beyond description to theoretical interpretation of the *kabsa* complex.

Kennedy's article on "*Mushāhara*: A Nubian Concept of Supernatural Danger and the Theory of Taboo" (1978a) is perhaps the most detailed of the previous works on *kabsa* (or *mushāhara* as it is called among the Nubians), describing with some specificity the complex of *mushāhara* beliefs and practices. In his synoptic summary of what he describes as the "enigmatic" nature of *mushāhara* customs, Kennedy concludes:

> It is apparent that these taboos are associated with the crisis rites of birth, circumcision, marriage and death. Examination of other elements of the life-cycle ceremonies reveals that the *mushāhara* customs, along with other prohibitions and positive rituals, are aimed at protecting people from dangerous spirit-beings who threaten fertility and life during these temporary states of sacred vulnerability. These spirit-beings for the most part are connected with the Nile and/or ghosts of the dead, and their main danger is a threat to fertility and to the reproductive areas of the body. Examination of such rites also reveals that the basic meaning of most of the ritual substances, appurtenances, and acts is their association with spirit beings, either through pleasing them or defending against them. Even the concepts of ritual pollution and cleansing have the meaning of neutralizing and dispersing spirits. (1978a:134)

As suggested in this summary, Kennedy highlights certain key elements in the *kabsa* complex, including ritual acts, life-cycle-related rites of passage, sacred vulnerability, threats to fertility and the reproductive organs of the body, and ritual pollution and cleansing. But, Kennedy's focus on *mushāhara* customs *as taboos* is, most certainly, a reflection of the ethnographic data collection process in this case. Namely, Kennedy was in charge of the analysis of a large amount of disparate ethnographic data collected by a number of fieldworkers during the course of a major relocation study of the Nubians in the early 1960s (Kennedy 1978b). *Mushāhara* was not a separate focus of investigation, but was discovered in the process of collecting data on pre-relocation Nubian ceremonial life. It appears that *mushāhara* was never systematically explored as a ritual in and of itself; rather, separate ethnographers made record of *mushāhara* customs whenever they happened to be mentioned by independent informants. Once all the data were in, Kennedy attempted to make sense of *mushāhara* customs, a task he obviously found quite difficult. As he explained: "It is not easy to find a key to these diverse observances. They are frequently isolated from one another in performance and people usually either could give no explanation for them or replied that their forefathers did it that way" (1978a:127).

Thus, Kennedy was forced to weave an interpretation of *mushāhara* around a highly disconnected body of data, collected largely by others, a task that would be difficult under the best of circumstances. Most important, the data on *mushāhara* collected in the Nubian project were derived largely from informants practicing *mushāhara* precautionary measures, rather than from informants who had actually been affected by *mushāhara* and could explain its various outcomes and remedies. Although preventive measures are an important part of the *kabsa* (*mushāhara*) complex, as we shall see, they constitute only a small part of the overall picture. Because Kennedy's data revolved around preventive rituals, therapeutic rituals were essentially overlooked, leading Kennedy to undertake an insightful, although somewhat partial analysis of *mushāhara* customs as "taboos."

Further, Kennedy, like Boddy (1989), focused his analysis on the reproductively oriented malevolence of spirit-beings, especially Nile spirits, against which the *mushāhara* customs are aimed. Kennedy concluded that:

> A constant feature of crisis rites is the use of Nile water for purification, while among the most prevalent ideas and emotions involved is the fear of pollution by blood, associated with sexuality and ultimately with fertility. The concept of ritual vulnerability thus seems to be based upon the idea that blood (particularly blood from the sex organs) subjects a person to great supernatural danger because it attracts powerful capricious spirits, who will prove a threat to fertility. (1978a:130)

As we shall see, spirits do *not* play a part in the *kabsa* complex among urban Lower Egyptian women. The differential importance of spirits is probably a reflection of geographical and/or cultural variation in the *kabsa* complex, with belief in blood-hungry spirits incorporated into this complex only among the Nubians and Sudanese. However, it remains unclear in Kennedy's study whether Nubians themselves believe they must carry out these *mushāhara* "taboos" to protect against otherworldly spirits, or whether they undertake these measures to protect against the polluting qualities of earthly human beings, as is the case for Lower Egypt.

Drawing on the work of Kennedy, Boddy (1989), in one of the most recent accounts of *mushāhara* among rural Sudanese village women, describes *mushāhara* in the glossary of her book as a "complex of practices, illnesses, and ideas concerning blood; specifically, genital blood associated with femininity and fertility" (Boddy 1989:xix). Indeed, Boddy characterizes *mushāhara* as a form of "genital hemorrhage" associated with the "crisis rites" (Kennedy's term) of childbirth, circumcision, and defloration. She states that a "woman experiencing blood loss from the genital region is particularly at risk from spirits (*zayran* and other *jinn*, including river sprites), which might enter through the pregnable orifice and, *possessing her, inflict sterility*" (Boddy 1989:101; emphasis added). Thus, Boddy, even more than Kennedy, ties *mushāhara* to spirit possession, which is the major subject of her ethnography.

Yet, in an impressive symbolic analysis, Boddy goes beyond the spirit possession link to attempt to account for the many different instances in which human beings induce *mushāhara* in a woman—for example, if they visit her when returning from a funeral, if they visit her after having butchered an animal or attended a male or female circumcision, if they are wearing gold when she is wearing none, or if they happen to be a female gypsy and come within view of the vulnerable woman. To explain these disparate cases of *mushāhara* induction, Boddy refers to:

> damage stem[ming] from ambivalence; it occurs when the essence of death is mixed with that of birth, or conversely, when the condition for immortality is combined with that for mortality. It also occurs when she who has shed residual, postpotent ("black") blood in childbirth absorbs the essence of potent ("red") circumcision blood; or when a normally reserved, dignified, and enclosed Hofriyati female weakened by childbed or circumcision is brought into ocular contact with the uninfibulated, unconfined, and by Hofriyati standards, undignified gypsy, the antithesis of ideal womanhood. (Boddy 1989:103)

Yet, as will be argued here, *pollution* is a more compelling explanation of *kabsa* (*mushāhara*) induction than symbolic *ambivalence*; for, in this context, blood, death, gold, and even gypsies all have polluting qualities that may result in unfortunate reproductive outcomes. Furthermore, because Boddy assumes a secondary symptom of *mushāhara*—namely, genital bleeding—to be its primary reproductive outcome, she does not account for the other reproductive misfortunes, including infertility, miscarriage, stillbirth, and failure of lactation, which she mentions as being *mushāhara*-related.

Perhaps the most elegant part of Boddy's analysis is her interpretation of threatened "boundaries," which derives in part from the ideas of Douglas (1966). Boddy argues that *mushāhara* involves the violation of essential boundaries—both genital openings and doorways, which are symbolically associated in the *mushāhara* context. These threatened boundaries, she maintains, are, in fact, threats to *fertility*. Fertility, Boddy argues, is a woman's "precarious gift"—one that must be protected by preventing *mushāhara*. Thus, although Boddy does not explicitly address the threat of *infertility* as the outcome of this condition, her message is implicit: namely, *mushāhara* is a condition of boundary violation that threatens fertility, a message that will be more fully developed in the analysis of the Lower Egyptian *kabsa* complex that follows.

Kabsa: Central Features

In order to understand how *kabsa* serves to threaten the boundaries and fertility of women in Lower Egypt, it is necessary to begin by highlighting some of the central features of *kabsa* and its relationship to reproductive rites of passage in general.

The Lunar Month

Kabsa is an event associated with the cyclical comings and goings of the moon. The alternative term *mushāhara* refers to something that occurs on a monthly basis, and is derived from the Arabic term *shahr*, meaning both "new moon" and "month." Essentially, *kabsa*, like the period of reproductive liminality, is time-limited. A ritual initiate is only susceptible to the effects of *kabsa* until the end of the lunar month following the initial rite of separation. With the new moon—and hence the changing of the Muslim calendrical month[5]—the potential for *kabsa* disappears, as does the period of danger for the ritual initiate.

Yet, it is important to note some heterogeneity of belief in this regard. Namely, some women claim that the potential for *kabsa* is not eliminated with the new moon but rather lasts for the duration of one calendrical month following the rite of separation (for example, the wedding night) or for a forty-day postmarital / postpartum period. Others believe that *kabsa* potential vanishes much sooner — after the first week or as early as the first day after the initial rite. However, the vast majority of Lower Egyptian women believe that *kabsa* potential lasts until the new moon appears. Thus, to prevent *kabsa* from occurring, some Egyptians schedule major events, such as marriage, circumcision, and weaning, close to the appearance of the new moon, and some women begin *kabsa* healing rituals shortly before the new moon appears.

Gender Specificity

Those who are susceptible to *kabsa* during the lunar month are almost always girls and women. In Egypt, *kabsa* is largely a female experience. Those who cause *kabsa* tend to be female, and those who fall victim to *kabsa* are almost always female, making this a highly gender-specific condition.[6] Without exception, the Egyptian girls and women who experience *kabsa* are in the midst of a liminal period involving a reproductive rite of passage. *Kabsa* is a problem only of the liminal period and only of liminal personae. Those who are considered to be vulnerable to the effects of *kabsa* are those experiencing the transition from unmarriageable girlhood to marriageable womanhood following circumcision; from virginal celibacy to marital sexuality following wedding-night defloration; from unproven reproductivity to potential reproductivity following miscarriage, stillbirth, or abortion; and from potential motherhood to proven motherhood following childbirth. In other words, *kabsa* most commonly affects newly circumcised girls, new brides, women who recently miscarried or aborted, and women who recently gave birth.

Separation and Boundary Maintenance

In Egypt, girls and women undergoing such reproductive passages are normally separated from the outside world for the duration of the transitional period. Ideally, the girl / woman remains at home, confined to her bedroom for a period lasting forty days.[7] Although she is allowed visitors, careful consideration should be given to their number and kind. Furthermore, she should remain immured within the boundaries of her room, letting others venture into the outside world for her.

In reality, such separation and boundary maintenance are rarely adequately achieved. The household demands placed on Egyptian women are considerable, meaning that a forty-day period of relative inactivity is an unaffordable luxury. In addition, housing pressures, especially in Egypt's urban areas, have forced large numbers of human beings to live in rooms together. Thus, a separate room and accompanying physical boundary maintenance for a reproductively liminal woman is a virtual impossibility among the poor in the urban Egyptian context. Given these current conditions, the likelihood of *kabsa* is greater than ever.

The reason that the reproductively liminal woman requires the protection afforded by structural boundaries (that is, the four walls of her room) is that her bodily boundaries are no longer intact. A reproductive ritual initiate is considered vulnerable through her "openness." This openness stems from a number of sources. If she is a newly circumcised girl, the very boundaries of her genital flesh have been penetrated by the circumciser's knife, scissors, or razor blade—exposing the raw surfaces beneath the clitoris and labia.[8] If she is a new bride, she has just undergone the wedding-night defloration called the *dukhla*, which derives from the Arabic verb *dakhala*, meaning, literally, "to enter." In this case, her husband's penis has entered her, breaking open the barrier to her reproductive passageway (that is, the hymen), which is always expected to be intact among Egyptian brides. If she is a woman who has miscarried, aborted, or just given birth, the entrance to the "inner room" of her body—the uterus, or *bait il-wilid*, meaning literally the "house of the child" in Egyptian colloquial Arabic—has been opened with the passage of the exiting fetus.

Thus, reproductive vulnerability lies in the necessary, celebrated exposure of that which is interior—the inner workings of a woman's reproductive body. Because such bodily penetrations are culturally condoned for the most part,[9] female vulnerability to external forces must be removed in other ways—namely, through the erection of walls, or physical boundaries around the secluded reproductive ritual initiate. Yet, these physical boundaries may fail to protect her. *Kabsa*, as we shall see, entails the violation of these physical boundaries; it is literally and symbolically a problem of control over "entrances."

Boundary Violation

Kabsa takes place when another individual unfortunately penetrates the physical boundaries of the ritual initiate's room, entering upon the open, ritually vulnerable girl or woman. These *kabsa*-producing entrances are almost never malevolently intended. *Kabsa* usually occurs by accident, although, on very rare occasions, it may be produced intentionally by a woman's enemy, by an infertile woman desperate to overcome her problem, or at the request of a woman who desires *kabsa*-produced birth control (that is, through intentionally induced infertility). Because such entrances are usually unintentional, however, both those who cause *kabsa* and those who suffer its effects are rarely aware of the exact circumstances of this ritual boundary violation. This is especially true if the "individual" who has entered the woman's room was an animal, as is occasionally the case.

Most important, those who cause *kabsa* are never "neutral," ritually speaking. Rather, those who unwittingly enter bring with them ritual danger—danger so profound that it disrupts the normal reproductive rite of passage, thereby preventing the normal stage of reincorporation.

The State of *Makbūsa*

A girl or woman who has suffered *kabsa* enters a state called *makbūsa*, also known as *mitshāhara*. *Makbūsa* is a state of "boundness," in which normal reproductive functions are eclipsed.[10] When one is *makbūsa*, she remains suspended in an extended period of reproductive liminality generally characterized by infertility. In other words, in this state of *makbūsa*, the woman's bodily openings "close" through the healing of genital wounds or the return of the uterus and cervix to their normal configuration; however, the inner workings of the female reproductive body become "bound," preventing future conception or appropriate lactation from occurring.

In most cases, the woman who becomes *makbūsa* has no idea that she has entered this state. Symptoms are generally absent, although, in rare cases, a woman may become listless and somnolent, experience breast engorgement or shaking, or suffer weight loss, becoming "thin and dry." Because of the typical lack of symptomatology, diagnosis of *kabsa* is nonspecific. Rather, in most cases, it is made by default when a woman fails to conceive or, in the case of a new mother, fails to lactate.

Because infertility is the primary outcome of *kabsa*, women who fail to conceive, either after marriage or after a previous reproductive event (miscarriage, stillbirth, abortion, childbirth), are generally suspected of being *makbūsa*. In fact, among most poor urban and rural Egyptian women, *kabsa* is the first cause of a woman's infertility to be considered. However, because definitive diagnosis is impossible, women only come to know whether they are, in fact, *makbūsa* by undergoing healing rituals designed to unbind them. If, after such a ritual, a woman becomes pregnant, she is considered to have been *makbūsa* and to have been unbound through the therapeutic act. Yet, because these rituals are etiologically specific, a woman may undergo the incorrect version of the *kabsa* healing ritual and may fail to overcome her boundness. When such failure occurs, a woman remains *makbūsa* until she discovers the correct "cure." Since this may never happen, it is possible for a woman to remain *makbūsa* indefinitely.

The Dangers of Polluting Boundary-Crossing

But the question remains: How can one human being cause another human being to suffer such a reproductive setback—a setback that is all the more acute because of the degree to which infertile Egyptian women are marginalized? In the case of *kabsa*, boundary-crossing in and of itself is not a sufficient cause; what is also necessary is the ritual pollution of the boundary-crosser, whose dangerous impurity infects the room and its vulnerable occupant, causing reproductive calamity. *Kabsa* is a condition that entails *both* pollution and boundary violation, phenomena that are related, according to Douglas (1966).

Because of their reproductive "oozings" (for example, menstrual blood, postpartum blood, vaginal secretions, breast milk), women are more likely to be impure and are usually the ones to cause *kabsa*. Nevertheless, *kabsa*-producing boundary-crossers can be of either sex and any age, as long as they are polluted in one of the following ways.

Polluted by Blood

Individuals who are "bloodied" or who have come in contact with blood comprise the major danger to ritually vulnerable women. Egyptians often say that "blood causes *kabsa* to blood"—an expression pointing to the fact that both individuals in the *kabsa* episode may have been exposed to blood. In the case of the ritual initiate, one's own blood has recently been shed through reproductively related events. In the case of the polluted boundary-crosser, the blood may be one's own or from another source.

In many cases, the individual who causes *kabsa* to occur is another blood-shedding woman undergoing a similar reproductive rite of passage. In Egypt, it is widely believed that (1) a reproductively liminal woman may cause *kabsa* to another reproductively liminal woman if she unwittingly crosses the threshold of the latter's room; and (2) two reproductively liminal women undergoing the identical rite of passage (for example, two new brides or two recently delivered women) *may cause kabsa to each other* in the event of boundary-crossing or even a chance meeting. Theoretically, both women should be secluded in their own rooms, preventing such contact from occurring. However, given the difficulties of boundary maintenance described earlier, such crossings and meetings are often impossible to prevent. Thus, in many cases, reproductively liminal women are not only *in danger* but are a *cause of danger* because of their bloodshedding.

Yet, bloodied boundary-crossers are of many other types. Those who are ritually polluted by their own blood include: menstruating women; circumcised boys and girls; men knicked in shaving; barbers or other persons carrying bloodied shaving tools; depilated women;[11] and animals (primarily cats) that have delivered a litter.

In addition, recent contact with blood—human, animal, or "vegetable"—is enough to produce *kabsa*. Contact with the blood of another human being is a major source of *kabsa*-producing pollution. Thus, it is believed that women who have attended their children's circumcisions or women who have held the new bride's "honor" (that is, the handkerchief or piece of white cloth stained by the blood of defloration) are often responsible for *kabsa* production. In fact, in Egypt, it is thought dangerous for someone to carry the bloodied handkerchief outside the bridal suite and then to return with it to the room—effectively polluting the bride with her own blood.

Contact with meat and butchered animals is also a major source of pollution. For example, individuals may cause *kabsa* by carrying fresh, bloody meat of any kind (including poultry and fish) or a slaughtered animal without its skin; by slaughtering an animal such as a chicken; or by visiting the butcher or a slaughterhouse.

Vegetable "blood" is similarly incriminated. Tomatoes, with their bloody complexion and juice, are the major culprit; in Egypt, it is widely believed that tomatoes cause *kabsa* if carried into a ritually vulnerable woman's room. Likewise, lemons, which are sometimes used in Egypt to cauterize bloody wounds, are thought to cause *kabsa* if carried across the sensitive threshold.

Polluted by Excreta

But blood is not the only bodily substance known to pollute. Many of the other bodily fluids—including primarily semen, sexually induced vaginal secretions, urine, and breast milk—are considered impure, a notion that is upheld by Islam (Boudhiba 1985). Thus, individuals who have failed to "purify" themselves, by washing away these fluids from their bodies or their clothing, are considered to be polluted and ritually dangerous.

It is not surprising, therefore, that *kabsa* is often attributed to women who have failed to purify themselves following sexual intercourse; husbands who have failed to purify themselves following sexual intercourse and then return to the rooms of their new brides; individuals of any sex or age who have just urinated and are soiled by urine; and lactating women, especially those who are weaning and whose breasts are still leaking milk.

Polluted by Death

Death is also a source of pollution, not only because of the fluids and secretions which ooze out of dead and dying bodies, but because of the very threat that death poses to the living. In Egypt, where mortality rates are relatively high and few individuals live until old age, deaths are frequent, and thus contact with death is often unavoidable. In fact, pollution by death is relatively common and need not involve actual physical contact with a corpse. According to Egyptians, individuals may become polluted by death in numerous ways; but, in each case, they may cause *kabsa* to the ritually vulnerable woman who, in most cases, has yet to bring life into the world.[12]

Cemeteries are one source of pollution. Individuals who have visited a cemetery or have even crossed a cemetery on a journey may cause *kabsa*. Funerals are similarly implicated; individuals who have participated in a funeral, a funeral procession, or even passed such a procession in the street are capable of causing *kabsa*. Likewise, individuals who have given their condolences to a dead person's family are considered capable of causing *kabsa*.

Actual contact with the dead is particularly polluting. This contact may be physical: for example, washing a dead body with a loofah sponge, carrying a dead body, or touching the dead body of one's parent, spouse, or child. Yet, even visual contact is enough to insure pollution. Thus, someone who has just seen a dead person is liable to cause *kabsa*.

Furthermore, contact with death need not be recent. It is believed by some that individuals in mourning may cause *kabsa* if they enter the room of a ritually vulnerable woman. Black, the symbol of death and mourning, is particularly dangerous. This is probably the reason why black eggplants, also known as the "brides of the field,"[13] are widely believed to cause *kabsa* if carried into the room of the ritually vulnerable woman.

Polluted by Wealth

Because the vast majority of Egyptians continue to live in poverty, wealth is viewed ambivalently. On the one hand, achieving wealth is something to be admired; but, on the other hand, wealth creates envy and frustration among those who are less capable of increasing their economic standings. Furthermore, in historical terms, the vast majority of Egyptian peasants have been oppressed by wealthy, often absentee landlords, who extracted not only the crops from their fields but the labor of sharecropping tenant *fallāḥīn*.

In Egypt, gold has traditionally been used as the major sign of wealth. In fact, individuals often flaunt their wealth by adorning themselves with expensive gold jewelry. This is especially true of wealthy women, who may wear at once gold earrings, rings, necklaces, and multiple bangles on both arms. Because gold creates envy and is also thought to attract harmful spirits (Boddy 1989), it is a source of ritual danger and is thought to cause *kabsa* if worn into the room of a poor woman.

This is especially true of the most "pure," expensive, twenty-four-karat Sudanese gold known as *dhahab bundu'i*, or "nutty gold," because of its typical configuration in the shape of nuts. Individuals wearing *dhahab bundu'i* are thought to cause *kabsa* if they enter the room of a ritually vulnerable woman. Likewise, individuals wearing gold jewelry containing diamonds and pearls—precious gems that are unaffordable except among the upper class—are thought to cause *kabsa*.

Perhaps most interesting, however, is the danger of pollution stemming from gold jewelry containing coins or human forms. In Egypt, small, gold British pounds are found in various kinds of jewelry, particularly drop earrings. These pounds contain the faces of the British nobility, who, in recent Egyptian history, represented the colonial oppressors. Similarly, pharaonic figures are the most common human form found in other types of jewelry. Although popular among tourists, such jewelry is rarely worn by Egyptians, perhaps because of the tyranny with which many of the pharaohs were said to have ruled Egypt.[14] Thus, when an individual wearing either a golden coin or a human form enters a ritually vulnerable woman's room, the latter will become *makbūsa*.

It is very important to note at this point that not all of the *kabsa*-causing polluting encounters cited above occur with equal frequency or are even known to all Egyptian women. *Kabsa* is not a monolithic complex, and the *kabsa* beliefs and practices of poor urban Egyptian women display a considerable degree of heterogeneity. Moreover, some Egyptian women distinguish between types of *kabsa*-producing events occurring among different categories of ritual initiates (for example, some forms may be specific to new brides and others to new mothers). Nevertheless, that new brides are considered maximally vulnerable to *kabsa* is reflected in the most commonly cited *kabsa*-producing "combinations" as follows: (1) a woman who has recently delivered a child enters the room of a new bride; (2) a menstruating woman enters the room of a new bride; (3) someone carrying a black eggplant enters the room of a new bride; (4) someone carrying meat enters the room of a new bride; (5) a weaning woman with milk in her breasts enters the room of a new bride; (6) a woman who did not purify herself after sexual intercourse enters the room of a new bride; (7) a newly circumcised child enters the room of a new bride; (8) a husband who has just shaved enters the room of a new bride; (9) someone coming from a funeral enters the room of a new bride; (10) two newly married women meet and cause *kabsa* to each other; and (11) two women who have just undergone childbirth meet and cause *kabsa* to each other.

Kabsa Rituals: Central Features

But are there measures that a woman can take either to prevent *kabsa* or to overcome its effects? In Egypt, *kabsa* rituals, both preventive and therapeutic, constitute a rich domain of ethnogynecological praxis. In every case, the intent of these rituals is to overcome the effects of polluting boundary-crossing—either through preventive measures to ward off pollution potential or through therapeutic measures of depolluting unbinding. With regard to the latter, *kabsa* healing rituals can be seen as alternative rites of incorporation, in which ceremonial acts of depollution serve to reincorporate liminal personae into the normal, healthy social body of reproductive women. In a sense, these depolluting rituals are also rites of reversal, for only when the deleterious effects of *kabsa* pollution are reversed can a woman begin her reproductive rite of passage anew, resulting in her ultimate incorporation into the world of fertile mothers.

Unbinding

That *kabsa* produces reproductive binding is apparent in *kabsa* rituals, which are thought to unbind or untie the state of *makbūsa*. In fact, the Arabic verb *fakka*, meaning "to unbind, untie, or unfasten" something, is invariably used to describe the many ways in which *kabsa*, occasionally referred to as causing a "knot," may be overcome.

Unbinding the effects of *kabsa* is a task that is not limited in Egypt to ethnogynecological specialists. Unbinding procedures are widely known among Egyptian women, especially among older women, and may be suggested to the infertile by both lay persons and healers alike. For example, mothers and mothers-in-law tend to be forthcoming with *kabsa* preventive techniques and cures and are often vigilant in attempting to ensure that their daughters(-in-law) do not succumb to this much-feared condition. When *kabsa* fails to be prevented, these same female elders are often insistent that their daughters(-in-law) undertake *kabsa* healing rituals that many young infertile women may find repugnant. Daughters-in-law in particular are often coerced by their mothers-in-law to unbind themselves, even when the former doubt the validity of this ethnoetiology, as is sometimes the case.

Gynocentric Rituals

In Egypt, *kabsa* healing rituals are gynocentric—they are undertaken *for women by women*, who serve as ritual subjects, coparticipants, and officiants. Although men are peripherally involved in supplying unbinding appurtenances, they themselves never participate directly in *kabsa* healing rituals, which, when prescribed, are generally recommended only by women, especially *dāyāt*. Likewise, the *munaggimīn* who occasionally diagnose *kabsa* through clairvoyant means are generally women. Thus, it can be stated with some certainty that *kabsa* healing rituals in Lower Egypt are a women's specialty, even though the *kabsa*-producers and ritual suppliers may be men.

That *kabsa* healing rituals are under female control is perhaps less a specific form of female social power than a reflection of the fact that women, as a group, have much to lose in the face of *kabsa*. *Kabsa* threatens women, not men. And, in Egypt, female infertility of any kind, *kabsa*-induced or otherwise, is not socially tolerated (Inhorn n.d.). Because *kabsa* can strike any woman of reproductive age, women are inclined to acquire knowledge about *kabsa* and are often willing to help others with the ritual healing practices that may become necessary in their own lives.

Ritual Syncretism

Given that women are barred in many ways from formal Islamic ritual practice, including participation in Friday communal prayers at mosques, it is interesting that *kabsa* rituals are virtually always carried out within the framework of the Islamic ritual cycle. In the vast majority of cases, *kabsa* rituals are undertaken during the exact hour of the Friday communal noon prayer—the most important one in the Islamic weekly cycle of thirty-five prayers. Although some minor variation in the timing of *kabsa* rituals can be found,[15] this syncretic association of non-Islamic traditional healing practices with Islamic prayer rituals is extremely significant and appears to be an invariant feature of the *kabsa* ritual complex.

Given that *kabsa* beliefs are non-Islamic and were probably present in

Egypt before the coming of Islam in the seventh century,[16] the syncretism of non-Islamic "folk" traditions with Islamic rituals is extremely troubling to more scripturally minded Egyptian Muslims, particularly reform-minded, male Islamists who wish to divest the religion of unorthodox, localized, particularistic accretions such as this. Yet, while religiously literate Islamists may find such folk beliefs to be heretical, religiously illiterate Muslim women, who represent the vast majority of the Egyptian female populace, regard this association not only as natural, but also as critical, since performance of healing rituals during the most sacred time of the week greatly increases their likelihood of success.

Furthermore, given men's lack of involvement in *kabsa* rituals *and* the disapproval of such practices by many religiously literate Muslim men, it may be exceptionally convenient for women to perform their religiously illegitimate rituals—which often involve immodest acts in sacred places and religiously forbidden usage of body parts and substances—in a time and place beyond the official gaze of men. Given that Muslim men usually congregate at mosques during the Friday noon prayer, women are uniquely free during this brief period to perform their "female-centered" activities, of which *kabsa* rituals are but one example.

The persistent practices of *kabsa* healing rituals at sacred times and places is a measure of poor urban Egyptian women's response to their subjectivity—as Muslims and as members of an emphatically patriarchal society. Although many women know that their *kabsa* practices are frowned upon by Muslim men, they demonstrate a subversive, resistant stance in their continuing pursuit of such unorthodox rituals and their active attempts to aid other women in unbinding a problem that may, in fact, have been induced by men.

Ritual Repetition of Formulaic Actions

Another feature of *kabsa* healing, which is shared with other Egyptian ethnomedical healing rituals, is ritual repetition of formulaic actions in odd-numbered patterns of three and seven and occasionally five and nine. For example, *kabsa* healing rituals, including visits to sites where these rituals are to be performed, are always carried out over three consecutive Fridays. Likewise, *kabsa* rituals often involve stepping over the polluting substance three, five, seven, and occasionally nine times. Furthermore, preventive thread *kabsa* bracelets and rings to be worn by new brides and new mothers are always tied into seven knots.

In addition, within each of the various types of *kabsa* therapeutic

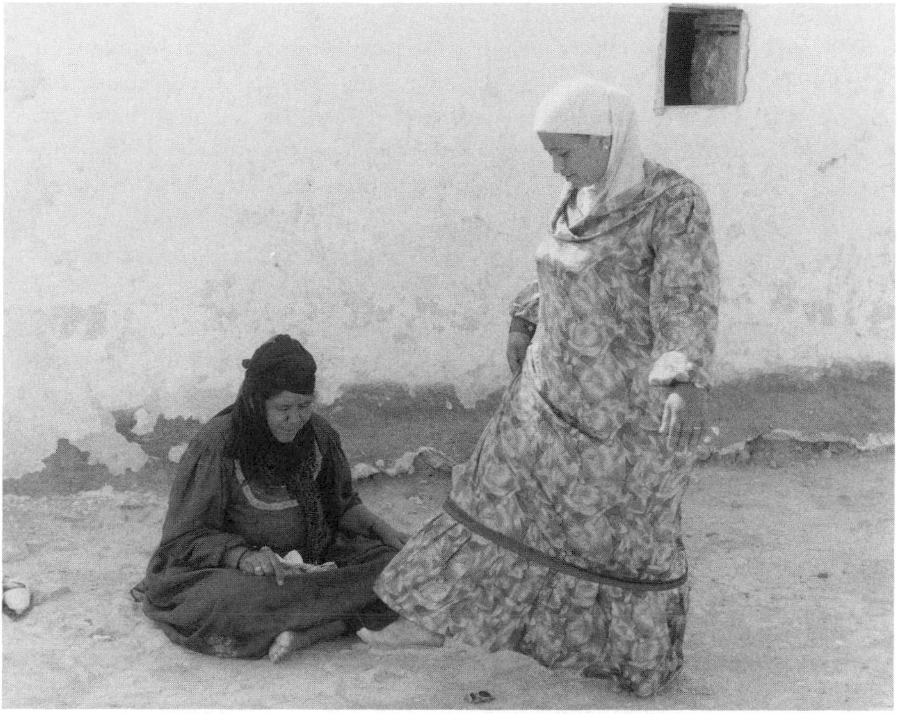

Photograph 5. A *makbūsa* woman stepping over the *mushāharāt*. (Photograph by Mia Fuller)

rituals, seven major formulaic ritual actions can be identified. These include (1) bathing with, (2) stepping over, (3) visiting and crossing through, (4) urinating on, (5) sitting on, (6) rubbing on, and (7) introducing into the vagina and/or mouth the pollutant.

The reason for odd-numbered repetitions and actions is related to Egyptian (and broader Middle Eastern) notions of good luck and protection, which are ensured through the avoidance of even numbers (Kennedy 1967; Pillsbury 1978). Thus, five-fingered hands are used as amulets of protection against the evil eye. Birth celebrations occur after seven days. Spirit placation ceremonies ideally last seven, or at least three, days. And, in the case of *kabsa*, one or more of seven formulaic ritual actions are to be repeated over three consecutive Fridays. In fact, most poor urban Egyptian women contend that rituals enacted only once or twice will fail to unbind *kabsa* effects.

Depolluting Consubstantiality

These formulaic actions are important in establishing depolluting consubstantiality: that is, making reproductive ritual initiates reexperience the polluting substance thought to have caused *kabsa* by bringing them into proximity with that substance or a symbolic representation of it. In many cases, consubstantiality, or the sharing of substance, is established between two humans, namely, between the woman who has sustained *kabsa*-induced reproductive problems, herein known as the "*kabs*-ee," and the actual polluted boundary-crosser who has caused *kabsa*, herein known as the "*kabs*-er" (or, in some cases, a "proxy *kabs*-er"). In other instances, substance is shared with a dead human, an animal, or an object with symbolically polluting qualities. In all cases, however, rituals of consubstantiality are thought to bring about a reversal or a negation of the original polluting event, thereby "making *kabsa* vanish" and releasing the woman from her state of boundness.

Most important, however, is the fact that these rituals of depolluting consubstantiality must be specific; ideally, they must be directed at the actual event thought to have caused *kabsa*, be it pollution by blood, excreta, death, or gold. Thus, when *kabsa* healing rituals are undertaken, they are always carried out with these causative categories in mind. For example, if a person who has come from a funeral is thought to have caused *kabsa*, the *kabs*-ee will likely be encouraged to undertake a ritual involving a visit to the neighborhood cemetery. Or, if a person carrying meat into the room is thought to have caused *kabsa*, the *kabs*-ee will often be told to step over a freshly slaughtered animal, often smearing her feet in its blood. Thus, ritual officiants who attempt to help the infertile woman unbind her reproductive capacities tend to direct their therapeutic efforts at the most likely cause of the problem. However, because the exact cause of *kabsa* is often unknown, healing rituals are often more speculative than specific, and alternate forms of ritual unbinding may be necessary, as seen in the initial story about Amina's *kabsa* problems.

Dual-Purpose Rituals

Furthermore, because the exact cause of *kabsa* is often unknown, many *kabsa* healing rituals are "dual-purpose"—that is, they are directed against more than one polluting substance. For example, because a *kabs*-er may be defiled by both blood and breast milk or both blood and urine at the time of *kabsa* production, ritual acts directed against *kabsa* effects often incorporate dual depolluting elements aimed at negating the effects of both substances.

This is why, for example, urination in or near cemeteries is one of the primary ritual acts of *kabsa* healing, or why coparticipants in *kabsa* rituals may "share" both blood and urine. Furthermore, this is why symbolic objects used in *kabsa* rituals are representative of more than one pollutant category and, in fact, may be seen as multipurpose agents of depollution in some cases.

Kabsa healing rituals are also dual-purpose in that they may undo the effects of both *kabsa* and *khaḍḍa*, or shock. This is particularly true of rituals in cemeteries, where exposure to the newly dead or skeletons is thought to unbind *kabsa* effects as well as provide therapeutic countershocking. Women who undertake *kabsa* bathing rituals are also encouraged to use cold water for the same reason, because, when dumped over the warm body, cold water exerts similar countershocking effects.

Ritual Forms

Given the odd-numbered association described above, it is interesting that *kabsa* healing rituals take five major forms.

preventive ritual behaviors

First, some *kabsa* rituals are preventive and involve simple behavioral guidelines and ritual acts carried out during the ritual initiate's liminal lunar month. These preventive behaviors and rituals are designed to protect the reproductively liminal woman from polluting boundary-crossing during the vulnerable transitional period. Although Kennedy (1978a) has subsumed these acts under the category of "taboo" behaviors, calling them "taboos" suggests a degree of social consensus and behavioral uniformity that appears to be lacking in Lower Egypt. Rather, *kabsa*-preventive measures are sometimes, but not always, practiced, given that many Egyptian women are much less aware of *kabsa* preventive rituals than therapeutic ones. Nevertheless, a number of preventive techniques appear to have some degree of social support among urban Lower Egyptian women and are practiced consistently enough that they merit attention, as shown in Table 2.

Of all of the behavioral measures to ward off *kabsa* effects, the use of preventive "*kabsa* bracelets" appears to have the most widespread support in Lower Egypt, particularly among women who are giving birth at hospitals and clinics. Hospitals, and especially maternity hospitals and clinics, are thought by many Egyptians to be thoroughly polluted places, given that they house other new mothers, women who are bleeding and "oozing" for various reasons, newly shaved physicians and other male visitors, and the

TABLE 2. Types of *Kabsa* Rituals and Their Performance by Ninety-six Infertile Egyptian Women in the Study Sample.

TYPE OF *KABSA* RITUAL (AND RITUAL ACTIVITIES)	PERCENTAGE OF WOMEN PERFORMING RITUAL*
Preventive Ritual Behaviors	
Behaviors of new brides	NS†
Bride should remain in her room during the first postmarital lunar month and restrict the number of visitors	
Bride should leave her room to meet her newly shaved husband and walk around him seven times	
If she markets, bride should walk into the market and back out again to negate polluting effects of meats and vegetables there	
Seven prepubescent (nonmenstruating) virgins or a postmenopausal *dāya* should make bride's bed	
Nonmenstruating (e.g., postmenopausal) woman should fashion seven-knotted thread around bride's finger	
Bride should wear an article of gold jewelry containing a human form or any article of 24-karat gold	
Bride should wear a small, leafy twig of Saudi Arabian caraway on a thread necklace	
Bride should wear a small piece of seven-leafed palm frond on a thread necklace	
Black eggplant or seven-leafed palm frond should be hung in the bride's room or over the doorway	
Behaviors of new mothers	NS†
Pregnant woman should deliver her baby at home (to reduce exposure to polluting boundary-crossings in hospitals and clinics)	
Pregnant woman delivering in a hospital or clinic should wear a seven-knotted *kabsa* bracelet for the duration of the first postpartum lunar month	
Postmenopausal woman should fashion a seven-knotted thread around new mother's wrist and the new mother should wear underwear and slip inside out	
Postmenopausal *dāya* should make a new mother's bed	
Newly delivered woman should remain in her room at home and restrict the number of visitors	
Behaviors of visitors	NS†
New brides should not visit new mothers and vice versa	
Menstruating women should not visit new brides or new mothers and should remain at home as much as possible until menses cease and vaginal purification (douching) has been undertaken	

TABLE 2. *Continued*

TYPE OF *KABSA* RITUAL (AND RITUAL ACTIVITIES)	PERCENTAGE OF WOMEN PERFORMING RITUAL*
Preventive Ritual Behaviors (continued)	
Women should bathe before visiting new brides and new mothers	
Gifts of meat should be placed outside of the doorway, where a new bride or new mother can come out to "meet the meat"	
Therapeutic Rituals with the Kabs-*er*	
Rituals of blood-sharing	5
Kabs-er cuts herself (usually her finger) and *kabs*-ee introduces blood into her own body by sucking on the wound or dabbing cotton in the blood and wearing it as a vaginal suppository	
Kabs-ee douses *kabs*-er's bloodied defloration handkerchief in water and drinks the liquid	
Rituals of excreta-sharing	6
Kabs-er urinates on the ground, then *kabs*-ee urinates on the urine to "wash away" *kahsa*-producing impurity	
Kabs-er and *kabs*-ee urinate on a patch of dusty earth, then fashion the moistened earth into one or two mud dolls (representing the desired child), which either or both women place in water, followed by mutual, purifying bathing with the water	
Both *kabs*-er and *kabs*-ee urinate in a collecting bowl, dip cotton in the urine, and introduce the cotton into their bodies as vaginal suppositories	
Both *kabs*-er and *kabs*-ee cut the other's finger following co-urination, then introduce the blood into their bodies as vaginal suppositories	
Sexually impure *kabs*-ee steps over sexually impure *kabs*-er seven times	
Rituals in cemeteries	3
Kabs-ee and *kabs*-er enter a cemetery together and *kabs*-ee steps over prostrate *kabs*-er seven times	
Kabs-er and *kabs*-ee co-urinate in or near a cemetery (e.g., on a pile of human bones in the cemetery, in front of the cemetery door), sometimes followed by fashioning a mud doll with the moistened earth, then placing the doll in water for mutual, purifying bathing	

TABLE 2. *Continued*

TYPE OF *KABSA* RITUAL (AND RITUAL ACTIVITIES)	PERCENTAGE OF WOMEN PERFORMING RITUAL*
Therapeutic Rituals with a Proxy Kabs-*er*	
Rituals of blood-sharing	32
Postmenopausal *dāya* (ritual officiant) places a small piece of proxy *kabs*-er's placenta or umbilical cord into *kabs*-ee's vagina "while the blood is still hot"	
Postmenopausal *dāya* (ritual officiant) drenches a piece of cotton with proxy *kabs*-er's delivery blood, then inserts cotton into *kabs*-ee's vagina (or tells her to insert it on her own), to be worn as a 24-hour suppository	
Kabs-ee ingests a small amount of blood from proxy *kabs*-er's delivery or cut finger	
Kabs-ee sits on or steps over (three or seven times) proxy *kabs*-er's "fresh" bloody placenta or umbilical cord	
Kabs-ee sits on proxy *kabs*-er's placenta, then dips cotton in placental blood to wear as a vaginal suppository	
Kabs-ee bathes with water in which proxy *kabs*-er's defloration handkerchief has been placed	
Kabs-ee steps over defloration handkerchief of a new bride seven times	
Kabs-ee licks defloration blood of a new bride	
Proxy *kabs*-er's circumcision blood is placed on cotton, which is worn by *kabs*-ee as a vaginal suppository	
Proxy *kabs*-er's menstrual blood is placed on cotton, which is worn by *kabs*-ee as a vaginal suppository	
Rituals of excreta-sharing	6
Kabs-ee steps over a small amount of proxy *kabs*-er's breast milk seven times	
Kabs-ee wears cotton dipped in proxy *kabs*-er's breast milk as a vaginal suppository	
Kabs-ee steps over a small amount of proxy *kabs*-er's breast milk, then dips cotton into it to be worn as a vaginal suppository	
Kabs-ee rubs proxy *kabs*-er's breast milk directly onto her own breasts and/or genitals	
Kabs-ee bathes with water in which proxy *kabs*-er's "unclean" items (e.g., semen-imbued underclothes or bedsheets) have been placed	

TABLE 2. *Continued*

TYPE OF *KABSA* RITUAL (AND RITUAL ACTIVITIES)	PERCENTAGE OF WOMEN PERFORMING RITUAL*
Therapeutic Rituals with Objects, Animals, and the Human Dead	
Rituals of blood-sharing:	
Blood of birth	33
Kabs-ee steps over a miscarried or stillborn infant three or seven times	
Kabs-ee bathes with water in which a miscarried or stillborn infant has been placed	
Kabs-ee boils a miscarried or stillborn infant in water, then "showers" with this water by dumping it over her head	
Kabs-ee steps over (or bathes with) a body part (e.g., brain) of a miscarried or stillborn infant	
If a fetus/dead infant cannot be found, *kabs*-ee steps over (or bathes with) an inanimate object representing a child (e.g., a doll made from stone, henna, metal, or mud or a baby toy) or the loofah sponge used to wash the body of a dead infant	
Kabs-ee wears a 24-hour vaginal suppository consisting of a feline placenta grilled to a peanut-like consistency, ground with wormwood, and wrapped in gauze	
Kabs-ee wears a 24-hour vaginal suppository of cotton dipped in feline delivery blood	
If a feline placenta or delivery blood cannot be "captured," *kabs*-ee should watch a cat deliver her litter	
If a feline placenta or delivery blood cannot be "captured," *kabs*-ee should sit on the placenta of another four-footed mammal (e.g., goat) or use its delivery blood in a cotton vaginal suppository	
Blood of slaughter	26
Kabs-ee visits a slaughterhouse to step over a slaughtered animal three, five, or seven times, wetting her feet in its blood	
Kabs-ee visits a slaughterhouse, dabs a piece of cotton in fresh blood of slaughter, then wears as a 24-hour vaginal suppository	
Kabs-ee visits a slaughterhouse and rubs the blood of slaughter on her breasts	
Kabs-ee visits a slaughterhouse, entering through one door and exiting by another	

TABLE 2. *Continued*

TYPE OF *KABSA* RITUAL (AND RITUAL ACTIVITIES)	PERCENTAGE OF WOMEN PERFORMING RITUAL*
Kabs-ee visits a slaughterhouse and stands under an animal's neck during slaughter, allowing the blood to gush onto her body	
Kabs-ee visits a slaughterhouse and steps over the blood of slaughter three, five, or seven times	
Kabs-ee eats raw meat from a newly slaughtered animal	
Kabs-ee's husband slaughters a chicken or duck, and *kabs*-ee steps over it or its blood three, five, or seven times, or rubs its blood on her breasts; afterward, she and her husband eat the animal	
Kabs-ee squeezes the blood from a piece of fresh meat and rubs the blood on her breasts	
Kabs-ee bathes with water in which fresh meat has been placed	
Kabs-ee ingests a piece of raw, spiced, bloody meat	
Kabs-ee steps over a piece of fresh, raw meat seven times	
Kabs-ee steps over meat or fish placed on the doorstep	
Blood of shaving	5
Kabs-ee steps over her husband's razor and other shaving tools or a barber's tools (razor, blade sharpener, scissors, comb) seven times	
Kabs-ee bathes with water in which her husband's or a barber's shaving tools have been placed	
Kabs-ee rubs her breast with her husband's or a barber's shaving tools	
Blood of defloration	3
Kabs-ee wears her bloodied defloration handkerchief or cloth as a 24-hour vaginal suppository, removes it, throws it into a busy intersection, then washes her genitals	
Kabs-ee bathes with water in which her bloodied defloration handkerchief has been placed	
Kabs-ee bathes with water in which her wedding certificate has been placed	
Rituals of excreta-sharing	15
Kabs-ee bathes with ablution water from a mosque	
Kabs-ee steps over a handful of seashells (usually clamshells) seven times	
Kabs-ee bathes with water in which seashells and pebbles from sea have been placed (making sure to cleanse genitals)	

TABLE 2. *Continued*

TYPE OF *KABSA* RITUAL (AND RITUAL ACTIVITIES)	PERCENTAGE OF WOMEN PERFORMING RITUAL*
Rituals involving death:	48
Inside cemeteries	
Kabs-ee enters a walled cemetery through one door and exits by another door	
Kabs-ee visits a cemetery without speaking until she returns home, remains at home for the rest of the day, and has sex in the evening	
Kabs-ee visits a cemetery with a postmenopausal woman to whom she does not speak	
Kabs-ee crosses a cemetery without shoes and urinates in front of the cemetery door upon exiting	
Kabs-ee bathes with seven glasses of water obtained from a spout inside the cemetery, pouring each glass over her head	
Kabs-ee bathes with a glass of ablution water taken inside a cemetery on the third Friday	
Kabs-ee strips naked and allows female gravekeeper to dump water over her body	
Kabs-ee urinates inside a cemetery between graves, on a broken tomb, on a stone, or on human bones	
Kabs-ee steps over a human bone, pile of bones, or full skeleton seven times	
Kabs-ee steps over a recently dead body seven times	
Kabs-ee steps over a new grave seven times	
Kabs-ee steps over the gravedigger's tools seven times	
Kabs-ee steps over a funeral bier in a cemetery	
Gravekeeper starts a small fire inside the cemetery and *kabs*-ee steps over it seven times	
Gravekeeper takes *kabs*-ee to a neglected tomb, where she peers in to see human skeletons	
Gravekeeper pours a pail of cemetery dust down *kabs*-ee's dress and she rubs dust on her breasts	
Outside cemeteries	20
Kabs-ee bathes with water and/or a loofah sponge used to cleanse a dead body	
Kabs-ee bathes with water in which clothes of a dead person have been placed	
Kabs-ee bathes with water in which a sheet used to wrap a dead person has been placed	

TABLE 2. *Continued*

TYPE OF *KABSA* RITUAL (AND RITUAL ACTIVITIES)	PERCENTAGE OF WOMEN PERFORMING RITUAL*
Kabs-ee bathes with water in which a collection of handkerchiefs owned by persons leaving a burial have been placed; handkerchiefs are then returned to owners	
Kabs-ee bathes with water in which a stone, brick, or bone obtained from a cemetery has been placed	
Kabs-ee bathes with water in which a green plant called "devil's leaves" obtained from a cemetery has been placed	
Kabs-ee sits on a funeral bier and has water poured over her head	
Kabs-ee steps over water used to wash a dead person seven times	
Kabs-ee steps over a dead infant or miscarried fetus in hospital or morgue seven times	
Kabs-ee steps over railroad tracks seven times	
With black eggplants	15
Kabs-ee bathes with water in which a mud doll fashioned from the soil of an eggplant field has been placed	
Kabs-ee bathes with water in which a black eggplant (sometimes skewered with a piece of wood) has been placed	
Kabs-ee steps over seven rows of black eggplants and tomatoes, fashions a doll from the dust of each field, places it in water and bathes with it	
Kabs-ee steps over a black eggplant picked fresh from the field and/or placed on her doorstep	
Kabs-ee visits and crosses over a field of black eggplants (which are said to turn rotten as the *kabs*-ee becomes fertile and pregnant)	
Kabs-ee urinates on or in a cored black eggplant, which is sometimes thrown into an intersection afterward	
Kabs-ee eats pieces of raw black eggplant obtained directly from an eggplant field	
Kabs-ee puts the core of a raw black eggplant into her vagina as a suppository	
Kabs-ee rubs a black eggplant on her breasts and genitals, throwing it into an intersection afterward	
Rituals involving gold	9
Kabs-ee steps over 24-karat gold seven times	
Kabs-ee bathes with water in which 24-karat gold has been placed	
Kabs-ee steps over 18-karat gold containing a human form (e.g., a coin or a pharaonic figure) seven times	

TABLE 2. *Continued*

TYPE OF *KABSA* RITUAL (AND RITUAL ACTIVITIES)	PERCENTAGE OF WOMEN PERFORMING RITUAL*
Kabs-ee bathes with water in which a gold earring in shape of a doll from Saudi Arabia has been placed	
Kabs-ee bathes with water in which gold containing a human form has been placed	
Kabs-ee bathes with water in which an article of gold has been dipped seven times	
Kabs-ee bathes with water in which silver jewelry containing a human form (e.g., a coin or pharaonic figure) has been placed	
Kabs-ee bathes with water in which gold jewelry with precious gems (especially diamonds and pearls) has been placed	
Kabs-ee bathes with water in which pearls have been placed	
Therapeutic Rituals with Mushāharāt	
Mushāharāt necklaces	27
Kabs-ee steps over a *mushāharāt* necklace seven times	
Kabs-ee bathes with water in which a *mushāharāt* necklace has been placed	
Kabs-ee rubs her breasts and umbilicus with a *mushāharāt* necklace, then dips it into a water-filled washbasin seven times, then ablutes herself with this water, then washes her umbilicus and genitals, then washes her entire body, but not in a bathroom (which is impure); afterward, she may dispose of the water by pouring it in three directions into an intersection	
Kabs-ee steps over or bathes with a *mushāharāt* necklace (as above), then uses a series of vaginal suppositories containing seven multicolored herbal substances for three or seven consecutive evenings, during which time sexual intercourse is prohibited	
Mushāharāt combinations	6
Kabs-ee steps over seven times or bathes with a *mushāharāt* combination containing three or more of the following items: beads, pearls, evil-eye amulets, old coins, animal replicas, human dolls, human figurines, shaving tools, seashells, human bones and/or skulls, multicolored grains, gold jewelry, palm fronds, black eggplants, tomatoes	

*This column does not total 100 percent because many women in the study sample undertook more than one *kabsa* ritual.
†No statistics are available on preventive ritual behaviors in the study sample.

dead. That a polluted individual may enter a new mother's hospital room during her vulnerable, "open" state is quite likely, given the lack of private rooms in most public hospitals and clinics in Egypt. Thus, it is widely believed that delivering one's baby at home decreases the likelihood of *kabsa* by reducing exposure to potential *kabsa*-causing boundary-crossings, and, as a result, many Egyptian women view hospital/clinic deliveries with a great deal of ambivalence and skepticism.[17] However, in cases in which hospital or clinic deliveries are necessary, a seven-knotted, thread *kabsa* bracelet, fastened on the wrist immediately upon delivery and worn by the new mother for the duration of the first lunar postpartum month, is thought to be protective against *kabsa* effects, as shown in Table 2.

THERAPEUTIC RITUALS WITH THE *KABS*-ER

If such preventive measures are not taken, or if taken fail to work for some reason, *kabsa* may occur, resulting in the bound state of *makbūsa*, which, to be overcome, requires therapeutic unbinding rituals. The most desirable means for a *kabs*-ee to become unbound is to undertake therapeutic healing rituals with the actual *kabs*-er, if this person is known and can be convinced to become a ritual coparticipant. Usually, the *kabs*-er is thought to be another woman living in the same household—most often a woman's sister-in-law (the husband's sister or husband's brother's wife) who is bloodied from a recent delivery or is menstruating and accidentally enters the new bride's room. However, persons other than sisters-in-law may also be identified—for example, another family member who brought meat into the woman's room or a neighbor who visited her after passing through a cemetery.

The purpose of coparticipatory rituals between *kabs*-ers and *kabs*-ees is for the *kabs*-ee to reidentify with the pollutant by which she was made *makbūsa* by the *kabs*-er, thereby making the effects of *kabsa* vanish. Furthermore, in the vast majority of cases, the *kabs*-er is a fertile woman; therefore, a subsidiary function of these rituals is to share substance with the type of woman the *kabs*-ee hopes to become—namely, fertile and "normal." For example, if exposure to the *kabs*-er's blood was thought to have caused *kabsa*, it is considered prudent to reexpose the *kabs*-ee to the *kabs*-er's blood. In such rituals, not only do the *kabs*-ee and the *kabs*-er share substance, but in many cases the *kabs*-ee's bodily boundaries are actually reviolated, or repenetrated, through the incorporation of the pollutant into the body itself. Especially notable is the introduction of the fertile *kabs*-er's blood into the *kabs*-ee's reproductive orifice, placing this pollutant in direct contact with the afflicted reproductive region and presumably enhancing the depolluting potential of this ritual act.

In addition, when two women have caused *kabsa* to each other, both becoming infertile as is sometimes the case, their sharing of bodily substances is thought to unbind both of them, making the effects of *kabsa* vanish and the period of liminality end. For example, if two women are thought to have caused *kabsa* to each other by virtue of some bodily impurity (for example, leaking breast milk or urine), it is thought best to overcome this problem through a ritual of co-urination. Co-urination is thought to negate the polluting effects of all nonsanguineous bodily fluids, because it represents the flushing effect of "water on water."

Thus, in an ideal world, the *kabs*-ee is able to identify her *kabs*-er, and coparticipatory rituals of the type described in Table 2 can be undertaken. Because they allow depolluting consubstantiality with the *actual* agent of *kabsa* production, these coparticipatory rituals are considered to be maximally efficacious, making them the ideal form of ritual reincorporation into the world of female fertility.

THERAPEUTIC RITUALS WITH A PROXY *KABS*-ER

However, because actual *kabs*-ers are so rarely known to the *kabs*-ee, rituals of *kabs*-er/*kabs*-ee coparticipation are often impossible to orchestrate. When actual *kabs*-ers are missing, it is widely acknowledged by Egyptian women that the next best strategy is to find a "proxy *kabs*-er"—one who is thought to be in, at the present moment, the *kabs*-er's condition when *kabsa* occurred. This proxy *kabs*-er, sharing significant polluting qualities with the actual *kabs*-er, may serve as a ritual stand-in in coparticipatory *kabsa* healing rituals.

As with actual *kabs*-ers, these proxy *kabs*-ers may be asked to share the products of their bodies, and especially their blood, in *kabsa* healing rituals. For example, if the *kabs*-er was thought to be a woman who had just given birth to a child and was both bloodied and lactating when she entered the *kabs*-ee's room, another new mother in the same condition can be found to stand in for the original *kabs*-er; her polluting bodily fluids are deemed sufficiently representative to be able to unbind the effects of *kabsa* in the *kabs*-ee. Indeed, women who have just given birth (and have therefore proven their fertility) are often sought out for proxy *kabsa* healing rituals in which their delivery blood or their bloodied placentas and umbilical cords are used by the *kabs*-ee in various ritual acts.

Because proxy *kabs*-ers are easier to locate than actual ones, the majority of coparticipatory *kabsa* healing rituals fall into this category. Furthermore, the variety of ritual forms is greater in this category, as is evident in Table 2.

THERAPEUTIC RITUALS WITH OBJECTS, ANIMALS, AND THE HUMAN DEAD

Some *kabsa* healing rituals occur without human coparticipants and involve acts of consubstantiality with the polluting substance alone or a symbolic proxy of it. Such noncoparticipatory rituals occur because in the vast majority of *kabsa* cases ritual coparticipants cannot be found to help *kabs*-ees unbind their reproductive capacities. In addition, *kabs*-ees, who by virtue of their prolonged reproductive liminality are often socially marginal, may be reluctant to recruit the services of fertile women in their efforts to overcome their infertility. Furthermore, *kabs*-ers or proxy *kabs*-ers may be unavailable or unwilling to perform the *kabsa* ritual, especially during the Friday noon prayer time when meal preparation is often taking place. Unwillingness may stem from several other sources, including disbelief in the *kabsa* complex, repugnance toward the necessary ritual acts, concern of husbands over Islamic orthodoxy, or fear of coparticipation in a ritual involving a reproductively marginal woman.

For all of these reasons, other avenues for overcoming *kabsa* may need to be considered. In fact, the vast majority of *kabsa* healing rituals are carried out by the *kabs*-ee alone, or with the help of an older ritual officiant, especially a postmenopausal mother, a mother-in-law, another female relative, or a female ethnogynecologist. Like the coparticipatory rituals already described, these solitary rituals are directed at the probable polluting etiology of *kabsa*; but, instead of overcoming *kabsa* through acts of depolluting consubstantiality with living humans, these rituals of consubstantiality involve sharing the substances of symbolically polluted inanimate objects, animals, and the dead.

Although these rituals demonstrate the greatest variety of forms, as seen in Table 2, they are similar to the coparticipatory rituals already described in that they tend to be quite etiologically specific, as follows.

Blood-sharing rituals with blood of birth. Given that individuals who have been "bloodied" in one way or another are thought to be the primary agents of *kabsa*, sharing of blood can be achieved by alternate means when *kabs*-ers or proxy *kabs*-ers cannot be identified or ritually enlisted. Because women who have been bloodied by birth and miscarriage are considered to be among the primary agents of *kabsa*, healing rituals involving stillborn infants and miscarried fetuses—the bloodied products of such women's bodies—are one of the primary ways in which Egyptian women attempt to overcome the effects of *kabsa* without the aid of actual or proxy *kabs*-ers. Not only do such rituals allow the sharing of polluting delivery blood, but they serve the important secondary purpose of putting *kabs*-ees in ritual contact with that which they most desire: namely, a human child. Even though the infants used in these rituals were never born alive, they are the closest physical representation of the desired outcome of the healing ritual, symbolizing the very reason for enacting such rituals among infertile women. Therefore, *kabsa* rituals with stillborn infants or miscarried fetuses are considered especially powerful and efficacious, given that most infertile women believe that they not only become unbound by them, but may also "catch something from the baby" (namely, imminent pregnancy).

Given the perceived potency of such rituals, an informal market in miscarried and aborted fetuses and stillborn infants exists among poor urban and rural Egyptian women. Instead of burying or disposing of these infants, women often keep them for ritual use. For example, women who have miscarried, either at home or in the hospital, may request that the fetus be saved and given to a family member or friend who is infertile for the purposes of *kabsa* healing. Even if the need for such a fetus is not immediate, the fetus may be preserved for several months, either in a plastic bag, a jar, or wrapped in cloth. In fact, many women undergo *kabsa* rituals with miscarried fetuses or stillborn infants who have been "pickled" (preserved in saline liquid in a pickled cucumber jar) or "mummified" (wrapped in gauze like a mummy). Furthermore, many *dāyāt* keep such "preserved" infants on hand in their homes, in case any of their infertile clients should require this form of *kabsa* healing.

However, the bloodied products of human delivery are not the only objects utilized in this form of *kabsa* healing. Some *kabsa* healing rituals use the bloodied delivery products of certain animals that are considered capable of causing *kabsa* by entering the room of a reproductively liminal woman. Cats are particularly suspect as *kabs*-ers, because, in Egypt, they tend to walk in and out of rooms at will (including the hospital rooms of new mothers). Thus, feline placentas—which are particularly difficult to obtain, given that mother cats quickly eat them (as well as those of humans in labor and delivery rooms in Egypt)—are sometimes used in *kabsa* healing rituals, as shown in Table 2. When a feline placenta cannot be "captured," feline delivery blood or the delivery products of other animals may be substituted.

Blood-sharing rituals with blood of slaughter. In addition to living cats, livestock that have been slaughtered for food are considered *kabsa*-producing by virtue of their blood which has been spilled. These "meat *kabsas*," as Egyptian women often call them, must be overcome through rituals in which the *kabs*-ee is reexposed to the blood of slaughter, insuring depolluting consubstantiality. In Egypt, it is thought best for the *kabs*-ee to visit a *madhbaḥ*, or slaughterhouse, where she participates in various ways in the slaughter of a domesticated animal (for example, a lamb, goat, cow, or water buffalo), as shown in Table 2.

Blood-sharing rituals with blood of shaving. Along with various animals, husbands are also considered dangerous to new brides and new mothers during the liminal postmarital/postpartum lunar month, because of their ability to cause *kabsa* via the blood of shaving. However, husbands themselves are uninvolved in overcoming this form of "shaving *kabsa*," because, as mentioned earlier, men do not actively participate in *kabsa* healing rituals. Rather, if this cause of *kabsa* is suspected, it is deemed necessary for the husband to provide his razor and other shaving tools (if he shaves himself) to his wife for the purposes of *kabsa* healing. If the husband is usually shaved by a barber, the barber's tools—including, if possible, his blade sharpener, scissors, razor, and comb—must be obtained, as shown in Table 2.

Blood-sharing rituals with blood of defloration. Similarly, husbands may cause *kabsa* to their new brides by deflowering them, leaving the room "polluted" (by blood and/or semen and/or vaginal fluids), and then returning to the bridal suite after having shown the bloodied handkerchief to family members. In so doing, husbands "enter" upon their new brides, causing *kabsa* by way of the bride's own blood on the husband's penis or on the defloration handkerchief, as well as by sexual pollution.

In Egypt, it is thought best for the *kabs*-ee to overcome this form of *kabsa* by performing a healing ritual using the bloodied handkerchief with which she was deflowered. However, because most Egyptian women consider their defloration handkerchief, which is the sign of their "honor" and that of their natal family, to be exceedingly precious, some women prefer to safeguard it, substituting instead their wedding certificates, as shown in Table 2.

Rituals of excreta-sharing. When a woman becomes *makbūsa* as a result of pollution by some other nonsanguineous bodily fluid, solitary *kabsa* healing rituals are also possible. The most common ritual employs seashells—typically, clamshells with, in some cases, the living mollusks. From a symbolic perspective, this use of clamshells appears to serve two purposes. First, clams come from the sea—in this case, the Mediterranean. Therefore, using clamshells in ritual bathing insures that the impurities causing *kabsa* are "washed away" in the vast Mediterranean waters. Perhaps more important, however, clams bear a strong resemblance to the female genitalia. Therefore, they can be used as a symbolic substitute for the woman whose genitalia were unclean when she caused *kabsa* to the *kabs*-ee.

Death rituals inside cemeteries. Of all the types of *kabsa* healing rituals, it may be the most difficult to enlist the participation of *kabs*-ers or proxy *kabs*-ers in death rituals involving visits to cemeteries, which are feared for their associations with sacredness, death, and harmful spirits. Therefore, in most cases, *kabs*-ees must visit cemeteries alone, where they undertake depolluting healing rituals either inside the cemetery proper or on its external periphery.

In the vast majority of cases, *kabs*-ees visit a cemetery during the Friday noon prayer time. If the cemetery is large and established and is therefore walled, the *kabs*-ee enters through a door on one side and exits by a door on the other, thereby "leaving *kabsa* behind" in this holy, pure place.[18] This "entry-exit" technique is notable, in that *kabsa* is a problem of unexpected "entrances." In all *kabsa* healing rituals involving visits to special locations—and especially to cemeteries—the emphasis on ritualistic entrances and exits connotes the fact that *kabsa*, a problem of polluting boundary-crossing, is "left behind" through a reenactment of boundary-crossing in a symbolically meaningful location.

But cemetery rituals may be more complex than simple acts of entry and exit. For example, the *kabs*-ee may be told to refrain from speaking from the time she leaves for the cemetery until the moment she returns home, then to stay inside her house for the rest of the day and have sex that evening. Or, she may be accompanied to the cemetery by a nonmenstruating (virginal or postmenopausal) ritual officiant, usually a family member, to whom she may not speak. In some cases, *kabs*-ees are instructed to cross through the cemetery without shoes and, on exiting, to urinate in front of the cemetery door.

However, in most cases, before exiting the cemetery, the *kabs*-ee is expected to perform various rituals, as shown in Table 2. Such rituals incorporate five of the key formulaic actions, including bathing with water, stepping over objects, visiting the gravekeeper, urinating on objects, and rubbing substances on oneself. However, two formulaic actions that do not take place inside cemeteries include "sitting on" polluting objects and "introducing into" the mouth or vagina some pollutant. Presumably, the penetration of death inside one's bodily orifices—by placing the genitalia on top of objects of death and especially by actually placing the substances of death inside one's body—is considered intolerably ominous.

Co-urination inside cemeteries—usually between graves, inside a tomb, or in front of or behind the exiting door—is also considered bad form, if not ominous, by some women. According to those who view cemetery urination as forbidden, the earth "can crack and swallow you, because this is the ground for dead people." Furthermore, because cemeteries are "clean" places where all of the dead have been "purified," cemetery urination represents a major form of sinful defilement.

It is also important to note that, in cases in which bones are involved, a willing gravekeeper must usually be found in order to provide them. Likewise, gravekeepers are the ones who assist *kabs*-ees in other "stepping-over" rituals, including those with dead bodies that have yet to be buried, new graves, or the gravedigger's tools. Thus, Egyptian gravekeepers are often major assistants in *kabsa* death rituals, especially when small remunerations are offered by ritual initiates. In fact, some *kabs*-ees begin their cemetery ritual by specifically visiting the gravekeeper, who asks, "Are you coming to get pregnant?"; when the *kabs*-ee answers affirmatively, the gravekeeper obtains the objects to be used in the ritual or takes the *kabs*-ee to the ritual location inside the cemetery.

Death rituals outside cemeteries. If the *kabs*-ee is unable or afraid to perform *kabsa* rituals inside the cemetery itself, rituals performed outside the cemetery may suffice, according to some Egyptian women. Despite their external location, these *kabsa* healing rituals, like cemetery rituals, are intended to reexpose the *kabs*-ee to the polluting qualities of death, primarily through bathing with water in which a symbolic object has been placed, as shown in Table 2.

In addition, *kabs*-ees may be encouraged to step over the spot where someone is known to have died. This seems to be the reason why women in

Egypt may step over railroad tracks in order to unbind themselves. Railroad tracks, in and of themselves, are not related to *kabsa*. However, railroad tracks *are* related to death in Egypt, primarily in terms of pedestrian fatalities.

Death rituals with black eggplants. Because black is the symbolic color of death in Egypt, the black eggplant—the only common vegetable whose hue is the color of death and mourning—is a primary cause of *kabsa* and is therefore used quite regularly in *kabsa* death rituals. As shown in Table 2, rituals directed at what Egyptian women call the "eggplant *kabsa*" incorporate six of the seven formulaic *kabsa* actions described earlier. Sitting on an eggplant is the only action that is not undertaken, given that destroying the object through sitting on it is not a desirable means of establishing consubstantiality.[19]

Following eggplant rituals, the ritual object itself is often disposed of by being thrown into an intersection. This is a means of signifying the removal of *kabsa* effects. Just as *kabsa* is "left behind" in the cemetery or "washed away" in the ocean, *kabsa* can be symbolically "thrown away" into intersections where passing cars and pedestrians will further obliterate its effects.[20]

Rituals with gold. For women who have been "bound by gold," *kabsa* healing rituals involve reexposure to gold forms that are thought to be particularly polluting. Ideally, some article of twenty-four-karat *dhahab bundu'i* is employed in such rituals. However, because twenty-four-karat gold is extremely soft, expensive, and uncommon among the Egyptian poor, it may be difficult to obtain. Therefore, other specific types of gold may suffice. For example, normal eighteen-karat Egyptian gold may be substituted, as long as it contains the form of a human (either the face on a coin or a pharaonic figure). Occasionally, when such gold cannot be obtained, women substitute silver jewelry with human forms or simply silver coins with faces on them. In addition, gold jewelry with precious gems, especially diamonds and pearls, may be utilized in *kabsa* healing rituals, given their association with *kabsa* causation. When gold jewelry is not available, pearls alone are sometimes substituted, as shown in Table 2.[21]

THERAPEUTIC RITUALS WITH *MUSHĀHARĀT*

Finally, some *kabsa* healing rituals utilize special *sacra*, or sacred objects that are polysemous, symbolically representing several major categories of *kabsa* causation. These objects, known by the collective title *mushāharāt*, are particularly effective when the cause of *kabsa* is entirely unknown, for they allow the *kabs*-ee to be brought into contact with symbolic representations of a number of substances. In many cases, these *mushāharāt* objects effectively summarize *all* of the major categories of *kabsa* causation and, in so doing, allow the *kabs*-ee to unbind herself in one highly efficacious ritual. Because of their polysemous potency and their usual origin in the holy cities of Medina and Mecca in Saudi Arabia, *mushāharāt* are considered quintessential unbinders of *kabsa* effects and are highly sought after by infertile Egyptian women.

In fact, in many cases, infertile women prefer to undergo *mushāharāt* rituals rather than the etiologically specific depolluting rituals of consubstantiality described above. Not only are the aforementioned rituals etiologically inexact and difficult to orchestrate, they are often objectionable to women, given the ritual enactment of immodest and sacrilegious acts (such as public urination), the alarming and distasteful sacralization of human body substances and parts (including fetuses and placentas), and the frightful merging in many cases of hoped-for birth with death. It is not surprising, therefore, that many women consider themselves lucky to bypass these rituals altogether by undergoing healing with *mushāharāt.*

Mushāharāt tend to be under the control of ritual specialists, particularly *sittāt kabira* and *dāyāt*. *Mushāharāt* themselves are generally of two types.

Mushāharāt *necklaces.* The vast majority of *kabs*-ees who undergo *mushāharāt* healing rituals in the homes of *mushāharāt* owners are requested to undertake the formulaic ritual actions of bathing with, stepping over, urinating on, and rubbing the breasts with a beaded necklace known as *mushāharāt.* These *mushāharāt* necklaces are usually obtained during the holy Islamic pilgrimage to the Saudi Arabian cities of Mecca and Medina and are therefore considered to be "of the Prophet Muhammad"—and, hence, especially sacred. Most *mushāharāt* necklaces of this type contain seven, relatively large (almond- to walnut-sized) beads, often of different colors, sizes, and shapes (including in many cases one phallic one). The beads are considered to be summary symbols of the various causal categories of *kabsa*, which is the source of their healing power. For example, *mushāharāt* necklaces usually contain a red, "bloody" bead (typically a carnelian) and a white, "milky" one called *labānna*. Likewise, a black bead symbolizes death, and several beads in the yellow-amber-orange-brown spectrum represent both gold and human bodily secretions, especially urine. *Dāyāt* and other healers who own these necklaces are often expert at

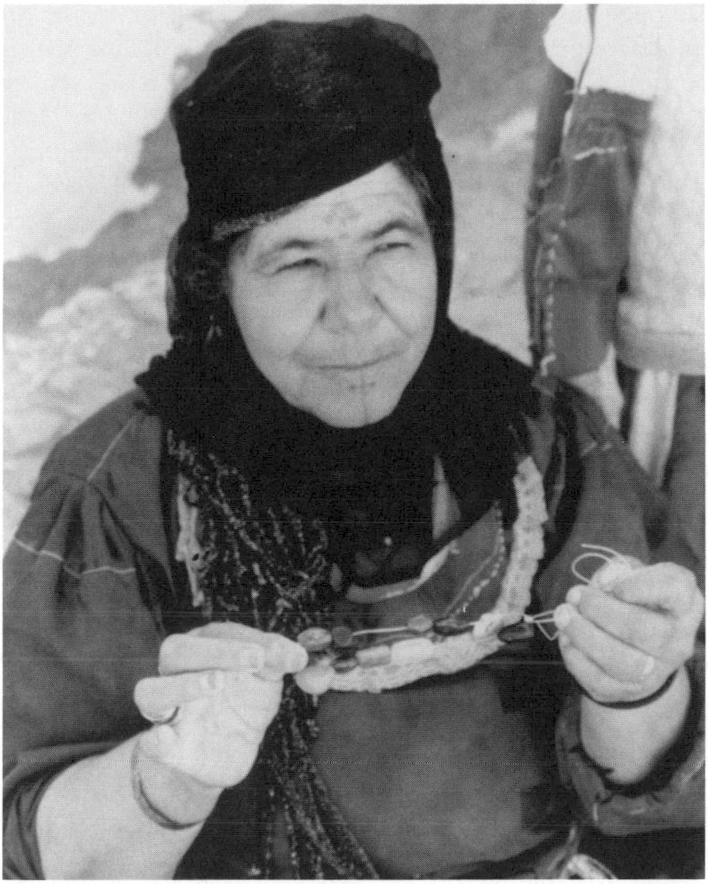

Photograph 6. A *sitt kabīra* holding her *mushāharāt* necklace. (Photograph by Marcia Inhorn)

explaining the symbolic meanings of these beads, although *kabs*-ees themselves are unlikely to possess such knowledge.

In addition to these beads, some *mushāharāt* necklaces contain additional objects that are also symbolic in character. For example, some *mushāharāt* necklaces feature old coins and metallic figures of faces or animals, presumably directed against the specific forms of gold and meat *kabsa*s. Likewise, the inclusion of seashells is certainly directed against the effects of *kabsa* from sexual pollution. Interestingly, some *mushāharāt* necklaces also contain a downturned hand or a blue-beaded eye, which are the major protective amulets against *ḥasad*, or "envy" (glossed as the "evil eye").

Although the formulaic ritual practices undertaken with these *mushāharāt* necklaces are identical to those already described, their performance may be more elaborate, as shown in Table 2. Furthermore, some healers who officiate at such *mushāharāt* rituals also request additional follow-up therapy consisting of a series of vaginal suppositories containing seven multicolored herbal substances that are similarly symbolic. For example, *kabsa* suppositories may consist of combinations of the following common herbs and plant substances: dates, caraway seeds, cinnamon, clove, alum, wormwood, fenugreek, frankincense, lavender, and long pepper. These colorful substances—many of which are recognizable as common spices—are to be ground into a fine powder, cooked until they thicken, wrapped in gauze (which may be dipped in olive oil), and then worn in the vagina for three or seven consecutive nights, during which time sexual intercourse is prohibited. If worn following *mushāharāt* necklace rituals, such vaginal suppositories are considered capable of unbinding the effects of *any* type of *kabsa*, according to the ethnogynecologists who prescribe them.

Mushāharāt *combinations.* However, not all ethnogynecologists who officiate at *mushāharāt* healing rituals own *mushāharāt* necklaces. Rather, their *mushāharāt* consist of an assortment of symbolic objects that, taken together, are also known as *mushāharāt.* Often kept together in boxes or on chains, these *mushāharāt* combinations are, like *mushāharāt* necklaces, meant to symbolize the major categories of *kabsa* causation and thus unbind the effects of any form of *kabsa.*

Mushāharāt of this type often include three or more of the following symbolically meaningful items: a large bead or pearl, evil-eye amulets in the form of a blue-beaded eye and/or a downturned hand, old gold or silver coins, animal replicas, human dolls, stone figurines of humans, razor blades and barber's tools, seashells, human bones and/or skulls, multicolored grains, gold jewelry, and, occasionally, black eggplants, tomatoes, and palm fronds.[22] Because such *mushāharāt* combinations tend to be more unwieldy than *mushāharāt* necklaces, *kabs*-ees are often requested to step over them, rather than to undertake the various other types of formulaic actions already described.

The Threatening Nature of *Kabsa*

As apparent from the ritual analysis presented above, overcoming the effects of *kabsa* through multifarious, often polysemous rituals of consubstantiality, which are intended to allow ritual subjects to be reincorporated into the social body of fertile women, attests to the power of belief in *kabsa* and the perceived seriousness of its reproductively incapacitating effects among Egyptian women. That women are seen as the vulnerable reproductive parties in the rite of passage to parenthood—and that women reproductively "bound" by *kabsa* must overcome its effects or be barred from achieving normal, adult personhood, according to widely accepted normative standards—attests to the precarious nature of women's fertility in Egypt and the social opprobrium that accompanies failures of women in the reproductive realm.

However, *kabsa* threatens not only Egyptian women. Indeed, its danger can be seen to extend to men, the Islamic body politic, and Egyptian society at large.

Given that men are accorded essential, life-giving powers through their fetus-carrying "worms," and that women are strictly marginalized as reproductive "receptacles," it is in some senses ironic that *kabsa*, a problem of women's reproductivity, is widely viewed as *the* principle cause of reproductive failure in Egypt. However, by "binding" women's reproductive bodies, making future efforts at conception and lactation futile, *kabsa* ultimately threatens to thwart the creation of *men's* most important product: a healthy human child. Hence, *kabsa* endangers not only female fertility, but male procreation as well. As such, *kabsa*, a quintessentially female problem, is widely feared by women for its power to destroy their lives by inhibiting *men's* most important achievement—for which they, as women, will be blamed. In this light, then, it is clear why Egyptian women are willing to undergo *kabsa* healing rituals that they may find revolting, frightening, and shameful and that may be frowned upon by men; for, in their world, much is at stake.

But *kabsa* threatens more than the reproductivity and associated social status of women and the procreative power of men. *Kabsa*, as fertility-incapacitating ritual pollution, indexes the potent danger of defilement to the Islamic body politic, a body that is implored to achieve and maintain "purity" in order to face God. Indeed, *kabsa*, as an elaborate complex of pollution and purification practices condemned by the religiously orthodox, actually signifies how truly dangerous pollution can be to Muslim women and the need for restoration of purity before such women may fulfill their crucial role in bearing Muslim believers. Thus, rather than subverting Islamic praxis, *kabsa* can be seen to *reinforce* it by instantiating the dangers of ritual pollution to the bodies of Muslim women and to the future of Islam itself. *Kabsa* rituals, in effect, are the perfect embodiment of the Islamic ideology of pollution and purification (Bourdieu 1977) — an embodiment which the religiously orthodox nonetheless fail to recognize.

To wit, *kabsa* pollution beliefs are intricately tied to, and even mirror, Islamic pollution and purity beliefs, which involve elaborate procedures to remove defiling substances from the body. As Bouhdiba (1985) explains,

> Islam teaches the art of remaining pure as long as possible and of expelling impurity as soon as one becomes aware of it. The life of the Muslim is a succession of states of purity acquired then lost and of impurity removed and then found again. . . . Whatever the body eliminates is impure and sullies the body. And that pollution must be cleansed each time. It is not sin that creates impurity, but man's very life involves pollution. This pollution concerns the functions of elimination and excretion, and nothing else. (1985:43)

In Islam, the body's excreta — including gas, menstrual blood, postpartum discharges, urine, fecal matter, semen, blood, pus, and breast milk — are considered impure and are even viewed with disgust (Bouhdiba 1985). Menstrual blood "arouses considerable revulsion," according to Bouhdiba (1985:51), and postpartum lochia and pseudomenstrual emissions are also cause for alarm. Thus, considerable, anxiety-producing attention is directed at the body and that which it discharges. "Eating, drinking, urinating, farting, defecating, having sexual intercourse, vomiting, bleeding, shaving, cutting one's nails. . . . All this is the object of meticulous prescriptions" (Bouhdiba 1985:55–56).

Such bodily self-monitoring and regulation are ultimately generated by fear — fear of being unworthy in the sight of God and his angels and, therefore, being subjected to the forces of evil. As Bouhdiba explains, "The impure man comes dangerously close to evil. In him existence precedes essence, making essence secondary, denying it in some sense, if only temporarily. The angels who normally keep watch over man and protect him leave him as soon as he ceases to be pure. So he is left without protection, despiritualized, even dehumanized. He can no longer pray, or recite sacred words, still less say the Quran. . . . His security, his *hasana*, is seriously in question" (1985:44).

Bouhdiba's analysis of the danger of pollution to Muslim believers accords well with Douglas's (1966) insights about the threat of pollution, and particularly bodily excretions, to the individual and, hence, social bodies. As she argues, "The body is a model which can stand for any bounded system. Its boundaries can represent any boundaries which are threatened or precarious. . . . We cannot possibly interpret rituals concerning excreta, breast milk, saliva and the rest unless we are prepared to see in the body a symbol of society, and to see the powers and dangers credited to social structure reproduced in small on the human body" (Douglas 1966: 115).

As Douglas has noted, a society experiencing itself as threatened by pollution will respond by expanding regulatory social controls over boundaries, including the margins of the body, such that points of potential infiltration by outside threats become the focus of intensive surveillance and regulation. Such attempts to protect both individual and social bodies from dangerous boundary violation tend to take the form of nervous vigilance over "entrances" and "exits," including the body's orifices. Thus, as Douglas (1966:124) argues, the threatened boundaries of the body politic are mirrored in the "care for the integrity, unity and purity of the physical body"—care which, in Muslim society, is manifest in elaborate ablution practices.

From this perspective, *kabsa* can be seen, both literally and symbolically, as a problem of control over sociophysical "entrances," particularly entrances into the reproductive bodies of vulnerable women. As we have seen, *kabsa* is a form of polluting boundary-crossing: a ritually violating entrance into the protective room of the sacredly vulnerable female ritual initiate, who is still "open" due to important bodily "entrances" (by defloration and circumcision) and "exits" (of nonviable fetuses and viable infants). Those polluted external intruders who cross the boundaries of her ritual sanctuary unwittingly "reviolate" her bodily boundaries with the pollutants which they exude. In so doing, they doom the reproductively liminal woman to a perpetual state of *makbūsa*, of which infertility is the predominant manifestation. Thus, in Muslim Egypt, it is understandable why nervous vigilance exists among women regarding polluting boundary-crossing into both "rooms" and "wombs" and why *kabsa* rituals are vigorously enacted to ritually protect the bodily orifices and to undo the damage of *kabsa* pollution through elaborate rituals of purifying consubstantiality.

Indeed, *kabsa*, more than any other culturally constructed illness category, indexes the danger of pollution to Egyptian Muslim society—a danger that has been underemphasized by anthropological scholars of the Middle East in their preoccupation with the dangerous spirits of possession. Furthermore, *kabsa* underscores the *range* of polluting danger—not only from women's menstrual and postpartum blood, which is typically isolated as a pollutant in scholarly discourse,[23] but from a number of substances which, together, are part of a complex symbolic system (Gottlieb 1988). Moreover, as a highly gendered illness category, *kabsa* indexes the danger of pollution *to women*, who are usually negatively assessed as the nefarious polluters of men (Buckley and Gottlieb 1988). What is more, in the *kabsa* complex, women not only adventitiously pollute other women with their bodily substances, but they *share* these substances in healing rituals, thereby harnessing their individual corporeal power for the greater good of the Muslim body politic.

But the question remains: Are *kabsa*-caused hindrances to women's reproductivity, men's procreative powers, and the purity and perpetuation of the Muslim body politic really threatening to Egyptian society at large—a society plagued by a purported "crisis" of overpopulation? It is clear that the current Egyptian and U.S. administrations view Egypt's problem as one of rampant "hyperfertility," not of depopulating infertility. This largely *externally generated*, neocolonialist discourse of excessive fertility has been spread to the Egyptian populace in recent years through educational and media campaigns that extol the virtues of limiting nuclear family size to two children.

Nevertheless, popular resistance to the Western message of overpopulation and fertility control—which may be threatening due to its genocidal overtones—is apparent in Egypt in a number of forms. These include repeated failures to meet population reduction goals (Stycos et al. 1988); a continuing high and steadily increasing average annual population growth rate of more than 2.7 percent (Faour 1989; Mitchell 1991); large average family sizes of nearly five children (Egypt National Population Council 1989); relatively low contraceptive acceptance and continuance rates among both rural and urban women (Inhorn 1994a; Morsy n.d.); and, most recently, vocal efforts by Islamist reform groups in Egypt to *increase* rather than to decrease the absolute numbers of Muslims, particularly in relation to Egyptian (and Western) Christian populations (Lane and Rubinstein 1991).

Furthermore, given the all-too-familiar experiences of reproductive failures and losses and infant/maternal morbidity and mortality, many poor urban and rural Egyptians feel the need to *increase* rather than decrease their numbers of children, despite Egyptian and Western governmental efforts to convince them otherwise. In such a climate—in which children are highly valued for numerous economic and symbolic reasons (Gadalla 1978; Inhorn n.d.)—infertility is simply untenable, as apparent in the large numbers of women who desperately seek treatment in both ethnogynecological and biogynecological settings throughout the country.

Thus, it is fair to conclude that reproductive threats of all kinds—

including potentially coercive population control initiatives and infertility-producing *kabsa* — are perceived as highly worrisome among an overtly pronatalist and increasingly religiously oriented poor Egyptian populace. *Kabsa*, as infertility-producing, polluting boundary violation, expresses in symbolically meaningful fashion the threat of limited fertility to the pronatalist Egyptian body politic — a body politic that, throughout history, has learned the harsh lessons of ***colonial boundary violation*** and continues to resist neocolonial efforts to curtail its growth through new regimes of fertility surveillance and control.

6. From Humidity to Sorcery

The Story of Habiba and Her Infertile Sister

Growing up in Damanhur, one of the provincial cities outside of Alexandria, Habiba was considered to be among the most "clever" of her twelve brothers and sisters. Although many of the girls in Habiba's neighborhood, including her seven sisters, did not attend school or dropped out in the elementary grades, Habiba's good marks earned the attention of her parents, and they allowed her to continue on to junior high. Habiba hoped to complete high school as well and to eventually become a teacher. However, with the engagement of her older sister, Nawal, Habiba's life was to take a different course.

Nawal became engaged to a young man from a well-respected farming family outside of Damanhur. When the young man's family came to visit Nawal's family to make the engagement arrangements, the oldest son, Gamal, saw Habiba and inquired about whether she might be available for marriage. Habiba had just turned fourteen and "even the idea of marriage" made her upset. She saw marriage as an obstacle to her educational goals, for she knew that no husband would want his wife to be in high school or to work as a teacher outside the home.

However, as it would turn out, Habiba had little say in what was to become of her. Her parents were happy to be marrying off two of their eight daughters to a family they considered very respectable. Although they realized they would be sending their daughters to a different way of life in a farming village, they deemed the marriage arrangements overall to be quite auspicious. Thus, when all was said and done and the plans were set, Habiba was married to Gamal and her sister Nawal to his brother.

As the months after their joint marriage passed, neither Habiba nor Nawal became pregnant. One of Gamal's married sisters, also living in the extended-family household, had borne several children in rapid succession. Thus, comparisons between her and the two sisters began to be made, and pressure began to be put on Habiba and Nawal to "do something" about their childless conditions.

In fact, it was highly suspected that Habiba and Nawal had caused *kabsa* to each other because they were married on the same day. Thus, their mother-in-law urged them to unbind each other by pricking each other's fingers and then sucking the blood, as well as urinating on each other's urine simultaneously. Furthermore, Habiba and Nawal performed a number of other simultaneous rituals to unbind the other forms of *kabsa*. In case someone had entered on them during their postmarital month wearing gold, they asked for gold from a number of different people, put it in water, and then bathed with this water during the time of the noon prayer over three consecutive Fridays. In case the *kabs*-er had come from a visit to a cemetery, they went to a cemetery, entered one door, urinated between two graves, and exited from another door. While in the cemetery, they also found a woman working there who made them take off all of their clothes so that she could dump water over them. After they had redressed, she brought some children's bones, put them on the ground, and asked Habiba and Nawal to step over them seven times. In addition, assuming the *kabs*-er might have been a menstruating virgin or a newly circumcised child, Habiba and Nawal found two such individuals, dabbed pieces of cotton in their blood, and wore the cotton overnight as vaginal suppositories. Similarly, suspecting the *kabs*-er might have been a cat, they found a cat delivering its kittens, dabbed some cotton in its delivery blood, and wore the cotton overnight in the same way. Likewise, Habiba and Nawal were told that they might have been made *makbūsīn* by the blood of their husbands' shaving. Thus, they obtained a barber's kit, placed it in water, and then bathed with this water at the time of the noon prayer over three consecutive Fridays. Finally, Habiba and Nawal were also warned about both meat and black eggplant *kabsa*s. So when a lamb was slaughtered in their household, they stepped over it seven times, and they also went to a nearby black eggplant field and crossed through it.

Having performed ten such *kabsa* healing rituals together, Habiba and Nawal came to realize that they probably were not *makbūsīn* after all, for none of the rituals succeeded in making them pregnant. Thus, they began searching for some other cause of their mutual childlessness.

First, they considered the possibility that at some point in the past both of them had experienced *khaḍḍa*, or a shock so strong that it had rendered them infertile. In order to make the effects of the shock vanish, they were advised by relatives and neighbors that a "countershock" was necessary—something that would frighten them badly. Thus, Habiba and Nawal were taken by their in-laws to the Damanhur General Hospital morgue, where they were shown the upper half of a body that had been badly mutilated in an accident. The morgue attendant also placed a dead infant on the floor and asked the two infertile women to step over it seven times. Afterward, when they offered the morgue attendant money, he told them not to pay him but rather to bring him a small coffin or sheets for the bodies of the indigent if either one of them was to become pregnant. Habiba and Nawal were also given the *ṭast it-tarʿba*, or pan of shock, by one of their neighbors who had obtained it while on the pilgrimage to Saudi Arabia. In this pan, they placed *ḥulba* (fenugreek), dates, and some seeds of unknown type purchased from the *ʿaṭṭār*, and they doused these ingredients in water before the pan was placed outside overnight. In the morning, they both drank the liquid and ate the contents of the pan in order to make a potential *khaḍḍa* vanish. They repeated this ritual for three days in a row. In addition, one of their husbands' younger brothers brought a snake without its poisonous glands into their home and, when Habiba and Nawal were least expecting, threw the snake at them. According to Habiba, Nawal was quite shocked, but the snake did not affect her in the least bit.

Obviously, Habiba and Nawal were not *makhḍūḍīn*, or shocked, because none of these countershocking methods helped them to overcome their infertility. Furthermore, by this point, five years of married life had already passed, and the situation in their household was becoming more and more tense. Although Habiba's husband was not pressuring her to have children and told her flatly that he disbelieved in these various *wasfāt baladī*, his parents and uncles felt differently and saw Habiba and Nawal as "useless"—two barren sisters who were depriving their precious menfolk of the children they deserved.

Thus, Habiba and Nawal were pressured into seeking expert advice on their infertility problems. First, they visited two *dāyāt*, both of whom recommended *ṣūwaf*, or vaginal suppositories, and *kasr*, or cupping, to cure potential utero-ovarian humidity and/or an open back. Habiba and Nawal agreed to the *ṣūwaf* in each case, but they refused to undertake *kasr* because they were told that their backs would be burned. The *ṣūwaf* prepared by the first *dāya* contained *shīḥ* (wormwood), grilled onions, and black glycerin, and consisted of small gauze bundles tied with a thread for easy removal. The *ṣūwaf* prepared by the second *dāya* consisted of black glycerin exclusively. Both *dāyāt* told Habiba and Nawal to wear one *ṣūfa* overnight for three nights in a row and to refrain from having sexual intercourse during this period. Each morning, they were to remove the *ṣūfa* and dispose of it by throwing it into an intersection. The first *dāya* explained that the *ṣūwaf* would "get rid of any infections or water in the ovaries." The *ṣūwaf* were effective in this regard, because both Habiba and Nawal experienced huge amounts of watery discharge from their vaginas after wearing each *ṣūfa*. They suspected that they had contracted such ovarian humidity from sitting on the cold floor all of the time and from working with cold water when they cleaned the family compound.

The second *dāya*, an old spinster famous for making the infertile pregnant, also recommended that Habiba and Nawal have their uteri "widened." She had performed manual vaginal examinations on both of them and had told them that they were both "tight." Habiba was certain that this diagnosis was accurate, because she had noticed that, after having sex with Gamal, "all the fluid comes out on a towel." Thus, Habiba and Nawal agreed to be treated by *mirwad*, or the "vaginal stick." The *dāya* took a long piece of thick wire with a piece of cotton on its end, inserted it into each of the women's vaginas, and "went round and round." Habiba was not certain that the *mirwad* did, in fact, widen her uterus, but "I felt it in my ovaries, and it hurt."

However, as with all of the other *wasfāt baladī* tried by Habiba and Nawal, neither the *ṣūwaf* nor *mirwad* resulted in pregnancy. Thus, Habiba and Nawal convinced their in-laws to take them on a *ziyāra*, or pilgrimage, to the mosque and tomb of Sayyid Ibrāhīm Dasūqī, a famous dead *Ṣūfī* in the provincial town of Dasuq in the governorate of Kafr al-Shaykh. There, the entire family made a number of different vows. Habiba prayed to God, promising him, "If it [pregnancy] happens, then I'll return with something to furnish the mosque itself, for example, a carpet, or I'll bring some money for the poor." In addition, Habiba's and Nawal's mother-in-law took the two sisters on a trip to Damanhur in order to consult with a famous *munaggima*, a woman widely renowned for her ability to tell fortunes accurately, to use her clairvoyant powers to locate missing objects, and, quite atypical for a female *munaggima*, to do and undo sorcery. When Habiba and Nawal visited the *shaikha*, she requested that each woman provide her with one of their own handkerchiefs and one of their husbands'. She told them that she would keep the handkerchiefs overnight and "see all that happens." When Habiba and Nawal returned to learn what the *shaikha* had seen, they were informed that Gamal's ex-fiancée, whom he had rejected, had done an *ʿamal*, or made a sorcery potion that she had poured over the family's doorstop "so that no one in the house will have children." On Habiba's and Nawal's wedding day, they had stepped over the *'amal*, making them infertile. After telling them this bad news, the *shaikha* requested £E 250 ($100) from each woman to "undo" the *'amal*.

Although Habiba and Nawal were convinced that the *shaikha* was correct about the *'amal*—given that she had told them other information about the family that she could not have known otherwise—they were unable to afford the exorbitant fees required by the sorceress. Their husbands' family also refused to pay, because, as their uncle put it, "If I were 100 percent sure you'd get pregnant after this, I would pay for you. But you can't be sure." The source of doubt in the family revolved around the fact that Gamal's married sister, who also lived in the household and had undoubtedly stepped over the *'amal*, had been able to have several children. Thus, Habiba and Nawal, both worried about the *'amal*, were without the necessary financial resources to undo it.

However, much to everyone's surprise, Nawal became pregnant shortly thereafter, having been married to her husband for nearly six and a half years. Although Habiba was extremely happy for Nawal, she felt doubly depressed by her own continuing state of childlessness. Furthermore, the final straw came when Gamal's uncle, upset with Habiba over her inability to provide his eldest nephew with children, called her a *dhakar*, or male. Extremely dismayed over this grave disparagement of her femininity, Habiba asked Gamal for money to make a trip to Shatby Hospital in Alexandria. In the popular magazine *October*, she had read that Shatby had a special infertility department where they were making "babies of the tubes." Furthermore, although Habiba had visited approximately ten physicians during the course of her seven-year conceptive quest, none of them had been able to tell her what was wrong with her, despite the fact that she had taken six years' worth of fertility drugs and had undergone one tubal insufflation, two D & Cs, and one cervical electrocauterization. Instead, four physicians had requested that Gamal undergo semen analysis and had informed Habiba that her husband's "worms were weak." Although Habiba and Gamal both accepted that Gamal might be slightly "weak," Habiba knew that something must be wrong with her, too, which is why she had persisted in her search for children for so many years.

When Gamal took Habiba to the hospital in Alexandria, the doctors ordered many expensive diagnostic tests, including one ultrasound, one diagnostic laparoscopy, two postcoital tests, a blood test for Habiba, and a semen analysis for Gamal. After these tests were completed, Habiba was scheduled for an operation called *hadīya*, or "GIFT" (gamete intrafallopian transfer)—but for a reason that the doctors did not divulge to either Habiba or Gamal. As Habiba explained,

> I'm the kind of person if I know what's wrong with me, I'll stay on until I'm cured. If the GIFT doesn't work, I'll repeat it. If they tell me about something else, I'll do it. I'll continue here. After that, I'll do nothing. We'll accept our luck. Maybe God doesn't want us to have children. It's his will. "God gives males to whom he wants and females, and makes infertile who he wants." He has his reasons. Of course, all life is written—your name and everything. Although it's written, you have to search. This is why God created medicine, and you have to try your best, then leave the rest to God.

Ethnogynecological Causes

As seen in the cases of Habiba and Nawal, *kabsa* is not the only possible ethnogynecological cause of Egyptian women's infertility. Rather, women such as Habiba and Nawal who fail to become pregnant are faced with a host of etiological possibilities, ranging from humidity to sorcery. In most cases, assessment of causation is characterized by mutability, multidimensionality, and a posteriori contextualization (Early 1982). In attempting to identify the source of their infertility, women engage in retrospective analysis of their personal histories, examining the multiple dimensions of their lives and areas of possible etiological involvement. Thus, such incidents as exposure to cold water or the experience of being severely frightened are identified and tallied, and as such areas are explored therapeutically and ruled out, alternative causes are considered. As a result, throughout their infertile careers, women rarely abide by a single cause, instead engaging in the active metamorphosis of their causal assessments as new information is considered and incorporated into existing illness narratives.

In addition, in considering causation, infertile women engage in a kind of causal ranking, based on notions of causal proximity, as this concept will be called here. Some causes of infertility are proximate, or "body-near," because they are viewed from the perspective of the individual and involve a failure of an individual's bodily parts and mechanisms. In this focus on the individual body and its breakdown, culpability for such corporeal failure, if assigned, often rests on the individual victim, who is deemed responsible in one way or another for "carelessness" and, hence, the body's decline. Among infertile women, three of the major ethnogynecological categories of infertility causation—*ruṭūba*, *dahr maftūḥ*, and *khaḍḍa*—constitute proximate causes of this nature, because, for the most part, they involve the endogenous location of harm within the body and self-inducement through lack of adequate corporeal attention. (*Khaḍḍa*, however, may be socially induced and therefore bridges the proximate and medial categories.)

Interestingly, biogynecological causes of infertility also tend to fall into this category, in that they are viewed as individual problems of bodily breakdown for which most women assume inordinate responsibility. Indeed, infertile women's tendency to upbraid themselves for their biogynecological problems—even if these problems were, in fact, unavoidable—is symptomatic of biomedicine's tendency to "victim blame" (for bad genes, bad behaviors, bad life-styles, and so on), leading to a sort of causal reductionism in which the disease becomes reified and the social, economic, and political factors involved in the production of disease are negated. The result is a narrow focus on the body as locus of disease and the need to assign culpability for that disease to the individual. Thus, when poor infertile Egyptian women retrospectively bemoan their corporeal "carelessness" leading to, for example, tubes blocked by vaginal infections they should have had treated, uteri they should have had "cleaned" following miscarriage, and *ṣūwaf* they should have removed in twelve rather than twenty-four hours, their self-reproach bespeaks the message of biomedicine, in which women and their bodies are often faulted.

Yet, ethnogynecology offers other, less condemnatory causal options. The causes of some of the major culturally constructed infertility categories, including *kabsa*, are viewed as medial, or "body-distant," in that they involve exogenous impingements on the physical body, due to the effects of relations within the social group. In other words, immanent in these causal processes are acts of "social communication" between bodies (Morsy 1993), acts which engender illness but over which the afflicted party may have minimal control. In this light, it is apparent that the medial causes of infertility in Egypt, including *kabsa*, *ʿamal*, the *ukht taḥt il-arḍ*, and, in some cases, *khaḍḍa*, tend to involve dyadic groups of two individuals, acting toward one another in ways that produce infertility in one or both parties. As in the case of *kabsa*, this behavior may be inadvertent, while in other cases, it may be volitional and malicious, with one individual serving as perpetrator and the other as victim. The term "individual," furthermore, must be defined in a culturally specific manner to include beings inhabiting the spirit world and animals, as seen in the case of *kabsa*.

In this chapter, the proximate and medial ethnogynecological causes of infertility will be examined. In the following chapter, we will explore the "ultimate" causes of infertility, which, according to both Muslim and Coptic Christian Egyptian women, lie exclusively with God, the Almighty, Beneficent Creator. Although infertile women such as Habiba may ponder the individual and social actions precipitating their illnesses, they subsume these levels of causality beneath the causal layer of ultimate importance, for, as they are quick to explain, it is God—and only God—who is responsible for the lives of humans in all their detail. From this perspective then, it is God who creates some humans fertile and others infertile and who creates the male and female fetuses that men pass to women's bodies. For those who do not succeed in procreating, the reasons are ultimately up to God, who may be testing a couple's patience and faith. Furthermore, God does not expect his believers to be passive in the face of adversity; rather, God created remedies for all afflictions, including infertility, and it is up to human beings to search for these remedies in a therapeutic quest guided by God himself. For many infertile women, part of this quest involves spiritual pilgrimages to holy sites, where they attempt to increase the strength of divine intervention through prayers, vowing, and saint-mediated intercession, to be discussed in the following chapter.

Thus, in exploring infertility causation, it is necessary to probe beneath the various layers of meaning through which women come to understand the causes of their afflictions. From this perspective, infertility causation can only be seen as multidimensional, because causes occurring at the proximate and medial levels must always be ultimately contextualized. Furthermore, understanding the multidimensionality of infertility causation as perceived by Egyptian women renders accessible explanations of illness that involve, simultaneously, ethnogynecological and biogynecological dimensions. Thus, when an infertile woman hospitalized for a uterine operation announces that she plans to "do the *mushāharāt*" immediately upon her release, she receives support for her belief in both the biogynecological, proximate (uterine tumor) and ethnogynecological, medial (*kabsa*-induced womb-binding) causes of her affliction.

Conceptualizing infertility causation in terms of causal proximity not only seems to come closer to Egyptian women's ways of thinking about illness, but also avoids dualisms in which illness causation is reduced to "either/or" terms. As Morsy (1981) has pointed out, the medical anthropological literature on the Middle East is replete with etiological dualisms, such that illness causation is usually deemed either "natural" or "supernatural" in nature (Early 1988; Greenwood 1981; Morsy 1993; Pillsbury 1978) or is attributed to "animistic" versus "animatistic" beliefs (Shiloh 1968). Such etiological dualisms, in turn, lead to related therapeutic dualisms, in which pluralistic ethnomedical healing systems are characterized as "Prophetic" versus "Galenic" (Greenwood 1981), "Arabian" versus "spiritual" (Myntti 1988a), or "natural" versus "spiritual" (Morsy 1993). Not only do urban Egyptian women not view illness causation and curing in such either/or terms, but they also see themselves as partaking of multiple healing traditions, which are available in the contemporary Egyptian setting because of its rich medical past. Thus, for infertile women, multiple ethnogynecological causes are open to consideration, and several ethnogynecological healing traditions present women with real options.

In terms of the ethnogynecological causes of infertility, many are precisely named, well-defined, and widely known among urban Egyptian women. Furthermore, several of these causes, like *kabsa*, lead to an illness category or condition that is also named. For example, just as a woman who has experienced *kabsa* becomes *makbūsa*, a woman who has been subject to *khaḍḍa* becomes *makḍūḍa*, and a woman who has been "tied" by an *ʿamal* becomes *marbūṭa*, all conditions associated with infertility. However, as Swagman (1989) has argued in his analysis of *fijaʿ*, or fright, in Highland Yemen, viewing these conditions as "culture-bound syndromes" seems misguided. Most of these conditions are not limited in their social address to Egypt or even the Middle East; fright illnesses such as *fijaʿ* and *khaḍḍa*, for example, are found worldwide. In addition, these conditions do not form an epidemiologically assessable "syndrome" based on a consistent set of symptoms; infertility, for example, is but one of the outcomes of *khaḍḍa*, or even *kabsa* for that matter. Rather, Swagman suggests the adoption of a "meaning-centered" approach to the analysis of conditions such as *fijaʿ*, arguing that "fright is a component of a culturally constructed illness model that is etiological and explanatory in nature; it is principally a manifestation of the cultural process of assigning meaning to disturbing illness processes" (1989:383).

Taking a meaning-centered approach to the analysis of Middle Eastern "folk etiologies" allows for "an epidemiology of meaning rather than an epidemiology of 'disease'" (Swagman 1989:383). Thus, we can see that *kabsa*, *khaḍḍa*, *ʿamal*, and the like are not "syndromes" per se, but rather ways of assigning causal meaning, usually retrospectively. For example, in the case of Habiba and Nawal, the two sisters were encouraged in discussions with female elders to look back on possible causal events precipitating their delayed childbearing. Neither woman manifested a specific set of symptoms other than childlessness, nor could they be sure that their childlessness was caused by any one identifiable ethnogynecological (or, for that matter, biogynecological) condition. Rather, diagnoses of various causal categories were made speculatively, after the fact, and were usually discounted altogether when treatments directed at these causes were deemed ineffective, or, when effective (at draining humidity, for example), still failed to produce the desired pregnancy. Thus, Habiba and Nawal, both afflicted by childlessness, were not suffering from any one culture-bound infertility "syndrome," nor did they view themselves in this way. Rather, for these women, and the still-infertile Habiba in particular, the quest for causal understanding of their infertility was a quest for *meaning*—of what particular event or set of events had led to their subsequent childlessness. This quest called for a rather systematic elimination of various causal possibilities through a strategy of repeated, empiric trials of ethnogynecological therapies. Ultimately, however, identifying the correct cause was much less important to these women than overcoming, through multiple therapies, the resultant childlessness, which, in their lives, had become socially intolerable.

Thus, to understand *ruṭūba*, *dahr maftūḥ*, and the other ethnogynecological causes of infertility to be described here, it is important to view them as etiological possibilities—causes of infertility which are known to many Egyptian women, which are considered when women pose the existential question "Why me?," and which are therapeutically countered in women's quests for conception.

Finally, it is important to note here that these causal categories, as well as their accompanying "cures," are not monolithic. Rather, among poor urban Egyptian women, the lack of precise uniformity of ideology and praxis surrounding illness has resulted in a certain indeterminacy in their typifications of such culturally constructed categories as *ruṭūba* and *'amal*. This is especially apparent in women's discussions of the *ukht taḥt il-arḍ*, or spirit-sister under the ground, whose very existence is debated among the urban poor and whose role in infertility causation is seen as quite questionable. Furthermore, for any particular ethnogynecological category of infertility causation, more than one therapeutic possibility may be suggested, resulting in a veritable profusion of ethnogynecological "infertility cures," as well as varying beliefs about what constitutes the most efficacious therapeutic praxis.

Thus, with any typification of the various ethnogynecological causes and cures of infertility found among the Egyptian urban poor, the risk of essentialism seems immanent. Nonetheless, in the descriptions that follow, areas of ambiguity and indeterminacy are highlighted to underscore both the presence and absence of cultural consensus among poor urban women, whose ideas about *ruṭūba*, *dahr maftūḥ*, and the rest are characterized by intriguing variation.

Draining Humidity

Ruṭūba, meaning "moisture," "dampness," "wetness," or "humidity," is considered by Egyptian women and the *dāyāt* and *'aṭṭārīn* who provide treatments for it to be one of the major proximate causes of infertility. *Ruṭūba* may affect virtually any part of the body and is considered to be the source of all rheumatism. However, when it affects the uterus, ovaries, or lower back (where the ovaries are thought to be situated and where the fetus is thought to be carried during the pregnancy), these parts of the body are thought to become filled and even engorged with moisture, preventing them from fulfilling their "catch-and-carry" functions described in Chapter 3. As one *dāya* explained, when *ruṭūba* is present in the ovaries themselves, they "slide around" in a yellowish discharge and will therefore not "catch" the man's worms or "hold" the child. In fact, *ruṭūba* is seen by many women as preventing pregnancy by "rejecting" or "killing" the husband's worms, "throwing everything out." Furthermore, *ruṭūba* is deemed responsible for creating a thick sediment that blocks the uterus, turns it on its side, or reverses it, all problems requiring correction if pregnancy is to occur.

As a proximate cause of infertility, women are thought to bring utero-ovarian *ruṭūba* upon themselves by exposing their bodies to the cold—especially to cold drafts, cold wind, and cold water. Specific behaviors incriminated in the contraction of *ruṭūba* include: washing the genitals or douching with cold water, thereby "catching a cold from down"; not protecting the genitals with underwear; sleeping naked or with the window open, thereby catching a draft; wearing clothing that does not protect the body from the elements; wearing wet clothing; standing in front of a fan wearing little clothing; working excessively in cold water; washing the floor with the skirt rolled up; sitting on a cold floor or cold tiles; walking barefoot in water or mud; and cleaning the roof in the rain.

Although the belief in *ruṭūba* is historically rooted in Galenic humoral theory, with its description of "cold, moist" conditions requiring "hot, drying" therapies (Dols 1984), understandings of *ruṭūba* have been transformed in contemporary Egypt into biomedically compatible terms. As many women explain, *ruṭūba* "is" a utero-ovarian infection, "is like" such an infection, or "causes" such an infection to occur, because both *ruṭūba* and pelvic infections are characterized by a liquid vaginal discharge. Thus, many women view the ethnogynecological term "*ruṭūba*" and the biogynecological term "infection" as being equivalent and, given the synonymous identity of the two conditions, as being amenable to either ethnogynecological or biogynecological therapies.

Most urban poor women who are infertile opt first for less expensive, more accessible ethnogynecological treatments for *ruṭūba*[1] — treatments that allow the humidity to be drained from a woman's utero-ovarian region. Such drainage is necessary if a woman is to be cured of *ruṭūba* and rendered reproductively fit. Such drainage can be accomplished through three mechanisms, as follows.

Ṣūwaf (Vaginal Suppositories)

By far the most common treatment for *ruṭūba* is administration of a series of vaginal suppositories, known collectively as *ṣūwaf* (sing.: *ṣūfa*).[2] *Ṣūwaf* means "wool" and refers to the fact that sheep's wool is occasionally (and probably originally) used to form the core of the suppository. However, in contemporary practice, other substances, including primarily cotton and gauze (forming a wrapper for the suppository), are also employed. Nevertheless, the collective term "wool" is still used by Egyptians to refer to this form of treatment.

Ṣūwaf are traditionally made and supplied to infertile patients by *dāyāt*, who often employ herbal substances obtained from *'aṭṭārīn*. *Ṣūwaf* are of four primary types, although great variation in specific ingredients can be found. These types include: (1) sugar-based suppositories; (2) perfumed suppositories; (3) grilled-onion suppositories; and (4) herbal suppositories with plant substances shown in Table 3.

Sugar-Based Suppositories

Many *dāyāt* prescribe suppositories composed of a sugar-based substance, in which cotton has usually been dipped, then wrapped in gauze. The most commonly employed substance is the syrupy liquid glycerin. Glycerin is glycerol, or hygroscopic trihydroxy alcohol, which is usually derived from the saponification of fats. In Egypt, glycerin can be obtained from pharmacies in either black or white varieties, with the black being more com-

TABLE 3. Herbs and Other Plant Substances Used in Ethnogynecological Treatments for Infertility.

LATIN NAME	ENGLISH NAME	ARABIC NAME	ETHNOGYNECOLOGICAL USE
Allium cepa	Onion	*Baṣal*	Vaginal suppositories for *ruṭūba*
Aristolochia clematitis	Birthwort	*Zarāwind*	Potable for female infertility
Artemisia genus	Wormwood	*Shīḥ, ifsantīn*	Vaginal suppositories, vapor sitz baths for *ruṭūba*, potable for female infertility, vaginal suppositories for *kabsa*
Astragalus gummifer	Astragal, milk vetch, tragacanth	*Kathīrā'*	Potable to strengthen ovaries
Boswellia carterii	Frankincense	*Lubān dhakar*	Vaginal suppositories, vapor sitz baths for *ruṭūba*, potable for female infertility, vaginal suppositories for *kabsa*
Carum carvi	Common caraway	*Kammūn armanī, kahramān*	Worn as *kabsa* preventive, in vaginal suppositories for *kabsa*
Cinnamonium camphora	Camphor	*Kāfūr*	Genital ointment for *ruṭūba*
Cinnamonium cassia	Cassia, Chinese cinnamon	*Salīkha*	Part of edible mixture for male infertility
Cinnamonium zeylanicum	Cinnamon	*'Irq il-ganāḥ, 'irfa*	Part of edible mixture for male infertility, vaginal suppositories for *kabsa*
Citrullus colocynthus	Colocynth, bitterapple	*Ḥanẓal*	Vaginal suppositories for *ruṭūba*
Combretum truncatum	Vegetable-glue plant	*'Asmah*	Part of edible mixture for *'amal* in women

Commiphora myrrha	Myrrh	*Murr*	Vaginal suppositories for *ruṭūba*
Conyza dioscoroidis	Plowman's spikenard	*Bārnūf*	Vaginal suppositories, vapor sitz baths for *ruṭūba*
Crocus sativus	Saffron	*Za'farān*	Vaginal suppositories for *ruṭūba*
Dracaena cinnabari	Dragon's blood	*Dam al-akhawain*	Potable for female infertility
Eugenia caryophyllata	Clove	*'Aranful*	Vaginal suppositories for *ruṭūba, kabsa*
Lavandula officinalis	Lavender	*Khuzāmā*	Vaginal suppositories for *kabsa*
Nigella sativa	Black cumin	*Ḥabbit il-baraka*	Vaginal suppositories for *ruṭūba*
Phoenix dactylifera	Male date palm	*Dhakar in-nakhl*	Vaginal suppositories for *kabsa*
Piper longum	Long pepper	*'Irq id-dhahab*	Part of edible mixture for male infertility, vaginal suppositories for *kabsa*
Pistacia lentiscus	Mastic	*Mistika*	Vaginal suppositories for *ruṭūba*, incense for *'amal* and *ukht taḥt il-arḍ* rituals
Prunus mahaleb	Perfumed cherry, mahaleb, St. Lucia cherry	*Maḥlab*	Vaginal suppositories for *ruṭūba*, potable for female infertility
Trigonella foenum-graecum	Fenugreek	*Ḥulba*	Vaginal suppositories for *ruṭūba, kabsa*, pan of shock for *khaḍḍa*, potable for female infertility
Triticum romanum	Emmer wheat	*Arasiya, sha'ar hindī*	Vapor sitz baths for *ruṭūba*, vaginal suppositories for *kabsa*
Zingiber officinale	Common ginger	*Zangabīl*	Part of edible mixture for male infertility

Information on Latin, English, and Arabic names from Bedevian (1936), Cowan (1976), and Manniche (1989).

mon in this form of therapy. Traditionally, Egyptian physicians prescribed glycerin suppositories for their infertile patients, and this remedy may have eventually made its way into ethnogynecological practice.

Occasionally, other sugar-based substances are employed instead of or in addition to glycerin. These include honey, molasses, sugar (crystals or cubes), *ḥalāwa* (the sticky boiled sugar and lemon mixture used for depilation), and *sukkar an-nabāt*, or the Egyptian equivalent of rock candy, which is crushed. Honey and molasses are also frequently used as a sort of "gluing" substance in herbal suppositories, to be described below.

Perfumed Suppositories

A much less common type of suppository consists of cotton imbued in strong perfume. According to *dāyāt* and women who have used them, such perfumed suppositories are useful not only for *ruṭūba*, but for refreshing a uterus that is "disgusted," especially after the menstrual period.

Grilled-Onion Suppositories

The most common type of vaginal suppository, however, appears to be one employing grilled onion as the core substance. Called *baṣal* in Arabic, onions (Latin name: *Allium cepa*) are a major crop in Egypt and are a common foodstuff as well. Onion juice has antibiotic, diuretic, and expectorant properties and, as a "hot" substance, is used in many Egyptian herbal remedies (Manniche 1989). According to Manniche (1989), onions were used in pharaonic Egypt in the form of a vaginal paste to "stop a woman from menstruating" (that is, to make her become pregnant). Today, onion-based suppositories are used for the same purpose—namely, to cause pregnancy by clearing the uterus of harmful, pregnancy-preventing moisture. By far the most common variety of suppository consists of a mixture of grilled (or boiled) onion and one of several varieties of the herb *shīḥ* (common name: wormwood; Latin name: *Artemisia* genus). Usually the onion and *shīḥ* are ground together, but occasionally the onion, if small, is left whole and the *shīḥ* is embedded in it. Other herbs may be added, and like sugar-based suppositories, the combination is typically wrapped in gauze and tied off like a teabag for easy removal.

Herbal Suppositories

The final variety of suppository, one that is almost as common as the grilled-onion type, is that consisting of a mixture of herbs, often in a honey, molasses, or vegetable oil base. The two most commonly used herbs, both separately and in combination, are *shīḥ* and *ḥulba*.

Shīḥ, or wormwood, is perhaps the most frequently employed substance in vaginal suppositories for *ruṭūba*. Although the wormwood genus, *Artemisia*, consists of thirteen varieties (Bedevian 1936), *A. herba alba* (known as *shīḥ*) and *A. absinthium* (known as *shīḥ rūmī*, "Byzantine wormwood," or *ifsantīn*, absinthe) appear to be the most commonly employed types. Actually, *shīḥ* has been used since pharaonic times as a medicinal substance, particularly as an intestinal helminthic (Manniche 1989). *Yūnānī* practitioners also used *shīḥ* with other herbs in hot oil to draw out excess body heat (Manniche 1989). Today, *shīḥ* is thought to draw out excess moisture from the body, which is why it is used in vaginal suppositories for *ruṭūba*. Contemporary *shīḥ* suppositories for *ruṭūba* are occasionally quite elaborate; for example, *one dāya*'s recipe consists of *shīḥ* mixed with henna and the egg of a bird, to be shaped like a doll, placed in gauze, and tied off like a tampon.

As with *shīḥ*, *ḥulba* (common name: fenugreek; Latin name: *Trigonella foenum-graecum*), has been used as a medicinal substance since pharaonic times, particularly for the treatment of gynecological problems (Manniche 1989). In ancient Egypt, *ḥulba* was used to induce childbirth, either taken orally or in the form of a vaginal suppository consisting of, among other things, incense, onions, beer, and fly dung. (The resemblance to contemporary grilled-onion suppositories, sans the dung and beer, is striking.) The seeds of *ḥulba* were found in the tomb of Tutankhamen, and the ancient Greeks believed *ḥulba* to be a "warming" herb, to be used for cold conditions (Manniche 1989). Today, *ḥulba* is used in hot teas to encourage lactation and to reduce menstrual cramping and in vaginal suppositories to effect against *ruṭūba*, a "cold, wet" condition. In fact, *ḥulba* is thought to "milk" a woman (like a cow), and, in the case of vaginal suppositories, to "milk all the harm" from a woman's body. As one *dāya* explained, "*ḥulba* burns a lot, so a woman can't do *ḥulba* suppositories very often. It opens everything inside until it reaches your back. So it gets the moisture out of your back, too."

Occasionally, other types of herbs, plant resins, and minerals obtainable from *ʿaṭṭārīn* are used in vaginal suppositories to drain *ruṭūba*. For example, infertile women are sometimes instructed by *dāyāt* and *ʿaṭṭārīn* to utilize what might be termed "symbolic suppositories" containing ground cloves, corn kernels, wheat, barley, rose water, and molasses—the seeds probably representing symbols of fertility. Furthermore, *aṭrūn* (also *naṭrūn*), or natron, a mineral substance extracted from the salt lakes of Egypt's Wadi al-Naṭrūn northwest of Cairo and once used in the pharaonic process of mummification, is available from Egyptian *ʿaṭṭārīn* and is occasionally included in vaginal suppositories. However, according to one *ʿaṭṭār*, *aṭrūn* is most effective as a treatment for infertility if ground and eaten and used simultaneously with a genital ointment consisting of *kāfūr* (common name: camphor; Latin name: *Cinnamonium camphora*), mixed with unidentified ground seeds in alcohol. Together, these substances will remove uterine *ruṭūba* if administered before bedtime.

Other herbs deemed useful in suppository form for draining *ruṭūba* and "opening" the uterus include:[3]

1. *Murr* (common name: myrrh; Latin name: *Commiphora myrrha*), an herb widely used since pharaonic times as a fumigant and medicinal, known for its ability to treat dysentery and diarrhea, relieve headaches, and soothe toothaches and backaches;
2. *Lubān dhakar* (common name: frankincense; Latin name: *Boswellia carterii*), an herb widely used since pharaonic times with *murr* as a fumigant and medicinal, known for its ability to treat respiratory problems (throat and larynx infections, phlegm, and asthma), to stop bleeding and vomiting, and to soothe burns;
3. *Ḥanẓal* (common name: colocynth; Latin name: *Citrullus colocynthus*), an herb native to the Egyptian desert and used since pharaonic times as a powerful hydragogue (that is, to expel water); also known as an effective laxative and expectorant and used to relieve headaches, aching joints, backaches, sciatica, and gout;
4. *ʾAranful* (common name: clove; Latin name: *Eugenia caryophyllata*), a common herbal spice, known since pharaonic times and used as a medicinal heart tonic, expectorant, anesthetic, stimulant, and organ strengthener (of the liver, kidney, and pancreas) and to relieve flatulence, dizziness, stomach cramps, and toothaches;
5. *Zaʿfarān* (common name: saffron; Latin name: *Crocus sativus*), a common herbal spice, known since pharaonic times and used as a medicinal to strengthen the liver and digestive system, to break down kidney stones, and to induce menstruation and relieve menstrual cramps;
6. *Ḥabbit il-baraka* (common name: black cumin; Latin name: *Nigella sativa*), an herb known since pharaonic times and used by the early Egyptian Copts in a remedy for itching skin;
7. The ground seeds of *maḥlab* (common name: mahaleb; Latin name: *Prunus mahaleb*), whose history as a medicinal in Egypt has not been carefully documented;

8. *Bārnūf* (common name: plowman's spikenard; Latin name: *Conyza dioscoroidis*), whose history as a medicinal in Egypt has not been carefully documented;
9. *Mistika* (common name: mastic; Latin name: *Pistacia lentiscus*), whose history as a medicinal in Egypt has not been carefully documented; and
10. An unidentifiable resinous substance called *fasūkh*.

These, with the exception of *fasūkh*, and other plant substances used in ethnogynecological infertility therapy are listed in Table 3.

All of these substances—from sugar to *shīḥ*—are utilized in vaginal suppositories because they are hydragogues; namely, they have an empirically demonstrated ability to expel water from the lower genital tract. In each case, *ṣūwaf* cause large amounts of water to be secreted and then discharged vaginally—an effective proof in the minds of most Egyptian patients and ethnogynecologists of the presence of utero-ovarian *ruṭūba* and the need for such treatment. Women who utilize *ṣūwaf* invariably report postsuppository watery discharges, which, in many cases, are sufficiently copious to drench towels and bedsheets. Not only do women feel "relaxed," "comfortable," and "dry" after such discharges have been released, but most believe that such discharges are indicative of complete utero-ovarian drainage. As they explain, *ṣūwaf* "release," "grab," "suck," "drink," or "draw out" all the uterine *ruṭūba* and accompanying discomfort, while at the same time "absorbing" infections, inflammations, and pus.

To be most effective, *ṣūwaf* must be administered in a specific manner. In most cases, *dāyāt* prepare, insert, and sometimes remove the *ṣūwaf* in their infertile patients, although some women are instructed to insert and remove the *ṣūwaf* themselves. Typically, this occurs over a three-day period immediately following the cessation of menses, when the woman is vaginally "purified" and the uterus is thought to be "open" and receptive to both medication and sperm. Most *dāyāt* insist that their patients refrain from sexual intercourse during this treatment period, although some allow patients to remove the *ṣūfa* for such purposes and then reinsert it afterward, manually douching in the morning. *Ṣūwaf* are typically worn either overnight for three nights or continuously for twenty-four hours, although great variation in this aspect of treatment can be found. For example, some women are instructed to wear *ṣūwaf* during the day only, to change *ṣūwaf* two or three times a day at designated hours, or to wear the same *ṣūfa* over a three-day period. In virtually every case, however, *ṣūwaf* are worn during the three or seven initial postmenstrual days, with the treatment cycle often repeated over three months.[4] As with *kabsa* rituals, the symbolic significance of the propitious numbers three and seven is readily apparent and is instantiated in a number of other ethnogynecological cures to be described here.

From the descriptions above, it is also apparent that *ṣūwaf* are similar to tampons (although tampons are unknown among poor urban Egyptian women), in that they are tied with a string for easy removal. Following removal, some women are instructed to discard the teabag-like *ṣūwaf* in a particular manner—for example, by throwing them under the bed or in an intersection. Problems occasionally arise, however, when women are unable to remove *ṣūwaf* by their threads. For example, one woman reported that a *ṣūfa* became "lost" in her uterus when a *dāya* inserted three *ṣūwaf* simultaneously into her vagina. Upon removal, only two were found, and the infertile woman experienced severe cramping, which sent her to a hospital emergency room. Because the woman was afraid to tell the physician what she had done (that is, undertaken a *wasfāt baladī*), no cause for the pelvic pain could be found, and she was discharged. When she failed to become pregnant after several more years, she underwent biomedical evaluation, which uncovered her bilateral tubal obstruction. She attributed her blocked tubes to the lost *ṣūfa* and regretted that her mother-in-law had forced her to make such a "mistake." Several other women reported similar stories, and some mentioned their concern that a lost *ṣūfa* might travel upward, eventually pressing against their hearts and killing them. (This fear is identical to that regarding the intrauterine device.)

Thus, Egyptian women themselves may fear the possibility of "ethnoiatrogenesis," or the deleterious effects of ethnogynecological remedies intended to be therapeutic. In the case of *ṣūwaf*, the possibilities of introduced infection, the exacerbation of existing infections, vaginal/cervical irritation, toxicity of absorbed herbal substances, and mechanical insertion/removal problems must be considered (El Malatawy 1985). However, such "complications" appear to be rare, making *ṣūwaf* an extremely popular and widely utilized form of ethnogynecological therapy for infertility in Egypt. In this study, for example, *ṣūwaf* were the second most common ethnogynecological therapy employed for infertility (following *kabsa* healing rituals), as shown in Table 4.

Kasr (Cupping)

Kasr, meaning both "breaking" and a "break" or "crack," is another extremely common form of ethnogynecological therapy for *ruṭūba* and for *dahr maftūḥ* as well. Although the name "*kasr*" is somewhat enigmatic, it appears to be associated with the "open" or "divided" back, for which *kasr* is frequently employed. Alternately, the term *ka'sāt hawā'*, or "cups of air"—a term signifying the removal of harmful air from the inner body—is sometimes used to describe the same procedure, although the term *kasr* is much more common.

Kasr is cupping, a pre-Islamic, Bedouin practice that was ultimately denounced by the Prophet Muhammad as heathen in origin (Ullman 1978). In fact, *kasr* forms part of the corpus of practices known as *ṭibb il-ʿarabī*, or "Arab medicine," which is derivative of pre-Islamic and prophetic medicine and is practiced today mostly by Bedouins in Egypt. However, *kasr* is not restricted to Bedouins; given its popularity and perceived efficacy in the treatment of gynecological, rheumatic, and muscular complaints, *kasr* is widely performed by both laypersons and ethnomedical healers throughout Egypt. As a result, many Egyptians, both male and female, have undergone *kasr* at one time or another in their lives.

When used for utero-ovarian *ruṭūba*, *kasr* is most often performed by *dāyāt*, often in conjunction with or immediately before or after *ṣūwaf* therapy. Even when performed separately, it is often undertaken under the same conditions as *ṣūwaf* treatment—that is, during the three post-menstrual days, while abstaining from intercourse, over three consecutive months. However, as with *ṣūwaf* therapy, the timing of *kasr* is variable. For example, *kasr* may be performed three times in one day, or three times a day for three days, or once a day over three consecutive weeks. Nonetheless, whenever *kasr* is performed, it often takes place early in the morning, before breakfast has been eaten.

Two items are necessary for the performance of *kasr*: (1) an object to be lit, usually a piece of cloth, such as a handkerchief or gauze, with or without salt wrapped in it, dipped in oil, gasoline, or alcohol, a candle, or a corncob; and (2) an object to serve as a sort of "suction cup," usually a glass jar, a pottery vessel, a silver or copper mortar, or a cup. When a small cup is used, the procedure is usually referred to as *ka'sāt hawā'* rather than *kasr*. In addition, some individuals who perform *kasr* advocate the use of raw dough or mud as a sort of "holder" for either a candle or a corncob. Thus, dough or mud is sometimes applied to the patient's skin at the site where cupping is to be performed.

When *kasr* is performed to remove utero-ovarian *ruṭūba*, the patient usually lies on her stomach with her lower back exposed. Oil may or may not be used to lubricate the patient's skin, and the lit object is situated upright so as not to burn it. Once the lit object is in place, the *kasr* vessel is placed immediately over the flame, thereby extinguishing it and causing vapor to rise. Adhered like a suction cup to the patient's skin, the jar is left in place for three to five minutes, after which it is removed, but with great difficulty. In fact, *kasr* is said to "grab," "suck," "collect," or "gather" the patient's skin, drawing out the cold internal humidity in the form of rising vapor. According to one *dāya*, "If there's lots of air, her skin reaches the top of the glass." Because of the vessel's tenacious hold on the patient's skin, redness and round bruises often form after the vessel is removed, even when post-*kasr* oil or alcohol is massaged into the skin.

As with *kabsa* rituals and *ṣūwaf* therapy, the number three is significant in *kasr* therapy as well. Not only is *kasr* usually performed three times over a series of three days, but *kasr* is traditionally applied to three standard locations on the patient's lower back: in the kidney area on both sides and in the lower middle back over the spine. Sometimes it is performed in seven locations: three on each side of the patient's entire back and one in the lower middle back over the spine. After *kasr* is performed on the back, most women are asked to turn over, so as to undergo the procedure on the abdomen. Usually, frontal *kasr* is performed over the navel and in the ovary region on both sides. If performed on front and back, the *kasr* cuppings form a "belt around the uterus," making a "lazy uterus alert" by "sucking" the air and humidity from it.

It is important to note, however, that some disagreement exists over the ideal location for *kasr* in cases of utero-ovarian *ruṭūba*. Many *dāyāt* argue that *kasr* should not be performed on the abdomen "over the ovaries," lest the ovaries become "spoiled" or "ruined" or the intestines accidentally get "sucked." Thus, they urge the restriction of *kasr* to the back, where, if performed correctly, the procedure can remove the *ruṭūba* which causes the ovaries to "slip around." Others argue that *kasr* should not be performed on the spine, which can be injured due to the lack of protective flesh. Still others argue that *kasr* should not be performed at all, because of its potential to cause internal damage.

Nevertheless, most *dāyāt*, and many laywomen as well, perform *kasr* for utero-ovarian *ruṭūba*. A humorally based "hot, drying" therapy renowned for its ability to draw cold humidity and air out of the body in the form of visible vapor, *kasr* is a popular treatment for infertility-causing *ruṭūba* and is undergone by numerous infertile women, despite the considerable pain of the procedure. In this study, for example, 36 percent of the infertile women who had undergone ethnogynecological therapy had received *kasr* for *ruṭūba* and *dahr maftūḥ*, as shown in Table 4. In a number of these cases, they had repeated the procedure over several treatment cycles.

TABLE 4. Ethnogynecological Causes of Infertility and Treatments Utilized by Seventy-six Infertile Egyptian Women in the Study Sample.*

ETHNOGYNECOLOGICAL CAUSE	ETHNOGYNECOLOGICAL TREATMENT	PERCENTAGE OF WOMEN USING TREATMENT
Ruṭūba (humidity)	*Ṣūwaf* (vaginal suppositories)	55
	Kasr (cupping)	36
	Tabwīkha (vapor sitz bath)	5
Dahr maftūḥ (open back)	*Kasr*	36
	Kawī (cauterization)	2
	Fatla (twining)	0
	I'fāl (locking)	6
Khaḍḍa (shock)	*Khaḍḍa* (countershocking)	17
	Ṭast it-tar'ba (pan of shock)	5
Miscellaneous proximate causes:		
Vaginal tightness	*Mirwad* (vaginal stick)	2
Uterine malposition	Anal corrections	1
Kabsa (polluting entrance)	*Kabsa* rituals	73
ʿAmal (sorcery)	Sorcery nullification	3
Ukht taḥt il-arḍ (spirit-sister under the ground)	Spirit appeasement	14
Miscellaneous medial causes	*Munaggimīn*'s treatment, including: *ḥugub* (preventive, therapeutic amulets), clairvoyant diagnosis, quasi-biomedical healing, prayer	14
God's will	Pilgrimages to mosque-tombs of *shuyūkh bil-baraka* (blessed *shaikhs*)	34
Unknown causes	Miscellaneous treatments	4

*Of the ninety-six infertile women in the study sample questioned, only seventy-six had utilized treatments for the ethnogynecological causes listed here. Twenty women had not availed themselves of ethnogynecological treatment.

Tabwīkha, or *Ḥammām* (Vapor Sitz Bath)

A much less common form of therapy for *ruṭūba* is called by the names *tabwīkha*, meaning "vapor" or "steam," and *ḥammām*, the Arabic term for "bath." In the therapeutic context, the term "vapor sitz bath" seems appropriate, given that women treated by *tabwīkha* squat over a basin of boiling water, aromatic herbs, and occasionally salt and/or oil. The steaming vapor that rises from the basin is thought to waft into the woman's vagina and uterus, given that her naked lower body is covered with a blanket used to trap the steam. Afterward, her hot, sweaty body is usually wrapped in the blanket, and she is encouraged to sleep this way for several hours.

As with *ṣūwaf*, herbs that are hydragogues are utilized in this vaporous mixture. The most commonly employed herbs are *shīḥ*, *bārnūf*, *lubān dhakar*, *fasūkh*, and *arasiya* (also known as *sha'ar hindī*) (common name: emmer; Latin name: *Triticum romanum*). *Arasiya*, a hard red wheat grown in Egypt since ancient times, was probably used in birth prognostications by pharaonic practitioners. Later, Hippocrates, the forefather of *Yūnānī* medicine, prescribed an infertility prognostication technique involving "fumigation" very similar to modern *tabwīkha* (Aiman 1984).

Like *ṣūwaf* and *kasr*, *tabwīkha* is also a "hot" therapy, which is why it is used to treat a cold condition such as *ruṭūba*.[5] However, *tabwīkha* is much less commonly employed for *ruṭūba* than either *ṣūwaf* or *kasr*. For example, in this study, only 5 percent of the women in ethnogynecological therapy had undergone *tabwīkha*, as opposed to 55 percent who had undergone *ṣūwaf* therapy and 36 percent who had undergone *kasr*, as shown in Table 4.

Closing the Open Back

Dahr maftūḥ, or an "open back," is considered by most poor urban Egyptian women to be a major cause of two common and related reproductive problems—primarily spontaneous abortion (miscarriage) and to a slightly lesser extent infertility. When a woman's back becomes "open," her internal reproductive organs, which are thought to be situated near the lower back, cannot "hold" anything—be it the fetus-containing sperm that must be "caught" to cause pregnancy, the menstrual blood necessary for fetal development, or the fetus itself, which is said to "stick" to the back during pregnancy while the "belly is full of water."[6] Thus, when open, the woman's back, which "endures everything during pregnancy," is said to become "light" or "slippery," allowing the conceptive products to "come down" or "slip out."

As with *ruṭūba*, women's backs become open (also termed "separated," "divided," or "cracked") through exposure to cold; for this reason, *ruṭūba* and *dahr maftūḥ* require similar therapies. However, women can also open their backs through overexertion—for example, by working too hard, carrying heavy objects, bearing too much weight on the head, or beating carpets too vigorously. Thus, during the early weeks of pregnancy, it is thought best for a woman to modify her normal work habits.

It is important to contrast the "openness" of *dahr maftūḥ* with that of *kabsa* — bodily disruptions that are of very different natures. Whereas women who experience *kabsa* are usually "open" for meritorious reasons (circumcision, defloration, childbirth, attempted childbirth), women who "open their backs" have brought this insalubrious condition on themselves. In the case of *dahr maftūḥ*, it is the openness itself which causes harm; the back that is open prevents pregnancy by failing to "carry" or "hold" the products of conception. In contrast, *kabsa* effects are *not* due to the openness of the genitalia themselves, but rather to the injurious penetration of pregnancy-preventing pollutants, which "bind" the reproductive organs. Furthermore, *dahr maftūḥ* is a proximate cause of infertility; it is considered to be endogenously located within individual bodies and has nothing to do with social relations. *Kabsa*, on the other hand, is a medial cause of infertility; bodily pathology is externally produced by social others who unwittingly harm the vulnerable *kabs*-ee. Nevertheless, both *kabsa* and *dahr maftūḥ* index what Boddy (1989) calls the "importance of interiority" and the need for "closure" of that which is "open." Indeed, the symbolism of opening/closing, binding/unbinding, locking/unlocking, and tying/untying is shared by several of the infertility causal categories in Egypt and is found elsewhere in the Middle East in descriptions of difficult health and social problems (Betteridge 1992; Bourdieu 1977).

Furthermore, the result of *kabsa* and *dahr maftūḥ* is the same: female infertility, which must be overcome through various ethnogynecological therapies. Women who have mistakenly opened their backs must undertake therapies to close their backs, lest they remain infertile. Backs can be closed in one of four ways, as follows.

Kasr (Cupping)

Kasr is thought to be the most efficacious therapy for *dahr maftūḥ* — even more so than in the treatment of uterine *ruṭūba*. In cases of *dahr maftūḥ*, *kasr* is usually applied only to the back, particularly the lower region, but occasionally on other sites as well. Applied in this way, *kasr*, a "hot" therapy, is thought to "close," "catch," "collect," or "bring together" the open back, and, in cases of cold-induced back pain, to remove it by way of heat. It is important to note, however, that *kasr* is being supplanted in some cases by mentholated plasters, which can be purchased from the pharmacy and are thought to be equally efficacious in healing open backs.

Kawī, or *Kayy* (Cauterization)

A related practice that appears to be much less common than *kasr* is one called either *kawī* or *kayy*, a traditional form of cauterization, or "branding," reportedly practiced in many other regions of the Middle East, where it is often called "*makwa*."[7] Dating to pre-Islamic Bedouin times and probably rooted in pharaonic medicine (Rosenberg et al. 1988; Ullman 1978), *kawī* is a component of contemporary Bedouin *ṭibb il-ʿarabī* in Egypt and is usually performed by senior Bedouin female healers.

Kawī involves placing a heated object, usually a nail or a small metal rod, much like a branding iron, on the patient's lower back, the site which is presumed to be "open." The procedure is very painful, burning the skin and leaving a permanent scar. Perhaps for this reason, it is much less commonly employed than *kasr* among urban Egyptian women. In this study, for example, only two women had undergone the procedure, and both regretted having done it, because of its pain and scar formation. As they explained, however, *kawī* "scares" the back into carrying the products of conception, and it also "tightens" relaxed nerves. For this reason, *kawī* is thought to be extremely useful for male infertility and impotence, both of which may be attributed to the "weak nerve" in the back that is essential in the spermatogenic production of worm-carried fetuses.

Fatla (Twining)

Another extremely painful procedure, usually performed by Bedouin women healers or *dāyāt*, is *fatla*, which means "twining" the open back to "twist" it together. In this form of therapy, a heated, threaded upholstery or other large needle is passed through the skin of the lower back in the spinal region. The thick thread (like the kind used in ear piercing) that is pulled through is tied and left in place for several days or weeks—usually until the flesh has swollen, pus has collected at the wound site, and the open back has been effectively "closed." Although two *dāyāt* participating in this study specialized in this procedure, none of the infertile women in the study sample had tried *fatla*, preferring instead to undergo the "locking" procedure described below.

I'fāl (Locking)

A much more common treatment for *dahr maftūḥ*—and the only one that is painless—is *i'fāl*, or "locking" the open back via an externally worn padlock. With *i'fāl*, a long piece of thread or an elastic or rubber band—all of which are expandable should the woman become pregnant—is fastened around the infertile woman's waist, and an iron padlock or locking iron ankle bracelet is fastened around it. Occasionally, ritualistic practices accompany this "locking" procedure. For example, a *dāya* may fasten the lock onto the woman's waist under the protective cover of a white sheet; or a blacksmith may fashion a special iron lock and key, which he fastens on a rubber band and "twists" around the woman's abdomen until her back is "closed"; or a nonmenstruating virgin may be requested to lock the padlock and keep the key. Timing may also be important. For example, some *dāyāt* recommend that locking should take place following *ṣūwaf* therapy and exactly at the time of the Friday noon prayer. In all cases, the woman is requested to wear the lock until she delivers a baby, at which time the lock either opens spontaneously, as some claim, or is removed by the keyholder.

Although five infertile women in this study had tried locking their backs, none of them had gone on to become pregnant. Therefore, in each case, they had removed the lock after several weeks or months, assuming that it was not helping them achieve pregnancy. However, locks are thought to be particularly beneficial for women who have experienced a previous spontaneous abortion and who need to close their open backs in order to "carry the child" through a current nine-month pregnancy.

Countering Shock

Among the Egyptian urban poor, a sudden fright or shock, known as *khaḍḍa* (or, less commonly, *fag'a* or *tar'ba*), is thought to cause a wide range of somatic symptoms and illnesses, including both male and female infertility. As with *fija'* in Yemen (Swagman 1989) and the "fright illness" of northwestern Iran (Good and Good 1982; Good, Good, and Moradi 1985), *khaḍḍa* in Egypt appears to be one of many fright/sudden shock conditions found in cultures around the world (Simons and Hughes 1985). In Egypt, *khaḍḍa* has been widely reported,[8] and is thought to differentially affect women, who are more susceptible to fright due to their "weaker" constitutions. Widespread belief in the deleterious effects of fright on the body is emblematic of popular theories of emotion and emotional distress in Egypt; namely, negative emotional states brought on by *khaḍḍa*, marital friction, occupational stresses, and a host of other problems of daily living are considered "core elements" in illness causation (Morsy 1993; cf. Good and Good 1982; Good, Good, and Fischer 1988). *Khaḍḍa*, as a sudden and emotionally distressing event, is thus a major precipitating factor in both male and female infertility. As poor urban Egyptian women state, "If you're upset, you can't get pregnant." Thus, among women, *khaḍḍa* "affects her *bait il-wilid* and her psychology and sometimes remains forever," and, among men, *khaḍḍa* "makes him impotent, and he's got no children in him anymore."[9]

Khaḍḍa is usually tied to terrifying occurrences, which are often brought on by an individual's own negligence. Falling down — for example, down a flight of stairs, off a low balcony, or, in the case of one woman, into a manhole in the street — is thought to be shock-inducing, as are "accidents" occurring through carelessness and ineptitude. But *khaḍḍa* is also socially induced, in that it may involve the direct or indirect actions of significant and insignificant others. Among women, being frightened by an animal or being surprised suddenly by another person may be enough to cause a significant shock. Among men, participating in a war, being involved in a car, truck, or train accident, or being arrested and sent to jail are thought to be significant, *khaḍḍa*-inducing experiences. Among both men and women, learning of a death in the family, witnessing something horrible, such as a death or a suicide, being burned in a fire, or receiving particularly bad news are all thought to bring on *khaḍḍa*.

When this happens, an individual of a sensitive disposition is thought to enter a state of shock known variously as *makhḍūḍ* (*a*) (meaning "frightened," "shocked," or "terrorized"), *mafgūʿ* (*a*) (meaning "pained," "afflicted," or "distressed"), or *matrūʿb* (*a*) (meaning "frightened," "terrified," or "afraid"). A person who is *makhḍūḍ* (*a*) may suffer almost immediate illness symptoms, often of a "nervous" variety. However, in many cases, those who have been shocked may only realize that they have entered the state of *makhḍūḍ* (*a*) when affected by some illness long after the original event. Such is the case with infertility; both women and men usually realize that they are *makhḍūḍīn* only when they are found to be infertile many years later. Thus, the diagnosis of a previous *khaḍḍa* is usually made retrospectively or, in many cases, is never made at all but is treated empirically instead.

To "make the *khaḍḍa* vanish," a "counter-*khaḍḍa*," and / or other special remedies for this condition are required. Among men, *kawī*, or hot-iron cauterization on the lower middle back, is often considered effective,[10] as is washing with water placed in their grandfathers' cooking pots. However, because women are viewed as particularly prone to *khaḍḍa*'s infertility-producing effects, they are thought to require the "strong" forms of shock therapy, which are of two basic types as follows.

Countershocking

The most common way of overcoming a *khaḍḍa* is through a second *khaḍḍa*, or a countershock, stronger than the first. Shocking a woman a second time is thought to cause unspecified bodily changes that eliminate the effects of the earlier *khaḍḍa* and increase her chances of conceiving. As one *dāya* put it, "A shock cancels another shock." The effects of shock in infertile women are typically canceled by frightening them in one of four ways.

DEAD BODIES

Death and particularly dead bodies are deemed frightening in and of themselves, and women who are *makhḍūḍin* are often exposed to the dead in order to be shocked. Infertile women are often taken to cemeteries and morgues for this purpose—and often for the dual purpose of unbinding *kabsa* effects. In these places of death, they are forced to view or touch the deceased, including the bodies of those recently dead, as well as bones and skeletons. Sometimes, bones or whole bodies are thrown at women, or women are pushed into tombs or onto the bodies of the dead. According to one woman, she was locked into a pitch-black hospital morgue, and a stone was thrown at her; although she was terrified by this incident, it did not succeed in making her pregnant.

ANIMALS

Animals are also used to frighten women. Typically, dead reptiles or rodents are thrown at the infertile woman or placed on her body while she is sleeping. In most cases, snakes are used, but some women report having had cats, fish, tortoises, rats, and cockroaches (which in Egypt become quite large) thrown at or placed on them. Other women are forced to view a large animal's slaughter for the same reason.

RAILROAD TRACKS

Although none of the women in this study were forced to undertake this form of counter-*khaḍḍa*, it is widely reported that infertile Egyptian women are sometimes coerced into lying flat on a set of railroad tracks, face down, while a train passes over their outstretched bodies. One woman in this study who refused to perform this type of shock therapy was forced instead to step over the railroad tracks immediately in front of a passing train.

SURPRISES

Finally, many infertile women are purposefully surprised by their husbands or family members in order to countershock them into pregnancy. Shotguns may be fired suddenly, or a person may jump in front of the infertile women from the corner of a darkened room. In one case, a woman reported that her husband grabbed her by the legs from behind, while she was standing watching the men pray at her neighborhood mosque. Not only did her husband surprise her, but he hurt her in the process.

Ṭast It-Tar'ba (Pan of Shock)

When available, the *ṭast it-tar'ba* (also known as the *ṭast il-khaḍḍa*), or "pan of shock,"[11] may be used instead of these countershocking methods to overcome infertility-producing *khaḍḍa*. Although some women contend that any copper basin or pan is suitable for this form of therapy, most insist that the special Saudi Arabian *ṭast it-tar'ba*, usually brought home by a pilgrim from the *hajj* to Mecca, is the only appropriate vehicle for this remedy. As a result, those who own the "real" *ṭast it-tar'ba* are usually sought out by others who are seeking shock therapy. The owners of these pans may eventually become specialized healers, much like the owners of the Saudi Arabian *mushāharāt*. In addition, many *dāyāt* own the *ṭast it-tar'ba*, given its popularity as a form of infertility therapy.

Generally, Saudi Arabian *ṭast it-tar'ba*s are flat, copper basins with religious inscriptions written inside and small objects, usually keys (symbolic of "unlocking" infertility and other shock-induced problems), dangling from the outside rim. With *ṭast it-tar'ba* therapy, various edibles — most often dates and occasionally raisins, *ḥulba* seeds, fava beans, sugar, or salt — are placed in the pan, with or without water or milk, and are left outside "under the stars" for one night, encompassing the dusk, evening, and dawn prayer times. Early the next morning before breakfast is taken, the infertile woman is requested to eat and drink the contents of the pan, including the dew that has collected. As with other therapies already described, women are often requested to repeat this procedure over three consecutive evenings, during the three prayer times, with three dates placed in the pan each time. In some cases, husbands, especially those who are suspected of being infertile, are also requested to join their wives in this therapy, and water from the pan may or may not be splashed on the infertile woman three times as well — supposedly to surprise her. Another variation on this theme is to separate the time of eating the dates from the drinking of the dewy liquid — the former in the morning and the latter in the evening.

Generally speaking, however, both eating and drinking from the pan are completed in the early morning hours.

One *sitt kabīra* who owned a *ṭast it-tarʿba* described the "best way" to treat infertility as follows:

> You get a big pot and put the pan of shock in it. And you put five to ten piasters or other small metal coins in the pan. Then you pour on it a large can of water, and you leave it out overnight "for the stars." This is on a Friday evening before the sunset prayer, so that you get the sunset prayer, the night prayer, and the dawn prayer. Early the next morning before sunrise, the woman undresses in the bathroom, and she drinks a helping from the pan full of water. All of this must be done before sunrise, because when the sun rises, it [the water; the cure] spoils. And then you pour the water all at once on her body. The water is cold, so she gasps, and the shock is removed totally.

Belief in *khaḍḍa* and in the therapeutic efficacy of both countershocking and the *ṭast it-tarʿba* in overcoming *khaḍḍa*-induced maladies is strong among the Egyptian urban poor. In this study, numerous women reported having been severely shocked at some point in the past and having considered this to be a possible cause of their subsequent infertility. Nearly one-quarter of all women had tried one or both types of shock therapy, as shown in Table 4. Unfortunately, however, none of the women experienced therapeutic success in countering *khaḍḍa*.

Vaginal Sticks, Malpositioned Uteri, and Therapeutic Comestibles

Although *ruṭūba*, *dahr maftūḥ*, and *khaḍḍa* are widely acknowledged as the most common proximate ethnogynecological causes of infertility, ethnogynecologists in Egypt may offer additional cures for miscellaneous proximate conditions, some of which are based on concepts and techniques derived from Egyptian biogynecology. These ethnogynecological therapies fall into three general categories as follows.

Mirwad (Vaginal Stick)

Mirwad can best be described as the "vaginal stick," given the way in which the *mirwad*, or "little stick," is used in this context. Some *dāyāt* believe that local therapy to the vagina—to "clean" or "widen" the vagina and, purportedly, the *bait il-wilid* as well—may be useful in overcoming infertility due to "narrow," "tight," or "dirty" reproductive organs. Although some *dāyāt* use their fingers for this purpose (a variation on their services as "deflowerers" of frightened brides), most use a metal "stick," varying in size from a piece of wire to an iron pipe or bar. The stick is typically covered with gauze or cotton and is used to scrape the vagina until it bleeds. Following this "cleaning" and "widening" which is repeated over seven days, *ṣūwaf* of soothing herbs or glycerin are inserted in the abraded vagina, and the patient is instructed to abstain from sexual intercourse, in part due to the pain.

Currently, ***mirwad*** is not a popular form of therapy for infertility in urban Egypt, as reflected in the fact that only two women in the study were offered and undertook the therapy in the homes of *dāyāt*. The most remarkable aspect of ***mirwad***, however, is that it mirrors very closely the popular biomedical therapy of dilatation and curettage (D & C), in which physicians purport to "clean" and "widen" the infertile uterus through a vigorous scraping of the interior of the organ with a metal instrument. Whether ***mirwad*** originated before the introduction of D & Cs in Egypt or practitioners of ***mirwad*** decided to provide an imitative, D-&-C-like therapy remains to be determined, since the history of ***mirwad*** in Egypt is undocumented. Yet, the lack of historical references to ***mirwad*** suggests that the ethnogynecological procedure is relatively new and may, in fact, be an example of a biogynecological therapy trickling down to the masses in a somewhat modified form.

Repositioning Malpositioned Uteri

Likewise, some *dāyāt* in Egypt offer uterine repositioning, based on the outdated notion still being perpetuated within Egyptian biogynecological circles that malpositioned uteri—including uteri that are retroverted, or "tipped back," and anteverted, or "tipped forward"—are a primary cause of infertility. As we shall see in Chapter 9, some Egyptian gynecologists continue to perform unnecessary surgery for these conditions on their infertile patients. As we shall also see, this notion of "tipped" and otherwise displaced uteri has thoroughly permeated popular thinking, to the extent that some *dāyāt* now claim to treat uterine malpositioning in infertile women.

Corrective techniques vary considerably from *dāya* to *dāya*. For example, Siham, the *dāya* introduced in Chapter 4, said she corrected uterine malpositions by making the infertile woman kneel on the floor, while she inserted her finger into the woman's anus and manually "raised" the woman's uterus. Other *dāyāt* accomplish the same results by inserting objects, such as hard-boiled eggs or dates, into the infertile woman's anus.

In a unique variation, one *dāya* said she instructed women to hammer a large, file-like nail into the ground, cover the nailhead with cloth, and then sit on the nailhead anally. The patient, who should be wearing a vaginal suppository of *ḥulba*, then swings her legs back and forth seven times. This therapy, the *dāya* noted, must be performed immediately after cessation of menses, when the vagina is "purified."

Therapeutic Comestibles

In addition to these mechanical therapies, a number of miscellaneous infertility remedies utilize edible or potable herbal substances. Potables tend to be prescribed for female infertility and edibles for male infertility, but some remedies are recommended for both husband and wife. These therapies are usually prescribed by *dāyāt* working in conjunction with *'aṭṭārīn*; some *'aṭṭārīn*, however, prescribe them directly.

POTABLES

Ḥulba, employed in *ṣūwaf* and the *ṭast it-tar'ba*, is also thought to be useful for female infertility when drunk as a hot tea first thing in the morning. Oral decoctions of *maḥlab* seeds or a mixture containing *lubān dhakar* and the seven kinds of *shīḥ* available from Egyptian *'aṭṭārīn*[12] are also recommended. *Zarāwind* (common name: birthwort; Latin name: *Aristolochia clematitis*), an herb used in pharaonic remedies to induce labor (Manniche 1989), is also recommended as a hot potable for women who are infertile or who have just given birth.

Another ancient Egyptian herbal remedy, known as *dam al-akhawain*, or "blood of the two brothers," is sometimes recommended as a therapy for female infertility. *Dam al-akhawain* is the herb "dragon's blood," obtained as resin from wounds in the bark of the *Dracaena draco* tree (Tackholm and Drar 1950; Bedevian 1936). Apparently, it has been used medicinally in Egypt since pharaonic times, and early *Yūnānī* practitioners believed it to be true dragon's blood because the color it yielded was so deep (Tackholm and Drar 1950). When used in contemporary infertility therapy, this resinous substance is crushed and boiled, producing a red liquid which is drunk. The remaining pieces of the resin are also supposed to be eaten.

Another potable remedy utilizes an herb called *kathīrā'* (common name: astragal, milk vetch, or tragacanth; Latin name: *Astragalus gummifer*) (Bedevian 1936). According to one *'aṭṭār*, when a spoonful of *kathīrā'* is added to one-half cup of milk with sugar, this thick mixture provides a powerful means of strengthening the infertile woman's ovaries.

EDIBLES

Whereas most of the potable remedies are intended for women, the edible ones are designed to strengthen infertile or impotent men. Generally, infertile men are encouraged to eat symbolically nourishing foods, such as pigeons, male rabbits, camel meat, stew made of the shanks of male breeding cattle, and various forms of honey (for example, mixed with male date palm or "country" butter and herbs). However, the advice of many Egyptian *ʿaṭṭārīn* is more specific. For example, one Alexandrian *ʿaṭṭār* provides a remedy consisting of twenty-one herbal substances, which he mixes and grinds to powdery consistency in his shop. A spoonful of this powder is to be placed in honey and *samna* and then eaten by the infertile man two times daily, once after breakfast and once after dinner. Not only does this mixture strengthen the "worms," but it is purported to improve sexual performance as well. Among the most important herbs in the mixture are: (1) *ʿirq id-dhahab* (common name: long pepper; Latin name: *Piper longum*); (2) *zangabīl* (common name: common ginger; Latin name: *Zingiber officinale*); (3) *salīkha* (common name: cassia; Latin name: *Cinnamonium cassia*); (4) *ʿirq il-ganāḥ* (common name: cinnamon; Latin name: *Cinnamonium zeylanicum*); and (5) *ʾaranful* (common name: clove; Latin name: *Eugenia caryophyllata*). According to the *ʿaṭṭār* who supplies this powdered herbal mixture, it can also be added to vegetable oil, wrapped in gauze, and fashioned into *ṣūwaf*. If used overnight for seven consecutive nights following the cessation of menses (and accompanied by sexual abstinence), it is considered to be an excellent treatment for female infertility.

Untying Sorcery

Ruṭūba, *dahr maftūḥ*, *khaḍḍa*, tight vaginas, and malpositioned uteri are all viewed by infertile Egyptian women as proximate causes of their infertility—that is, as etiologies of this problem that are largely endogenously located within individual women's bodies and, in the case of *ruṭūba*, *dahr maftūḥ*, and sometimes *khaḍḍa*, are brought on by women themselves through irresponsible forms of behavior, including exposure to cold, overexertion, and carelessness leading to frightening experiences. In all cases, treatments for these causes of infertility are also somatically oriented, in that the woman's body itself is manipulated, most often through therapies that are localized to the "reproductive region" between the waist and the upper thighs.

However, as noted earlier, not all ethnogynecological causes of infertility in Egypt are viewed as being so proximate, so localized, so amenable to treatment. As seen in the case of *kabsa* and sometimes *khaḍḍa*, infertility causation may be social relational in nature, in that the body may be socially affected by the inadvertent behavior of another person. Similarly, two of the other major causal categories of infertility in urban Egypt—acts of sorcery made by one's living enemies and the actions of angered spirit-counterparts, who are believed to inhabit the subterranean world—are immanently social in nature, indexing the extent to which disharmonious relations may impinge on one's physical well-being.

ʿAmal, or sorcery, is believed to be the second most common medial cause of infertility following *kabsa*, the latter of which is considered much more frequent. *ʿAmal* means, literally, "doing," "making," or "work"—sorcery being the "work" that is "done" or "made" in this case.

Unlike in some societies described in ethnographic literature where sorcery and sorcery accusations are rampant and serve as an effective means of social control, sorcery is not a particularly common occurrence in Egypt, although it is widely recognized as a cause of harm among the rural and urban Egyptian poor and has been reported from many other parts of the Middle East as well.[13] Because of its relative infrequence, most Egyptians do not consciously guard themselves against *ʿamal* as they do, say, against *ḥasad*, or the evil eye. Nevertheless, it is considered wise to cultivate cordial relations with one's neighbors, in-laws, and family members and to protect one's personal property and bodily waste products from use in potential sorcery bundles.

Among the Egyptian infertile, both men and women, *ʿamal* is a causal possibility that must be considered, for it is known to cause infertility, impotence, and infertility-related marital and sexual discord between husbands and wives. Typically, an enemy or a jealous or aggrieved individual—most often a jilted fiancé(e), an individual who has secretly been in love with the now-married victim, or, according to some Muslims, a Christian in love with a Muslim man or woman who is forbidden as a marital partner[14]—employs the services of a male *munaggim* specializing in sorcery in order to make an *ʿamal* directed against the victim. Essentially, the desire of the enemy is to influence the outcome of the envied marriage by causing sexual and reproductive problems that will lead to marital dissolution.

The "bad" *munaggimīn* who make *ʿamal*s usually compose sorcery bundles containing some item belonging to the victim or some item containing the victim's essence—for example, a piece of hair, a piece of clothing, a handkerchief used to wipe the nose or brow, or the piece of cloth bloodstained by the victim's "honor." However, an *ʿamal* may take many other forms involving some part of the victim's identity. For example, it may consist of an object or piece of paper with the victim's name written on it; or it may comprise a simple handshake between the perpetrator and the victim in which the *ʿamal* is written on the former's palm and effectively "touches" the victim; or an *ʿamal* may be "written into" the ululation on the victim's wedding night; or it may consist of a potion containing the victim's essence, which is poured into the victim's food or drink or over the doorstep. *ʿAmal*s consisting of objects are typically wrapped in cloth and buried, primarily under the threshold to the victim's home or in a cemetery, where the *ʿamal* effectively "pollutes" this pure place. Occasionally, the object is thrown into the sea or put into a fish that is thrown back into the sea, where it is believed to vanish forever. Or, if the *ʿamal* is written on a piece of wood, it is pounded into the ground. In each case, however, the point is to conceal the *ʿamal* from ready perception, making it impossible to locate without the active intervention of a skillful diviner. Once located, the *ʿamal* must be "untied" or "dissolved" through counteractive techniques undertaken by a knowledgeable *munaggim*.

Until the sorcery act is nullified, however, the *ʿamal* causes the victim to enter a state known as *marbūṭ(a)*, meaning "tied up" or "bound." As with the *kabsa*-caused binding of a woman's womb, the *ʿamal* is thought to cause a harmful "tying" of the victim's emotions and/or body, such that normal affective, sexual, and reproductive relations between spouses are inhibited. For women, their wombs may become tied, resulting in continuous bleeding and their failure to become pregnant. More often, however, an *ʿamal* affects women's emotions in such a way that they become repulsed by their husbands and disgusted by sexual intercourse, leading to their failure to conceive. The same is true of men who are *marbūṭin* and who may view their wives as hideous and undesirable. When this happens, the husband and/or wife are repelled by one another, both sexually and emotionally, and fighting and even divorce, the desired goal of the perpetrator, may ensue.

As one infertile woman affected by such an *ʿamal* explained,

> When he comes near me, I feel suffocated. We feel bored with each other, and we fight. Sometimes I don't feel attracted to him, and sometimes I want [sexual] relations and he doesn't and vice versa. I don't know exactly what happened, but I think maybe an *ʿamal* is responsible for the problems between us in sex. Maybe a relative of mine—for example, if I had a fight with anyone or if there is anyone who is jealous—maybe she had this *ʿamal* made and put it

> on a tree or in a grave. Here in Egypt, some people make *'amal*s and tie the man, and he can't come near his bride. They bring a *shaikh* and he reads Qur'an and does other things, and the man sees if his organ is okay. He enters on the bride, and, if not, they find him a stronger *shaikh*.

As suggested by this woman, in urban Egypt, *'amal*s are thought to be most commonly directed against men and are intended to affect their sexual performance. The most common symptom of *'amal* among males is their failure to achieve or maintain an erection, a problem that leads, indirectly, to infertility. For many men, the *rabṭ*, or "tying" of sorcery, is felt as early as the wedding night, when the bridegroom is "just like a woman" and is "unable to go near" his new wife. Emasculated, the new groom who is *marbūṭ* may suffer from the sorcery effects indefinitely, or until the causative *'amal* is undone. Until that time, the impotence is likely to lead to infertility through the "relaxation" of the sexual organ and the resultant lack of intercourse and ejaculation.

Because so many young Egyptian men experience impotence and related infertility problems during the first days, weeks, or months of marriage—which, according to disbelievers, results not from *'amal* but from sexual inexperience and resulting fear, guilt over hurting their virginal wives, or repressed homosexuality—the need for sorcery nullification in this population of young Egyptian males is great and is thus an extremely important and lucrative activity for male *munaggimīn* in Egypt. In fact, most male *munaggimīn* specialize in serving this young male population, just as most female *munaggimīn* specialize in the nonsorcery-related infertility problems of young Egyptian women.

*'Amal*s are usually discovered through a divinational process in which the *munaggim* asks the victim a series of uncannily penetrating questions. As noted earlier, *munaggimīn* are often called *'arrāfīn*, or "knowing ones," because of this psychic ability to divine information that would not be accessible to average human beings. Although many Egyptians believe that *munaggimīn* resort to trickery in order to appear psychically gifted, some *munaggimīn* are considered to be truly endowed with extraordinary psychic powers and are sought out for their ability to locate and retrieve sorcery bundles or to divine other means by which the sorcery was made. Furthermore, some male *munaggimīn* refuse to "make *'amal*s," specializing instead in their retrieval (which is said to be done by the *munaggim*'s spiritual "servants") and "untying."

When a *munaggim* diagnoses *'amal* as the cause of a client's infertility or infertility-producing impotence, he will usually suggest one or more of five ritual "untying" activities, which are most often undertaken by both husband and wife in some combination.

Urination

As with women who have suffered *kabsa*, men who have been the victims of sorcery are often instructed by *munaggimīn* to urinate in or on some object in an attempt to untie an *'amal* that has caused impotence and/or male infertility. In most cases, the husband urinates into the mouth of a live fish called *armūt*, which is known in Egypt for its ability to avoid capture by most fishermen and which, after being caught and swallowing the husband's urine, is thrown back into the Mediterranean where the *'amal* "vanishes." Or the husband urinates on a piece of red-hot metal of the type used in *kawī*, such as an ax blade, an undertaker's shovel, a piece of lead pipe the same length as the husband's penis, or an iron hitching post; such urination is said to "cool off" the object and "dissolve in water" the *rabṭ* represented by it. Following these urination rituals, many men are said to "go home and become a man" (that is, perform sexually).

Potions and Foodstuffs

Because victims of sorcery often unwittingly eat or drink the malevolently intended *'amal*, *munaggimīn* who are hired to untie the *'amal* often ask victims to eat or drink various potions or special foodstuffs or, occasionally, to rub the potion on their penises before having sex. Soft-boiled eggs, upon which the *munaggim* has "written" special formulas to undo the sorcery, are one such popular remedy. Bottled syrups and oils may also be supplied by the *munaggim* with instructions to rub the oil onto the penis precoitally or to drink the potion each morning for seven days, followed by sex every evening. Sometimes seeds, to be dissolved in water and drunk each morning, or tablets and injections are also dispensed. Honey and *samna* mixtures are also popularly prescribed for men, who are usually requested to eat one spoonful every morning for seven days.

Ḥugub (Amulets)

The use of a *ḥigāb* (pl.: *ḥugub*), or an amulet prepared by a *munaggim*, is one of the most common mechanisms by which sorcery is undone. Both husbands and wives may be given a *ḥigāb*, which usually consists of a piece of paper, sometimes folded, upon which indecipherable formulas or purportedly religious verses (sometimes written backwards) have been inscribed. *Munaggimīn* usually also provide special instructions on how the *ḥigāb* is to be utilized. In general, one or more of seven formulaic actions are prescribed, similar in some ways to those already described for *kabsa.* Namely, the husband and/or wife may be told to: (1) bathe one's body and/or the floors of one's home with water (or rose water) in which the *ḥigāb* has been immersed; (2) drink water in which the *ḥigāb* has been immersed; (3) wear a *ḥigāb* on the breasts, in the case of women, or under the armpits or in the underwear, in the case of men; (4) sleep on a *ḥigāb* placed under the pillow; (5) hold a *ḥigāb* for fifteen minutes or more while the Qur'an is being read by the *munaggim*; (6) step over a *ḥigāb* seven times; and (7) burn a *ḥigāb* with resinous *mistika* as *bakhūr* (incense) for the purposes of domestic fumigation. In most cases, either seven *ḥugub* are "written" or the patient is told to cut one *ḥigāb* into seven pieces and to perform one or more of these formulaic actions over the course of seven days at sunset, or over three consecutive Fridays at the time of the noon prayer. In rituals involving water, women are often told to throw the water afterward into an intersection, as described previously for *kabsa*.

Herbal Remedies

Some *munaggimīn* also work with or double as *'aṭṭārīn*, prescribing for women herbal remedies to be used in bath water, to be eaten or drunk, or to be worn as vaginal suppositories. Although women tend to be suspicious of the *ṣūwaf* prepared by male *munaggimīn* because of the anxiety over semen described in Chapter 4, some *munaggimīn* are careful to prescribe *ṣūwaf* containing herbs only, often the same hydragogues already described for *ruṭūba.* Such *ṣūwaf* are usually dispensed with a *ḥigāb* written by the *munaggim* for use in one of the seven ways described above. Occasionally, however, *ṣūwaf*, a *ḥigāb*, and edible/potable mixtures may be prescribed simultaneously. For example, one *munaggim* prescribed the following combination: (1) an edible combination of *ḥummuṣ* (chickpeas) and black *'asmah* (common name: vegetable-glue plant; Latin name: *Combretum truncatum*), mixed with hairs, one spoonful every morning before breakfast; (2) the juice of a large Egyptian onion, taken at the same time; (3) a *ḥigāb*, written directly onto the woman's shirt; and (4) three *ṣūwaf* of unknown ingredients.

Home Purification

Finally, many *munaggimīn* are equally concerned about ridding the couple's home of the *'amal* that has affected it and the marital relationship of its occupants. To do so, they usually recommend some purifying ritual for the home itself, performed by the wife, who uses the same water to wash her own body or to drink. In most cases, *munaggimīn* advise the woman (1) to sprinkle the entire apartment with pieces of a *ḥigāb*, lentils, various herbs, or salt, then (2) to wipe all surfaces of the apartment with water, and then (3) to dump the used water in front of her doorstep or in an intersection, thereby transferring the water beyond the threshold of the household. All of these procedures are necessary to make the residual effects of the *ʿamal* disappear from the couple's home.

Appeasing Spirit-Sisters

Human beings are not the only ones capable of inflicting infertility on others. Among poor urban Egyptian women, a controversial theory holds that normally peaceable spirit-counterparts, living in a shadow world beneath the ground, may become upset with their earthly sisters, rendering them temporarily infertile. Until a misbehaving woman "appeases" her spirit-counterpart, usually through the provision of sumptuous victuals, her relations with the spirit will suffer, and she will remain frustrated in her attempts to bear a child.

According to those who abide by this theory, the world under the ground is inhabited by a race of spirit-beings who are imperceptible to humans. Most Egyptians consider these spirit-beings to be *jinn* or *ʿafārīt*, the mischievous, often evil spirits mentioned throughout the Qur'an. However, others consider these spirit-beings to be subterranean *malaika*, or angels, equivalent to the heavenly angels above. These spirit-beings are said to be of both sexes and of all ages and marry and live in families, thereby mirroring the human world. They are considered to be attracted to water and frequently inhabit the areas underneath toilets, baths, and shower drains (which is why the privacy of the bathroom is considered slightly dangerous, a danger that can be diminished by saying God's name and uttering formulaic phrases when entering and exiting). In fact, some call these spirits the "toilet angels."

Those who believe in this spirit world argue that each woman has a *qarīna*,[15] or spirit-counterpart, who lives underground and is identical "like a twin" or a woman's "reflection." As one woman put it, "If I'm happy, she's happy. If I'm sad, she's sad. If I'm upset, she's upset. If I'm married, she's married. If I have no children, she has no children." This spirit-counterpart is usually referred to as the *ukht taḥt il-arḍ*, or "sister under the ground," and she is viewed as having the best interests of her earthly sister at heart. In fact, some view her as the guardian of her earthly sister and her sister's children. Or, as one woman put it, "Even though they're *jinn*, they're our friends."

Nonetheless, the *ukht taḥt il-arḍ*, as either spirit or angel, can become angered by her human sister when the latter misbehaves. In retaliation, the *ukht taḥt il-arḍ* may cause bodily injury to her human counterpart (or her children), usually in the form of imperceptible "beatings" or "pinchings" that can render women infertile or cause miscarriage among the pregnant. When a spirit-sister "touches" her human counterpart in this way—rendering her reproductive organs temporarily damaged—she invariably leaves some physical mark on the victim's body, primarily bruises or other visible scars.

Yet, a normally peace-loving spirit-sister must be aroused to act this way. Invariably, the *ukht taḥt il-arḍ* becomes vicious only when she is upset by her human sister's "above-ground" actions. Specific actions known to infuriate the *ukht taḥt il-arḍ* usually occur at night, which is the time of greatest spirit activity, and generally involve an encroachment on the spirit's underground habitat. These disturbing actions include pouring hot water down the toilet or on the floor without saying God's name, thereby scalding the spirit-sister; tapping, stamping the feet, or jumping on the floor, thereby knocking her around; or beating a cat or one's children. The physical abuse of one's children is said to be particularly upsetting to the *ukht taḥt il-arḍ*, because, as a woman's twin, she has identical children of her own.

In addition, the *ukht taḥt il-arḍ* reacts poorly to her human sister's states of emotional distress or imbalance. These include crying and brooding; fighting with one's husband; wearing black and being very morbid; hating one's mother-in-law; being haughty, proud, or vain; being generally ill-mannered; becoming easily disgusted with other people or their children; going to sleep at night on an empty stomach or while still upset from a fight; not eating because of a loss of appetite or refusal of food; or screaming or crying at night, especially while alone in the bathroom.

Having said as much, it is important to reiterate an earlier point about the controversy surrounding the very existence of *akhawāt taḥt il-arḍ*, as well as their role in human affairs. First, many poor urban Egyptian women entirely disbelieve in—or at least seriously doubt—the existence of subterranean spirit-counterparts or spirits of any kind. According to these women, belief in spirits or their ability to influence earthly life is "nonsense" and a "product of the imagination."

As one skeptical *dāya* pointed out,

> There is nothing called *jinn*. Counterpart, my foot! In my life, I've never seen an *'ifrīt*, and I go at the beginning and the end of the night. And I've seen bombs and soldiers and shooting and all this, but I've never seen *'afārīt*. It's all lies. There is no *'ifrīt* except the human being. I've never seen, nor my grandmother, nor my sister [both *dāyāt*]. Only uneducated people believe in things like that. If I know a person, I go and prevent her from doing it [spirit appeasement], because she will spend her money on stupid things.

Another woman argued, "This is all nonsense. Faithful people don't mix with people under the ground; only infidels do. What is nonsense is that we mix with them. They exist and only appear to the unfaithful. Lots of people think *akhawāt taḥt il-arḍ* and *ikhwān taḥt il-arḍ* can become upset, but Shaikh Shaarawi [the popular televised cleric] said that's not true and that all this is nonsense."

Second, even women who are willing to believe in the existence of spirit-counterparts question whether these counterparts are *jinn* or *malaika* and whether they are inherently good or bad. As suggested above, the "spirit versus angel" question is a point of great contention. Some women insist that the *ukht taḥt il-arḍ* is an angel and, as such, is incapable of causing harm to humans because she "comes from God to protect humans from evil." Others insist that angels are found only "above" and that subterranean beings are necessarily *jinn* or *'afārīt*, making the *ukht taḥt il-arḍ* a *jinnīya*, or female spirit. Others argue that angels live "above" as well as "below"—with humans "in the middle"—and that both heavenly and subterranean angels are capable of causing harm to humans. For example, some women argue that heavenly angels become upset when the dead child they are expected to guard is buried face down, thereby "giving its back to God." According to these women, unless the child is turned upright, its angels will prevent the dead child's mother from becoming pregnant again. The most common view, however, is that the *ukht taḥt il-arḍ* is *not* an angel, but is rather a *jinnīya*; as such, she is neither inherently malicious nor inherently beneficent, but she has the *potential* to cause harm if unduly irritated by human action.

Third, the notion of a subterranean world "mirroring" the human world is a point of great debate. Some women argue that *jinn* do *not* necessarily live underground, but rather inhabit empty, "godforsaken" places, such as deserted cemeteries. Others contend that a subterranean spirit world does exist, but that it does not mirror the human world. Rather, oppositions and reversals are found there, such that, when a woman is happy, her spirit-sister is angry and vice versa. Or, instead of having spirit-sisters, human females have spirit-brothers and human males have spirit-sisters.[16] According to some, a woman's *akh taḥt il-arḍ*, or "brother under the ground," can cause problems for a woman, including infertility, simply if he feels jealous regarding the human woman to whom he is "married." Such jealousy is thought to be aroused when a woman is passionately in love with her husband (or vice versa); when she is very coquettish, spending much time admiring her own beauty; or when she combs her hair during the Friday noon prayer when she should be attending to spiritual matters. Still others argue that a woman may have *both* a jealous spirit-brother and a perturbable spirit-sister, whose responses to her actions may affect her future fertility.

Fourth, even women who acknowledge the existence of spirit-counterparts may doubt their causal role in human infertility. Although women may be "earth-touched" by the *ukht taḥt il-arḍ*, the damage is too slight, according to some, to cause an affliction as serious as infertility. Others argue that the *ukht taḥt il-arḍ* does not *cause* infertility as a result of anger, but rather *becomes* angry because her human-sister is incapable of producing children. As a result, the infertile woman deprives her spirit "twin" of subterranean children.

Finally, it is exceedingly important to note that a major point of *agreement* surrounds the issue of spirit possession. Among poor urban Egyptian women, the vast majority believe that these spirit-counterparts are incapable of "possessing" a woman, rendering her *malbūsa*—literally, "worn" by a spirit. Because spirit-counterparts are seen as being mostly "human-friendly," they have no interest in causing permanent spirit affliction, which can only result when other "evil" spirits take over a human being's mind and body. Thus, a woman who is *malbūsa*, or possessed, is very different from a woman who is simply "on the outs" with her angry spirit-sister.

As one woman explained, "The *ukht taḥt il-arḍ*, she's a *jinn*, a bad soul. She can hurt your body, even make marks on your body, and she can prevent you from getting pregnant. But, to be *malbūsa*, this is something else. This is when you're worn by a *rūḥ* [soul]. Then you're sick, 'touched' in the mind, not normal. You must do a *zār* [spirit placation ceremony]. But this is something different."

Another woman explained, "There are *'afārīt* that enter your body sometimes and cause problems that are solved only when you go to a certain kind of *shaikh*. He 'brings him [the *'ifrīt*] out' and makes him talk through the body of the woman so that he says what he wants. Then the *shaikh* sends the *'ifrīt* away, and she does what he wants. This takes place if she's very ill, sick, and there's no hope with medicine or doctors. She is *malbūsa.*"

Another woman agreed that "a woman who is *malbūsa* is very sick. She can't move and just sleeps on the ground and she's not herself mentally. They say it's from spirits. People do the *zār* for her, and if it's right, it will work to make her better, and if not, it won't."

Thus, according to poor urban Egyptian women, spirit possession can cause infertility only in the most indirect of ways, in that women who are possessed are severely "affected" mentally and physically and are incapable of fulfilling normal social roles, including reproductive ones. According to them, infertility is rarely, if ever, attributable to possession alone, but rather arises from a host of other etiological possibilities, including the "touch" of a temporarily angered spirit-counterpart described in this chapter. As one experienced *dāya* concluded rather succinctly, "Being *malbūsa* has nothing to do with pregnancy."

That most poor urban Egyptian women do *not* attribute infertility to spirit possession is a fact of their existence that appears to diverge considerably from the lived experience of other infertile Middle Eastern women. To read the ethnographic literature from rural Egypt (El-Hamamsy 1972; Morsy 1978a, 1978b, 1993), Morocco (Greenwood 1981), Sudan (Constantinides 1985; Boddy 1989), and Tunisia (Creyghton 1977), one could almost conclude that all infertile women are spirit possessed. Indeed, in discussions of spirit possession and of the famous "*zār* cult" which offers relief to spirit victims, women who are infertile or in some other way "reproductively impaired" are often represented as major devotees of these spirit-possession cults. Of the three major ethnographies dealing with health and illness in the Middle East (Boddy 1989; Crapanzano 1973; Morsy 1993), all deal to a great extent—if not exclusively—with spirit possession, and all link spirit possession to female infertility, including in poignant case reports.

Undoubtedly, some women who are infertile—and perhaps particularly those who are living in relatively closed, rural communities—claim spirit possession as a socially acceptable "sick role" when other therapeutic and explanatory options have been exhausted. As Morsy has noted, spirit possession may have a compensatory value for "persons who are particularly susceptible to social stresses and conflict" (1978a:602). In her study of rural Egyptian women, she found that infertile women actively sought the sick-role label of spirit possession to "justify their deviant situation of being childless in a society that places primary emphasis on female reproductive and maternal functions" (1978a:602).

Yet, in a more recent account, she notes,

> Both women *and* men in positions of relative powerlessness, when granted the social sanction of the sick role, are allowed temporary deviance from culturally prescribed role expectations and/or transgression of their positions of relative powerlessness. Yet, the low incidence of 34 cases of *'uzr* [spirit possession] in a combined group of 368 adult men and women suggests that the "making social" of claims to this culturally sanctioned strategy of indirect control is subject to structural constraints. When I expressed surprise upon hearing from a local healer that he only diagnoses "not more than four or five" new cases of possession illness per year, he responded: "What more do you want, otherwise the whole village would come to a standstill." (Morsy 1993:146)

It is possible that Middle Eastern ethnographers' obsession with possession[17] has shaped the description of Middle Eastern illness categories in such a way that possession is overdetermined as a cause of affliction in general and that the link between possession and infertility is overstated—with other, alternative etiologies being left totally or largely unexplored. Judging from the urban Egyptian case, possession plays a decidedly minimal role in the lived experiences of infertile women, whose "management of everyday life" (Early 1988), including their health problems, revolves around a number of other pressing issues, both biogynecological and ethnogynecological in nature.

Among the poor urban Egyptian women in this study, none had ever considered herself to be spirit-possessed, nor had any of them ever sought such a "compensatory" sick-role label. Furthermore, only one woman had ever participated in a *zār*—not to cure her infertility, since she was adamant that she was not "possessed," but rather to "calm her nerves," which had become frazzled by her increasingly difficult marital situation. Thus, according to the women in this study, the *zār* was not an appropriate therapy for treating infertility, although several of them had been encouraged by elderly relatives or greedy *munaggimīn* to participate in or mount a *zār* to help with their infertility problems. (In fact, the mention of the *zār* as an infertility "treatment" often brought derisive laughter.)

Rather, in terms of therapy, infertile women who believed in the spirit-counterpart etiology described alternative ways of "satisfying," or "making up" with these angered spirit-beings. As they explained, female *munaggimīn* tend to specialize in spirit appeasement, given that they are thought to be able to diagnose such "spirit-counterpart problems." Clairvoyant diagnosis of angered spirits takes many forms. Some female *munaggimīn* read palms or cups or make diagnoses and predictions after "sleeping on" patients' handkerchiefs or photographs. Others use the "line-of-questioning" or "opening-the-Book" approaches undertaken by male *munaggimīn*. Some simply make diagnostic pronouncements without formal diagnostic methods or questioning, while others may do this after first asking the patient why she has come.

When female *munaggimīn* actually invoke patients' spirit-sisters in order to understand the spirits' requests, their ways are often much more dramatic. For example, some of them cover their faces with religiously inscribed veils and speak from under them after being given the patient's money-filled handkerchief. Others smoke the *shīsha*—inhaling honey-imbued tobacco through a large, standing water pipe, which is normally viewed as a male activity—and then speak in altered voices, such as those of a child. Once invoked, an infertile woman's angry *ukht taḥt il-arḍ* makes her "request" to the *munaggima*, who informs the infertile woman of what her spirit-sister desires. Sometimes, the *munaggima* may act normally, making the spirit's request in a matter-of-fact manner to the patient. In other cases, the *munaggima* may be "worn" by the spirit and may seem to be possessed. She may cry and contort her body, making statements such as, "I'm mad at you, because you slept without eating, and I wanted to eat. Now I want food."

Once these requests by the *ukht taḥt il-arḍ* are heard, efforts must be made by the infertile woman to "make up" with her spirit-sister by satisfying these demands. Generally, spirit requests are fulfilled in one of two ways.

Animal Sacrifice

The primary way to pacify an angry spirit-sister is to slaughter one or more small animals in her honor. Generally, the animals to be slaughtered are fowl (chickens, roosters, or pigeons), but occasionally rabbits are also sacrificed. The *ukht taḥt il-arḍ* may request only one animal or a number of different ones, usually of specific colors and sexes. For example, one woman's *ukht taḥt il-arḍ* asked for the following male animals: three large rabbits (black, beige, and gray), two roosters (red and white), one black chicken, and three pigeons (black, brown, and red). In addition, the spirit requested a large number of other food items, including one kilo of cracked wheat, one kilo of tomatoes, black pepper, *samna*, three kinds of yogurt, sugar, brown coffee, and tea, as well as three candles (red, white, and yellow). Likewise, a woman whose husband's *ukht taḥt il-arḍ* was jealous of her, thereby preventing her from having children, was told by a *munaggima* that the spirit-sister wanted the following combination of animals and foodstuffs: a pair of red pigeons, a black chicken, an egg, a carton of yogurt, corn, wheat, fava beans, and lentils, to be left in a pan overnight with a white candle lit in the center of it.

It is important to emphasize that obtaining all of these items is usually quite difficult for poor women and their husbands, who may be unable to afford the ceremony. Furthermore, it is extremely important to note that, unlike all other ethnogynecological therapies for female infertility, sacrificial ceremonies of this sort usually involve the active participation of women's husbands—probably because female *munaggimīn* realize that it is the husbands who must be willing to finance these expensive ceremonies. Compared to most other ethnogynecological therapies, which usually range in price from one to one hundred Egyptian pounds (forty cents to forty dollars, and mostly within the lower end of the spectrum), the spirit appeasement ceremonies prescribed by female *munaggimīn* are quite expensive. In the first example cited here, the items themselves cost two hundred pounds (eighty dollars), and the *munaggima* requested an additional one hundred pounds (forty dollars) for her services. In the second example, the husband and wife had yet to undertake the ceremony because of their inability to cover the costs of the designated animals and other items, as well as the *munaggima*'s fees, which were one hundred pounds for the husband and one hundred pounds for the wife.

If a couple is able to afford such a ceremony, they must obtain the animals and any additional items requested by the spirit, although the slaughtering of the animals is usually performed by the *munaggima*. Each *munaggima* performs the slaughtering ceremony in a particular, distinctive fashion. For example, the *munaggima* may (1) slaughter the animal over the patient's head, so that the gushing blood lands on her, (2) slaughter the animal and smear some of its fresh blood onto the patient's skin, (3) slaughter the animal and provide some of the blood to the patient to apply to a cotton vaginal suppository, (4) slaughter the animal and smear its blood under the patient's bed and on her doorstep, or (5) slaughter the animal and write a *ḥigāb* for the patient with its blood. The slaughtering, furthermore, may be carried out in a special location, such as on the patient's doorstep or in a bathroom lit by candles. Likewise, the slaughtered animal(s) may be disposed of in a special manner. For example, the husband and wife may be instructed to (1) eat the animal(s) by themselves, (2) give the animal(s) to the poor, (3) bury the animal(s) in a special location, often with bread and salt, (4) throw the animals into the sea, or

(5) give the animal(s) to the *munaggima* herself for disposal. Because of the tendency of female *munaggimīn* to take the slaughtered animals with them following a sacrificial ceremony, many Egyptians suspect that female *munaggimīn* undertake these animal sacrifices so that they can obtain meat as well as money.

Provision of Milk, Sweets, and Other Gifts

Although most spirit-sisters are appeased through animal sacrifice, they may on occasion request other gift items that appeal to their appetites and aesthetic sensibilities. Milk and sweets, such as sugar cubes or the popular Egyptian sweet rice pudding, *ruzz bil-laban*, are often requested together, and the infertile woman may be instructed to drink some of the milk before leaving it out in a bowl, usually overnight. Scented soaps and perfumed essences, such as licorice or rose water, are also commonly requested, and the infertile woman may be instructed to wash the floors of her house with these fragrant ingredients. Or she may be instructed to fumigate the house with sweet-smelling *bakhūr*, or incense. Occasionally, some spirit-sisters may request more expensive gifts, such as new white headscarves or dresses. Others, however, are less demanding, asking for henna or candles or the opportunity to eat "bread and salt" together with their earthly sisters. Because bread and salt are considered in Egypt to be among the most basic items of human subsistence, "eating bread and salt together" is a metaphorical statement used to emphasize the bonding of individuals, including humans to their spirit-counterparts. In other words, those who have eaten bread and salt together are said to be nearly as close as those related by "blood" in a society in which kinship ties supersede all others.

However, in most cases, the material demands of spirit-sisters are great and, in many cases, the monetary demands of the female *munaggimīn* who invoke these spirits are even greater. Because *munaggimīn* tend to be the most costly of all ethnogynecologists and because they are suspected of being charlatans by many Egyptians, infertile women who have been diagnosed as having spirit-counterpart problems are often reluctant to carry out the expensive appeasement measures described above.

Dismissing the Evil Eye

Finally, in concluding this discussion of the ethnogynecological causes of and cures for infertility among the Egyptian urban poor, it is important to dismiss *ḥasad*, the "evil eye," as a significant causal factor. Like spirit possession, the evil eye is invariably mentioned as one of the leading supernatural causes of ill health among populations throughout the Middle East and in the Pan-Mediterranean region; and, given the pervasiveness of evil-eye beliefs, their historical depth, and their religious acceptance, this attention is probably merited.[18] In Egypt, the health-demoting consequences of *ḥasad*, or the envious glance of a covetous person, have been well documented, particularly with regard to children's health (Fakhouri 1972; Millar and Lane 1988; Morsy 1980b, 1993; Nadim 1980; Pillsbury 1978). However, with little exception,[19] poor urban Egyptian women do *not* deem *ḥasad* to be responsible for infertility. As one woman put it rather succinctly, "It can hurt your kids, and it can affect your material things, including food and money. But it is *not* related to pregnancy." Unfortunately, however, when children fall ill, evil-eye accusations are often directed against vulnerable infertile women, who, by virtue of their childlessness, are deemed inherently and inescapably envious (Inhorn n.d.; Morsy 1980b, 1993). The ineluctable result is stigmatization and ostracism of infertile women within the community, a misfortune that compounds their already difficult pilgrimages for pregnancy.

7. Divinity, Profanity, and Pilgrimage

Farida's Story

Farida was born in a village in Upper Egypt and, as a young woman, was considered very comely. When an educated man from the community asked for her hand in marriage, Farida's poor parents were delighted, since they considered the groom's education and government position to be sources of great prestige and security for their daughter. Farida and her husband had their own daughter within the first year of marriage, but, within the second year, Farida's husband divorced her to marry an educated colleague with whom he had fallen in love. Farida, an illiterate teenager, was asked to sign her name to some papers, without ever realizing that she had endorsed the consent agreement to her divorce.

As a divorcée with a young daughter, Farida's chances of remarriage were poor, even though she was considered the young beauty of her small village, where she had returned after her husband left her. However, several years after her divorce, Farida's brother returned home on military leave with a friend from the army named Hesham. When Hesham saw Farida, he could not take his eyes off her, and he asked Farida's brother if she was married. Told that she was a divorcée with a three-year-old daughter, Hesham was thrilled to learn of Farida's availability and, much to Farida's family's surprise, asked whether he might marry her. The family, and Farida, agreed to the marriage, which took place twelve years ago.

Since then, Farida's daughter, Mirvat, has grown to become a young woman, and Farida and Hesham, an Alexandrian police inspector, have grown to love each other very much—despite Farida's secondary infertility and her continuing inability to provide Hesham with his own children. Although Farida has been pregnant three times in twelve years, each pregnancy ended in late miscarriage, due to "tumors" in her uterus. These tumors have caused Farida to bleed between periods, preventing her and Hesham from having an active sex life. Farida feels that she has deprived

Hesham of both sex and children, which are his right as her husband. She has told him to remarry, although she is actually fearful of this. But she contends that she could remain in a polygynous marriage as long as her co-wife lived in a separate room. However, Hesham says he will never remarry. He feels sorry for Farida and takes heart in knowing that at least Farida is able to become pregnant. He has continued to tell her throughout their marriage that she and Mirvat are enough for him, and he has treated Mirvat as his own daughter. Furthermore, on his policeman's salary, Hesham will never be able to afford remarriage. In fact, Farida was forced to work at a nearby shoe factory in order for the family to eat three meals a day and to support her therapeutic quest. This "search for children" has taken Farida to four doctors, two hospitals, and several ethnogynecologists, who have advised *kabsa* and *khaḍḍa* healing rituals, performed *kasr* on her open back, and supplied her with grilled onion and *shīḥ* suppositories.

However, Farida has put most of her energies into praying to God and "his people" for a child. She has made many *ziyārāt*, or "visits"—more than she can count—to Alexandrian mosque-tombs and shrines dedicated to *shuyūkh bil-baraka*, or blessed saints whose "power is very strong." According to Farida, "You ask them for anything, and they just grant it." When Farida visits the shrines of these *shuyūkh*, she prays to God "normally," and then she makes a vow to the *shaikh*, saying, "If you help us and let us keep a child, we'll get you a small carpet or put some money in your box." According to Farida, the *shuyūkh* have God's divine grace, or *baraka*, and they can therefore help human beings get their prayers answered. Most recently, on a *ziyāra* to the tomb of Shaikh Abu Nur in the Alexandrian neighborhood of Bahair, Farida, desiring a free operation for her "tumors" at Shatby Hospital, asked, "If they keep me inside the hospital to operate on me, I'll put five pounds in your box." When she went to the hospital for an examination later that week, she was astonished to hear the doctor utter the words, "You're staying" (for the operation), and she knew that her prayer-request had been answered.

Yet, although Farida believes that these *shuyūkh bil-baraka* have interceded on her behalf in the eyes of God, she is also quick to note that her ability to become pregnant and deliver a living child is ultimately "God's will." As she explains, "It's God's will that I have such problems inside [her body]. He could easily not have caused me all this. But God is showing me his omnipotence, because I get my babies, created beings, shaped as human beings, and I can't get them to live. God is showing me it's up to him. But, of course, he's leading me to treatments."

God, His People, and Infertility

As a good Muslim, Farida accepts the fact that the events of her life—including her early divorce and her ongoing reproductive trials and tribulations—are "God's will" and are caused by God for reasons that only he can know. Like most poor urban Egyptians, Farida is religiously illiterate but religiously pious, turning to her religion to sustain her through times of trouble and to seek understanding for her misfortunes. Infertility, like other major health problems, is widely acknowledged by Egyptians as the type of misfortune for which religiously based interpretations are to be sought. Thus, it is not surprising that infertile Egyptian women—very few of whom are formally religiously educated—not only take great solace in their religion and their faith in God, but also attempt to explain their particular reproductive problems according to the nature of their beliefs in God and God's role in their lives. The same can be said of the ethnogynecological and biogynecological specialists who treat these women. According to them, other possible explanations of infertility, including both ethnogynecological and biogynecological ones, are proximate to the ultimate reality—that is, that infertility is a condition "from God," which he bestows upon certain human beings for a reason. This reason is something that infertile Egyptian women admittedly ponder; but, as they are quick to note, they ask the question "Why me?" without intending to question the wisdom or righteousness of God's creation of them as infertile. This is a reality that they accept and that they attempt to overcome with God's help, since he, too, created medicine for this purpose.

As Farida points out, it is God who guides women on their therapeutic quests and who, if he should decide, leads them to the correct "treatment." "Treatment" is broadly defined by most (although not all) poor urban women as comprising both biogynecological and ethnogynecological remedies, even though they are aware that both doctors and the "Sunni people" (religiously literate, orthodox Islamists) frown on ethnogynecological remedies, although for somewhat different reasons. Yet, the poor infertile women who "search for children" in Egypt tend to abide by and protect their beliefs in *kabsa*, *ruṭūba*, *dahr maftūḥ*, *ʿamal*, and the other causes of infertility that Egyptian biogynecologists and many Islamists reject. Furthermore, these women see their ethnogynecological attempts at overcoming these problems as quite legitimate in the eyes of God, who urges his followers to "seek" so that he may guide them. Thus, women's interpretation of the nature of "God's medicine" is much wider than that of the members of the medical and religious establishments in Egypt, who advocate only "modern" medicine. And as "good" Muslims, these women do ***not*** see their instrumental visits to *shuyūkh,* and especially *shuyūkh bil-baraka* who can help heal them, as being sacrilegious in any way.

According to most poor urban Egyptian women, *shuyūkh bil-baraka* are the "true" *shuyūkh*, individuals living or dead who are "chosen" by God and blessed with his divine grace. These *shuyūkh*, most of whom are *Ṣūfī* saints, are not seen by women as God's "partners," but rather as intermediaries, who intercede on the behalf of human beings so that their prayers to God may be answered. This is why Farida makes *ziyārāt*, or pilgrimages, to the *shuyūkh*'s tombs, where her prayers for the healing of her reproductive problems have a better chance of being heard.

Thus, to fully understand the nature of Farida's and other Egyptian women's "searches for children," it is necessary to understand how women's religious convictions and beliefs about God and "his people" play a major role in their therapeutic quests. In many cases, women's religious faith takes them on healing pilgrimages that are "not so holy" in orthodox religious terms, combining as they do the sacred and the profane. Yet, such religiously inspired therapeutic pilgrimages must be seen as part of the larger fabric of Egyptian religious life and especially the religious life of women, who are often ignored in such discussions.

Religion and the Egyptian Body Politic

To begin, it is important to understand that, in Egypt, the body politic is a predominantly Muslim body, with approximately 90 percent of all Egyptian Muslims. Muslims in Egypt are almost exclusively of the majority Sunni branch of Islam, with Shi'a sects virtually absent in the country. In addition, approximately 10 percent of Egyptians are Christians, mostly Egyptian Orthodox Copts, who complain that their numbers are underrepresented in national censuses.

Both Muslims and Coptic Christians are monotheists, believing in one God, Allah. However, Muslims view Jesus as a prophet, rather than as the son of God, and acknowledge Muhammad, who received God's word in the form of the Qur'an, as the final prophet. Unlike Coptic Christians, who worship Jesus as the Lord, Muslims ascribe no human incarnations to God. To Muslims, who are the focus of this discussion, Allah is the one God, the Supreme, the Omnipotent, the Compassionate, the Merciful.

Belief and faith in God, his power, his wisdom, and his mercy are ideologies shared by all Muslims, regardless of sectarian differences and degrees of religiosity. Muslims call themselves "believers" in God, and they attempt to follow the Sunna, or the "straight path" forged by the Prophet Muhammad, whose exemplary life is described in the Hadith, a collection of his sayings and deeds. Islamists, or those Egyptians who are extremely devout, or "Sunni" as they are called in Egypt, are characterized by their efforts to follow as closely as possible Islamic scriptural ideals as stated in the Qur'an and Hadith.

Although the vast majority of Egyptians are not "devout" in this sense, most are "religious" in that they profess belief and faith in God, attempt to undertake the "five pillars" of Islam (namely, profession of faith, prayer, almsgiving, the fast of Ramadan, and pilgrimage to Mecca), and strive to avoid wrongdoing and practices that are *ḥarām*, or sinful, according to the tenets of Islam in general and Islamic jurisprudence in particular. Yet, it is also important to note that most Egyptians, both men and women, are not religiously educated in a formal manner, especially those who are illiterate and who are therefore unable to read the Islamic scriptures. In Egypt, it is estimated that approximately 37 percent of adult males and 66 percent of adult females are illiterate (Omran and Roudi 1993), effectively barring the majority of Egyptian Muslims from the acquisition of religious knowledge, except through nonprint media (for example, television and radio broadcasts, audiocassettes, and so forth). Furthermore, because Egyptian women are essentially barred from many of the "formal" practices of Islam—including Friday communal prayer services at mosques, where religious clerics offer interpretive sermons—they are less likely than men to be well versed in religious matters.

Yet, despite their lack of formal participation in orthodox religious rites and their lack of religious education, most poor urban women in Egypt consider themselves to be religiously pious and guided by God, whom they see as playing a profoundly important role in their lives. To understand the nature of women's religiosity and its influence on their religious praxis, including their healing pilgrimages, it is necessary first to typify poor urban Egyptian women's religious beliefs—beliefs that have rarely been privileged in academic discourse.

Women's Religious Beliefs

Despite abundant and far-reaching scholarship on Islam, scant attention has been paid to Muslim women's religious observance, including the nature of their religious beliefs and the transformation of their beliefs into practice. As Fernea and Fernea (1972) note, Western scholars in particular have been guilty of assigning Muslim women to a "residual category," failing to study either their public or private religious lives and portraying them, erroneously, as less devout than men. Not only has the impact of Islam on women's lives been ignored, but few if any scholars have seriously examined the impact *of women on Islam* in their roles as female saints, functionaries, curers, and early contributors to the Islamic scriptures (Ahmed 1989; Dwyer 1978). This lack of academic privileging of Muslim women's religious experience, practice, and influence—and the presumption that women are somehow subordinate and peripheral in religious as in other matters—has seriously hampered the anthropology of Islam, according to Tapper and Tapper (1987). They state:

> We maintain on the one hand that men's day-to-day observance of apparent "orthodoxy" is far from unproblematic, and on the other that it is wrong to assume *a priori* that women's religious "work" is less important than or peripheral to that of men. Not only do women too practice the central, day-to-day rites of Islam, but in their performances they may carry a religious load often of greater transcendental importance to the community than that borne by men. We maintain that any anthropology of Islam will be inadequate unless it gives full consideration to both women's and men's religious ideas and practices and the relation between them. (1987:72)

Although various scholars have advocated additional research on Islam as *lived* by both men and women, the links between Islamic orthodoxies and gender, and the specific kinds of everyday Islamic religious praxis, including gendered praxis, typical of particular local contexts (Delaney 1991; Early 1993a; Eickelman 1982; Eickelman and Piscatori 1990a; Fernea and Fernea 1972; Tapper and Tapper 1987), relatively little ethnographic work of this nature has been carried out.[1] This is as true for Egypt as it is for other parts of the Middle East, with the result that little is known about how Egyptian Muslim women practice their religion or how this practice relates to their beliefs in divinity.

Certainly, a gendered corrective is called for, but one that does not essentialize women as a monolithic, "unorthodox" religious force, opposed in belief and practice to the "orthodox" world of Muslim men. Among poor urban Egyptian women at least, their religious convictions are often shared with men, who may, in fact, play a pivotal role in educating their wives, mothers, and daughters about religious matters. Furthermore, in urban Egypt at least, the popularization and commercialization of Islam—

through well-received television and radio shows and a thriving market in religious audiocassettes—has brought Islam to the masses, leading to the increasing religious education of illiterate women and perhaps to the increasing homogenization of their religious knowledge.

But what are poor urban women's religious beliefs? And how do they pertain to their understanding of infertility? As we shall see, women's beliefs in and about divinity could not play a more central role in their understanding of misfortune, of which infertility is but one example. Ultimately, it is women's beliefs in God and his role in their lives which informs *all* aspects of their pilgrimages for pregnancy, pilgrimages which they view as divinely inspired.

God as Creator

First, most poor urban Egyptian women see God, who is referred to as male, as the creator of the universe and of all life in it. Egyptian women are fond of saying that "God is everything" and "everything is from God." All creation, including the creation of human beings, is ultimately in God's hands; or, as Egyptian women say, "human beings are incapable of creating even a fingernail." Most important to this discussion, God is seen as orchestrating human procreation. Not only does God decide who will be fertile and who will be infertile, but he also imbues each fetus with a soul and decides which ones will be male and which will be female. The proof of his creative force, according to women who know the approximate translation,[2] can be found in the following Qur'anic verse (42:49–50):

> Unto Allah belongeth the Sovereignty of the heavens and the earth. He createth what He will. He bestoweth female [offspring] upon whom He will, and bestoweth male [offspring] upon whom He will;
>
> Or He mingleth them, males and females, and He maketh barren whom He will. Lo! He is Knower, Powerful."

Thus, human procreation is divinely guided, and, as such, it is ultimately beyond human control. Speaking of procreation, one woman explained, "He creates pregnancy. He creates children. And he makes liquid water into a fetus." Or, as another put it, "He's the one who created children from the beginning to the end. It's with his power. He's the one who gives the fluid to the husband, and God is the one who is creating the baby inside us, and he makes the baby move, for example, its fingers and everything."

Because God ultimately controls procreation, it is his decision to give children or not to give. Thus, women who use birth control may still become pregnant because God wants this. Likewise, a husband and wife may never have a child, because God wants this, too. These decisions are his and his alone, because God is the ultimate creator. Women express this variously, with formulaic phrases such as, "It's in God's hands," "God decides," "God has his reasons," "It's God's judgment," "It's when God wants," "God permits," "It's God's wish," "It's God's will," and "God gives his permission." Or, as they are particularly fond of saying when referring to their own inconsequential role in such matters, "There is nothing in our hands."

Predestination

Thus, God, who is omnipresent, is the one who decides everything, and these decisions are made by him before an individual's life begins. Once born, an individual's destiny has already been determined. As many poor urban Egyptian women explain it, on the tree of life, each person has a leaf, upon which his or her life is written; included on the leaf is the time of birth, if and when marriage will occur, if and when children will be born, and how and when a person will die, at which time the leaf falls from the tree.

Because each individual's life is "written" by God (with the help of his angels) in this manner, life occurrences can be seen as being under God's control, according to his wishes and his will. Events are not random; rather, they occur at predestined times according to a plan, the purpose and meaning of which can only be known by God. For example, if God does not allow a woman to become pregnant, God knows that her time for motherhood has yet to come. Furthermore, he has his reasons for waiting—for example, to prevent the birth of an abnormal child or one who will grow up to lead a bad life. God has his reasons for everything he does, including "approving the timing" of life's events. This is the nature of God's wisdom and judgment. Thus, women who fail to become pregnant can often be heard to remark, "My time hasn't come yet."

Human Volition

Yet, just because life is "written," human beings are not passive creatures, devoid of volition and will. God expects human beings to exercise their minds and to make choices, including decisions about how to lead their lives. As one woman explained, "God is the one who decides your life, but he gave you a brain, and when he gave you a brain, he showed you good and bad. It's the person himself who decides to go the right or wrong way."

Although humans have been divinely endowed with intelligence and morality, God is seen as making the "important" decisions about humans' lives, overruling and reversing human decisions at any time, for reasons known only to him (since he does not "reveal his secrets"). As one woman explained, "You can think and imagine and wish for lots of things, and God may have in mind something totally different for you. We have a saying, 'The worshipper is in a state of thinking, and God does the action.'" Another commented, "Each person has twenty-four wishes, but God doesn't grant them all. There is always something missing, including possibly children." Others argue that the more a human being wishes for something, the less likely God is to grant that wish. Therefore, those who are "dying for" children do not get them, and those who do not want children get too many. One woman put it this way: "Those who have children suffer from responsibility, and those who don't search. Neither is happy. It's his [God's] ability and greatness that no one should question."

Although God decides the "important" matters of humans' lives, he is seen as disapproving of human passivity and indecision. Therefore, it is argued that God expects those who are sick to seek treatment. Infertile women take this notion very seriously. As one woman stated, "God prevents us from having something, but he shows us the way to get it. It says in the Qur'an, 'Try my worshippers, and I will try with you.'" Another explained, "He's the one who decides and gives. The human beings have nothing in their hands. It's God who makes the doctors. He creates the medicine, and he's the one who showed us to go to doctors." Or, as another woman put it, "If you try to help yourself, God will help you. That's why God gave medicine."

But, if and when "medicine" takes its effect is God's decision. God may choose to heal or not to heal, to give life and take life away. As one woman explained,

> It's written that God created medicine and said, "Search for medicine, and I will help you." But you have to think about it, too. For example, someone has a bad sickness and with treatment, he doesn't get well. And he goes back to God with his prayers, and there is something written in the Qur'an, "Wish from God and have faith in Him, and He can make you well from anything you can't get over." Some people get well; these are the ones who have *real* faith in God. It doesn't matter that you don't have faith if you don't get well. A woman can be very close to God, but that's a fact she has to live with.

Thus, in matters of life and death, sickness and health, God is seen as having the "final word." Final outcomes, such as irreversible infertility or even death, are always under his control and "out of the hands" of humans. God may grant or deny human wishes for wellness, cause or alleviate human suffering. These are his choices, and his alone. Although humans may attempt to overcome their problems — and, in fact, are expected to do so — they cannot, ultimately, overcome God's will regarding their health and well-being.

Whether God creates all medical problems, however, is a point of some debate. Although it is widely believed that God creates all medical conditions, just as he provides all remedies, some women contend that their medical conditions, such as blocked tubes, are the result of irresponsible actions, or "human failing." Speaking of her own medical condition, one woman remarked, "He's not the one who causes, for example, blocked ovaries. That's the negligence of humans. If one of my ovaries is blocked, that's because when I delivered a baby, I didn't do a D & C." However, a woman expressing the majority opinion stated, "Just like anyone born without vision or fingers, she's born with blocked tubes. He has power in everything. He can make all women pregnant if he wants to, and he can prevent all women from being pregnant if he wants to."

God's Reasons for Human Suffering

When deciding who will have blocked tubes and who will not, who will bear children and who will remain barren, who will live and who will die, God is not whimsical. All of the decisions made by God, even when they cause human suffering, are made for a reason and are meaningful. For example, in his actions, God may be reminding human beings of his power, strength, and omnipotence. Or he may be setting an example, so that human beings may learn from one another. Or he may make human beings suffer for something so that, when they finally receive it, they will be grateful and caring. Or he may deprive individuals of happiness in their earthly lives so that they will be rewarded in Paradise or suffer less on the Day of Judgment. As one woman stated, "A needle prick in life lightens some suffering in the afterlife."

Or God may be testing human beings. According to most poor urban Egyptian women, infertility is best viewed as a test of both patience and religious faith. When God fails to grant a husband and wife a child, he is testing their faith in him and their ability to endure hardship — just as he tested Ibrahim (Abraham) and Zakariya (Zacharias) in the days of old, giving them children when they were elderly and their wives were barren or postmenopausal.[3] Indeed, God is thought to have tested the Prophet

Muhammad himself, whose first wife, Khadija, was the only one to bear living children. Although 'A'isha, one of the Prophet's wives, was infertile, she was deemed "the Mother of the Worshippers of God" by the Prophet and was held in great favor by him (Fernea and Bezirgan 1985).

According to poor urban Egyptian women, when God tests husbands and wives in this way, he seeks to determine: Will they continue to believe in me, even if I allow years to pass without granting them a child? Will the wife give up her quest for therapy? Will the husband divorce his infertile wife in haste? Do they have faith in my ability to help them overcome their problem?

According to one woman, "He tests the strength of their faith and the slavery of humans to him, to see if they will be patient or not. He can give a person a child after twenty years. He means something by infertility, but we don't know what it is." Commenting on infertile women's often frenetic "searches for children," another woman argued, "Women are *not* patient. They make themselves into *'aṭṭārīn*. They fill themselves with herbs and spices they think will help them get pregnant. But this is all nonsense. A few months go by and they tell the woman, 'Get up and do something. Have a D & C, a tubal insufflation.' But if she does ninety-nine operations and God doesn't want her to have children, she never will."

Those who are impatient or without faith will never be granted a child by God. But whether God punishes humans for their misdeeds by depriving them of his gift of children is a point of great contention. According to most women, infertility is a test but *not* a punishment. They argue that God only punishes in the afterlife and that during one's earthly life, God is forgiving and merciful. As one woman stated, "God never does anything bad like that. He's all goodness. He's big. He never harms. He's generous. He forgives. God has his own wisdom."

Those women who disagree with this view tend to be ones who feel that they (or their husbands) are, in fact, being punished for their mistakes and improprieties. These include, *inter alia*, failing to pray; refusing an arranged marriage; commiting adultery, premarital sex, or prostitution; engaging in malicious gossiping or wishing harm to one's enemies; using birth control before having children; being tyrannical or abusive to one's spouse; divorcing a spouse and abandoning one's children; interfering with a sibling's wedding plans; and committing a heinous crime, such as beating, raping, or killing someone.

Obviously, there are levels of difference between these misdeeds, with greater misdeeds being punished more severely, according to those who view God's punishment in this way. For example, a woman who underwent three abortions shortly after her marriage to a coercive husband who eventually divorced her is certain that her continuing infertility in her second marriage is God's way of punishing her. "I cry all the time now that I did them," she lamented. "I'm afraid from God that I'm going to hell. But I think I was too young then, and I did as I was told by my husband."

Furthermore, God is seen as punishing those who doubt his wisdom. Thus, infertile women who lament their fate and ask repeatedly "Why me?" are considered unlikely to receive God's favor of children. As one woman explained, "God gets angry and will never give you."

Indeed, as apparent in the Qur'an, God regards children as a great favor to believers, extolling the virtues of children in his proclamation, "Wealth and children are the adornment of earthly life." Yet, he reminds believers that wealth and children are also human beings' greatest temptations, and he cautions that good deeds are more deserving of reward in his eyes.

Thus, according to poor urban Egyptian women, religious faith and devotion to a merciful and compassionate God are the only *true* hope for overcoming a problem that he created, for reasons that only he can know. For Egyptians, who attempt to surmise these reasons without questioning their divine inspiration and authority, ultimate causes of and solutions to infertility problems lie with God himself, who helps his worshippers in their quests to overcome the more proximate and medial causes of infertility that he creates. Thus, it is God who decides the outcome of each woman's therapeutic quest, including if and when conception will occur.

However, because the gift of fertility is ultimately incumbent upon God's divine wisdom and will, convincing God of one's worthiness as a (re)productive member of society and as a parent is viewed by many Egyptian women as an essential part of the "search for children." How one seeks to demonstrate one's worthiness depends to some degree on one's religious orientation, level of religiosity, and religious education. For poor urban Egyptian women—who tend to be minimally schooled, religiously illiterate, "religious" but not devout, and who often do not pray regularly, because of their lack of knowledge of the formulaic prayer verses and the culturally grounded belief that prayer is an activity restricted to men and older women—leading an upright life is seen as the best demonstration of one's worthiness in the eyes of God and one's ongoing devotion to him. Many women attempt to pray informally, if not frequently and correctly, and generally attempt to be good Muslims by following widely accepted religious codes of behavior. For some, the experience of infertility also makes them more religious, given their conviction that they and their husbands are being "tested" by God in order for him to determine the sincerity and strength of their faith and patience.

However, for many of these women, an exceptional demonstration of one's devotion, belief, and faith in God involves *ziyārāt*, or "visits" (pilgrimages), to holy places associated with the dead *shuyūkh bil-baraka* favored by God for their goodness and piety.

Healing Pilgrimage

In the western Nile Delta region of Egypt, thousands of Muslim pilgrims make *ziyārāt* to the many shrines, some large, some quite small, dotting the urban and rural landscape. Most of these shrines contain the tombs of dead saints, and some, especially the relatively famous ones, host magnificent mosque-tomb complexes. Most of these shrines are associated in some way with a dead "pious one" (Eickelman 1989)—a *sayyid* (a descendant of the Prophet Muhammad); a renowned cleric who is regarded as pious for the quality of his learning; a founder or descendant of a founder of a *Ṣūfī* religious brotherhood; or a "holy" person, male or female, known for exceptional religiosity and the demonstrated ability during his or her lifetime to perform "miracles." For the masses of rural and urban poor Egyptians who visit these sites as pilgrims—given that pilgrimage of this sort tends to be a class-based phenomenon (Biegman 1990)—these dead *shuyūkh*, as all Muslim religious notables are called, are believed to radiate *baraka*, a living form of beneficial power associated with divine blessing, grace, or holiness, which is transferrable to their descendants, followers, and visitors (Biegman 1990).

Belief in the miraculous *baraka* of saints, the formation of "cults" involved in the veneration of such saints, and the subsequent movement of thousands of miracle-seeking pilgrims to and from saints' shrines are considered to be among the major hallmarks of North African Islam (Crapanzano 1973; Eickelman 1976; Eickelman and Piscatori 1990a; Gellner 1969). Although Egypt is usually not regarded as part of this North African complex, scholars of Egypt have documented the existence of similar cults of saints, primarily *Ṣūfīs*, dating back to at least the sixteenth century (Gilsenan 1973; Gran 1979). From the beginning, these cults were involved in healing, especially among the poor and among women, whose conditions had worsened with the development of protocapitalist market conditions in the country (Gran 1979).

Today in Egypt, the poor, and poor women in particular, continue to worship dead, miracle-working saints, whose tombs, if relatively accessible, they may visit on a regular basis. Indeed, in Egypt, it is women—not men—who are most actively involved in saint veneration and who are therefore the primary participants in the salvation-oriented *ziyārāt* to local and regional saints' tombs. The essentially "female character" of local pilgrimage in the Middle East (Betteridge 1983)—and men's accompanying embarrassment and even disdain regarding this activity—has been noted by a number of scholars working in various regions of the Middle East (Crapanzano 1973; Dwyer 1978; Mernissi 1977; Tapper 1990). Yet, with a few notable exceptions, the character of female participation in saint worship and pilgrimage has been poorly studied, in part because of lack of interest and in part because of the inaccessibility of these activities to Western male researchers (Betteridge 1989). In her examination of why Muslim women more often than Muslim men are concerned with shrine visitation and why such women's visits are often disparaged by men, Tapper notes:

> In academic studies of Muslim societies, men's ideals, beliefs, and actions have usually been privileged above those of women; typically, this bias confirms and reinforces the bias against women that is intrinsic to Muslim cultural traditions themselves. If questions of gender are to be investigated, it is essential to analyse a notion such as *ziyaret* that has a prominent place in practised Islam, and to consider implicit behaviours that are associated with it. (1990:237)

That Tapper's essay on gender and pilgrimage in Turkey is the only one of its kind in a recent volume devoted to *Muslim Travellers* (Eickelman and Piscatori 1990b) is typical of the androcentrism in Middle Eastern pilgrimage studies. Likewise, the nexus between healing and pilgrimage, which often go hand in hand, is overlooked in that volume, and has been underprivileged in general as a topic of serious Middle Eastern scholarship. Although it is easy to find passing references to women's involvement in healing pilgrimages to saints' shrines,[4] extended discussions are virtually absent in the ethnographic or other social scientific literature. To wit, in the only major work on Middle Eastern *Ṣūfī* healing, Crapanzano (1973), who studied the psychotherapeutically oriented Hamadsha order of Morocco, essentially discounts the experiences of women, including what appears to be their active participation as "patients" in both the Hamadsha healing rituals themselves and in pilgrimages to the Hamadsha saints' tombs. For example, Crapanzano mentions the problem of "barrenness" in passing five times, citing it as one of the primary reasons why *women* seek Hamadsha healing and journey to the Hamadsha *zawiya*s, or lodges, and to the saints' mosque-tombs located in a distant, rural area. However, his psychoanalytically oriented discussion of the Hamadsha "system of therapy" focuses exclusively on *male* role conflict and mentions nothing of the conflicts faced by infertile women unable to continue the male line in this monogenetically oriented society.

Among women in Egypt and elsewhere in the Middle East, healing, as well as the solution of other difficult life problems, is a primary impetus for *ziyārāt* to saints' shrines (Betteridge 1983, 1992; Dwyer 1978; Early 1993b; Mernissi 1977; Morsy 1993). Such healing, furthermore, may be multifaceted. On the one hand, belief in *baraka* and the abilities of *baraka*-bestowing dead *shuyūkh* to perform miraculous cures, including the restoration of fecundity to the infertile, brings hope to those whose health problems seem intractable or who have failed to find relief in other therapeutic venues. In addition, the activities of the pilgrimage itself—including the respite from everyday routine, the exhilaration of travel to a spiritually "magnetic" center (Preston 1992), the cathartic effects of unburdening one's "private heartaches" (Tapper 1990) on a nonjudgmental but responsive holy one who can be requested to act on one's behalf, the ability to be part of a sympathetic, experienced community of female sufferers who often congregate at these shrines (Mernissi 1977), and the ministrations of the living *shuyūkh bil-baraka* who often attend to these shrines and who pray and write healing *ḥugub* for suffering pilgrims—are part and parcel of the healing process. Thus, even if miraculous cures do not eventuate, the pilgrimage itself may bring relief and "psychological relaxation," as well as spiritual renewal through contact with divinity (Betteridge 1983).

Furthermore, as Mernissi (1977) has noted, Middle Eastern women's pilgrimages to holy sanctuaries are "power operations," means by which subaltern women can seek control over their sexuality and fertility in societies that tend to be emphatically patriarchal. The *empowering* effects of pilgrimage stand in stark contrast to women's *disempowering* encounters with physicians and hospitals, which, as we shall see in the following chapters, are often subordinating, frustrating, even humiliating experiences for poor Egyptian women. Speaking of Moroccan women's similar experiences, Mernissi states:

> In the . . . hospitals, women hold a classically powerless position, condemned to be subjects, receptacles of impersonal decisions, executors of orders

> given by males. In a public hospital, the doctor is the expert, the representative of the bureaucratic order, empowered by the written law to tell her what to do; the illiterate woman can only execute his orders. . . . Moreover, the hospital is a strange, alien setting, a modern building full of enigmatic written signs on doors and corridors. . . . In comparison to the guardians who stand at the hospital's gates and its offices, the saint's tomb is directly accessible to troubled persons. . . . The task of the saint is to help her reach her goal. She will give him a gift or a sacrifice only if he realizes her wishes, not before. With a doctor, she has to buy the prescription first and has no way of retaliating if the medicine does not have the proper effect. It is no wonder, then, that in spite of modern health services, women still go to the sanctuaries in swarms, before they go to the hospital, or simultaneously, or after. Saints give women vital help that modern public health services cannot give. They embody the refusal to accept arrogant expertise, to submit blindly to authority, to be treated as subordinate. . . . Visits to and involvement with saints and sanctuaries are two of the rare options left to women to *be*, to shape their world and their lives. And this attempt at self-determination takes the form of an exclusively female collective endeavor. (1977:103–4)

In Egypt as in Morocco, pilgrimages to saints' tombs allow women to reaffirm, if only temporarily, control over their lives and their personal well-being through actions that are autonomous from men. Typically, *ziyārāt* to the mosque-tombs of blessed *shuyūkh* are journeys that women make alone, allowing women the opportunity to demonstrate their activism and independence. Furthermore, travel may be arduous; among Alexandrian women, for example, four of the five major pilgrimage centers they visit are located in distant cities and require that women face and overcome the importunities of public transportation. Thus, even though women's *ziyārāt* often require money from husbands and, in most cases, permission to travel by husbands or other family members, the pilgrimage typically remains an exclusive female activity, with shrines often serving as protected "female turf" (Betteridge 1983).

For the poor Egyptian women who make pilgrimages to these shrines, their journeys are typically instrumental quests, motivated in large part by their desire to obtain solutions to and relief from major problems plaguing their lives or those of their loved ones. For many infertile women, the quest for divine intervention through pilgrimages to holy sites is considered an integral part of the search for children, and, for some, is a component of their overall quest for therapy that may be repeated many times during their "crisis years" (Dwyer 1978) as potentially reproductive, but infecund women.

In the view of infertile women, there are two compelling reasons for making such pilgrimages. First, many poor Egyptian women believe that mosques and other holy places are "houses of God" and that God is more likely to hear and answer their prayers in a "pure" place where he is certain to be present. Thus, Egyptian women tend to distinguish between "normal" prayer at home and prayer in a pilgrimage center. Essentially, women believe the shrines of saints to be better settings for making their direct, "prayer-requests" to God. For infertile women, these prayer-requests are usually quite straightforward—namely, women ask their merciful God to grant them a child.

However, after registering their direct prayer-requests to God, women make a second, "indirect" prayer-request to the *shaikh bil-baraka* to whom the shrine is dedicated. As women understand it, *shuyūkh bil-baraka*, who are "dead but alive," are "close to God" and can therefore serve as divine intermediaries by helping to ensure that God hears and considers the original prayer-request. Furthermore, praying to *shuyūkh* who are known to be close to God is a way of obtaining some of the *shuyūkh*'s *baraka* itself, which, in essence, is like receiving God's grace. The desire to obtain *baraka* from holy *shuyūkh* is a major reason why many Egyptian women prefer to make their prayer-requests at pilgrimage centers. With this transfer of *baraka*—usually obtained through the circumambulation of the saint's tomb and touching of the cloth covering his grave—women feel empowered and believe that their chances of being rewarded by God are ultimately much greater.

Furthermore, women typically vow to compensate the *shaikh bil-baraka* for his intercessional role. These vows tend to involve tangible promises of material repayment for the *shaikh*'s spiritual and material assistance—but if and only if a woman's prayer-request is granted. For example, a woman whose infertility problem was linked to her husband's impotence visited a famous Alexandrian mosque-tomb after having gone for an entire year without having sexual relations with her husband. In the mosque, she first asked God to help her with her problem, and then she asked the same of the *baraka*-bestowing *shaikh*, promising to return with "whatever amount of money" she could afford if he interceded on her behalf. As she explained, "as soon as I arrived home, we had sex."

Such "reciprocity" to *shuyūkh* on the part of poor infertile women takes many forms. Some women promise that they will return to the pilgrimage site annually, often at the time of the saint's *mūlid*, and they may promise to make an annual contribution as well. Other women promise to bring small gifts to the shrine, such as toys to be distributed to poor children, or paint to refurbish the shrine, or candles, cloths, and handkerchiefs to illuminate and decorate the grave, or new prayer-rugs for the mosque floor. Still others promise to hire a *shaikh* to read the Qur'an or a religious singer to praise the Prophet.

Partly because of the contractual nature of the vowing process and partly because of the worship and veneration of intermediary figures (which is anathema to Islam, constituting, as it does, the supreme sin of *shirk*, the association of other beings with God), women's pilgrimage activities in Egypt and elsewhere in the Middle East are considered quite controversial by orthodox religious forces, as well as by many men, who eschew what they view as the self-serving quality of such activities (Betteridge 1989; Tapper 1990). As Tapper (1990) sees it, it is the content of women's exchanges in particular—which are neither "pure gifts" nor forms of market exchange—that may explain why *ziyārāt* are derided by men with such "dismissive hostility." She notes:

> Ironically, precisely because the women's activities blur the kinds of exchanges which are well-defined and prestigious in terms of orthodox religion . . . women confirm, to men and themselves, their distance from the sources of both supernatural and secular power. In each case the exchanges associated with women's movements outside the home become a further expression of women's marginality and dubious orthodoxy, while their inferior gender status becomes a self-fulfilling ideology in itself. (Tapper 1990:253)

Yet, for poor infertile women, their strictly *quid pro quo* transactions with dead *shuyūkh*, who receive "payment" only *if* they solve a woman's problems, are preferrable to the often "useless" and exorbitantly expensive encounters with other healers, who tend to exact compensation before their "cures" are ever realized. Furthermore, as seen in the previous chapter, the fees demanded by healers for their services may be well beyond the means of poor women and their husbands, who are often forced to delay therapeutic intervention until sufficient funds for treatment can be secured. The same is true of biogynecologists in Egypt, who rarely offer "sliding scales" of payment for poor patients and who charge in one office visit what a poor family may expect to earn in an entire month. Thus, vowing to saints—and the inherently individualized process of determining appropriate, affordable, cash and noncash repayments, "according to one's means"—makes immanent sense to poor women, whose access to monetary funds are usually quite restricted.

Furthermore, part of the appeal of pilgrimage in Egypt lies in the presence of living *shuyūkh bil-baraka*, who frequent pilgrimage centers and are thought of as healers in their own right. Some of these *shuyūkh* are descendants of the dead *shuyūkh* enshrined in their tombs. At shrines dedicated to *Ṣūfīs*, many are members of the saint's brotherhood, and some are considered to have acquired the dead *shaikh*'s *baraka* through years of devoted service to the perpetuation of his memory. For troubled pilgrims, these living *shuyūkh* may offer a number of special services, such as the reading of the Qur'an "over" them, the writing of religious *ḥugub*, and the pronouncement of special *ṣalāwāt*, or healing prayers. Some *shuyūkh* may not speak, but may initiate bodily contact, such as the touching of pilgrims' hands, bestowing their own *baraka* on the afflicted in this manner. Many of these *shuyūkh*, furthermore, preside over collection boxes, where pilgrims make their devotional alms and repay the saint for miraculous services rendered.

Muslim Pilgrimage Centers in Northwestern Egypt

For women in Alexandria and the northwestern Nile Delta region of Egypt, there are five major pilgrimage centers, comprising large mosque-tomb complexes located in Cairo, Alexandria, and two provincial cities in between. Although *ziyārāt* to these major centers are desirable, they are often impractical for women, who journey instead to lesser shrines, which, nonetheless, may offer more specialized healing. For many poor women, *ziyārāt* to the "big" shrines offer once-in-a-lifetime opportunities to visit other cities, particularly Cairo, which is an infrequent destination for the Alexandrian poor. In Cairo, the number of shrines is tremendous (Biegman 1990), but Alexandrian women generally recognize two as being of supreme importance, with the three other "big" shrines being located closer to home. These pilgrimage centers can be described as follows.[5]

Mosque of Sayyidnā al-Ḥusayn (Cairo)

The mosque of Sayyidnā al-Ḥusayn is one of Cairo's principal pilgrimage centers and is one of two in which entry is forbidden to non-Muslims.[6] The head of Ḥusayn, one of the twin sons of Fatima, the Prophet Muhammad's daughter, is said to be buried here. Because of this, the mosque is a major pilgrimage site for Egyptians, as well as for Shi'a Muslims from around the world, who revere Ḥusayn and his father Ali (the fourth caliph and son-in-law of the Prophet) as Shi'a martyrs. For the Shi'a community, the celebration commemorating the *mūlid*, or birthday, of Ḥusayn is one of the most important events in the calendar year of religious celebrations and is held for two weeks around the mosque in Cairo. For the urban and rural poor of

Egypt, who are predominantly Sunni Muslims, the mosque is also a major pilgrimage center throughout the year, given its dedication to the Prophet's grandson.

Mosque of Sayyidah Zaynab (Cairo)

Many pilgrims who visit the mosque of Sayyidnā al-Ḥusayn also visit the mosque dedicated to his sister, Zaynab, who fled to Cairo and who died and was buried at the site of this mosque. As with the mosque of her brother, the mosque of Sayyidah Zaynab is restricted to Muslims, and, similarly, it is the site of a major *mūlid* celebration, which lasts two weeks and which is attended by both non-Egyptian Shi'a and Egyptian Sunni Muslims.

Mosque and Tomb of Sayyid Aḥmad al-Badawī (Tanta)

In the provincial city of Tanta, located on the major agricultural highway between Cairo and Alexandria, the mosque-tomb of Sayyid Aḥmad al-Badawī, a thirteenth-century founder of a still operative *Ṣūfī* brotherhood, is a major pilgrimage center, attracting as many as two million visitors during the *shaikh*'s *mūlid* alone. Because of the *shaikh*'s founding of the Badawiyyah (also called Ahmadiyyah) *Ṣūfī* brotherhood, the magnificence of his large mosque-tomb, and his spectacular *mūlid* celebration, which follows directly after the major cotton harvest and is the largest in the Delta region, this pilgrimage center is one of the most active in northern Egypt and is the subject of two recent scholarly works, including an ethnographic film called *El Moulid* by the Egyptian-born anthropologist Fadwa El Guindi and a text entitled *The Hidden Government* by Reeves (1990).

Mosque and Tomb of Sayyid Ibrāhīm Dasūqī (Dasuq)

In the agricultural town of Dasuq, located northwest of Cairo and southeast of Alexandria, the mosque-tomb of Sayyid Ibrāhīm Dasūqī, an eminent *Ṣūfī shaikh* and student of Sayyid Aḥmad al-Badawī, is another major pilgrimage site, second only to that of al-Badawī's in Tanta. The *shaikh* to whom this large mosque is dedicated was born into an Egyptian *Sūfī* family and studied under Shaikh al-Badawī, reaching such a high state of knowledge that he was encouraged to start his own brotherhood, known as the Dasūqiyyah (also Burhamiyyah). His *mūlid* is second in size only to that of Aḥmad al-Badawī in Tanta and follows directly after al-Badawī's.

Mosque and Tomb of Abū 'l-'Abbās al-Mursī (Alexandria)

For Alexandrians, the mosque and tomb of Abū 'l-'Abbās al-Mursī, located on the shores of the Mediterranean in central Alexandria, is their primary pilgrimage site, renowned for its elegant minarets and domes, which are located over the tomb of Shaikh al-Mursī and three other venerated *shuyūkh* who are said to be buried there. Like Aḥmad al-Badawī and Ibrāhīm Dasūqī, Abū 'l-'Abbās al-Mursī was a *Ṣūfī shaikh*, leader of the Alexandrian Shadhili brotherhood. Although less spectacular than the aforementioned *mūlid*s, the *mūlid* of Abū 'l-'Abbās al-Mursī is a major attraction for Alexandrians and for those who come as pilgrims from the northwestern Nile Delta region of Egypt.

Minor Pilgrimage Centers

In addition to these five major pilgrimage centers, a number of smaller mosque-tombs and shrines serve as minor pilgrimage sites and are known among local inhabitants for their small *mūlid* festivals. In Alexandria, for example, at least five other mosques, including those dedicated to the *shuyūkh* Sidi Gabr, Sidi Busiri, Sidi Kamal, Sidi Bishr, and Sidi Abari, are considered holy sites for *baraka*-seeking Muslim pilgrims. Likewise, the tomb of Abu Dardar, located in the old section of Alexandria, in the center of a major thoroughfare, is considered especially holy because of the fact that the tomb for this religious figure was built at the exact site of his death. Instead of moving the tomb, the Ministry of Transportation opted to build a tramline around the small structure, which is encircled by tracks.

For Alexandrian women, furthermore, the small mosque of Sitt Naima, located in the ancient Manshiyyah section of Alexandria, is especially important. Sitt Naima was one of God's "chosen" women, considered capable of curing other women's health problems. Today, her *baraka*, which is obtained by drinking or rubbing one's body with the ablution water of her mosque, is considered useful in overcoming *kabsa* problems in particular. For this reason, many infertile women visit Sitt Naima's mosque in the hope of unbinding their wombs.

In fact, many smaller shrines have become renowned by virtue of their "specialization" (Betteridge 1992; Biegman 1990). Although saint/shrine specialization in the Middle East has been poorly studied, Betteridge (1992) has shown how specialized shrines develop their own body of legend and lore to account for their specialized character and capabilities. Typically, specialties in miracle-working are related to the hagiography of the saint and the correspondence between the saint's troubled biography and the facts surrounding the petitioner's plight. Thus, "shrines of conception" (Betteridge 1992) may be devoted to saints whose own lives or those of their mothers were plagued by infertility and miraculous reversals of this problem. Likewise, shrines devoted to women saints often specialize in the problems of mothers and children as they negotiate the difficulties surrounding marriage, maternity, and the threats of premature mortality.

Many of these specialized shrines may be quite modest in appearance, usually consisting only of a small, square building covered with a round, conical, or pointed dome (Biegman 1990). The dome typically marks the room where the grave, contained in a sarcophagus, is found. The sarcophagus is usually covered with a green or white embroidered cloth and is surrounded by a cage-like grill made of wood or metal. Around the sarcophagus, there is typically enough room for pilgrims to walk, sit, pray, or even lie down, and the bars of the grill may be spaced so that pilgrims' hands can reach the tomb inside.

Some shrines, furthermore, are characterized by their "sacred geography" (Preston 1992)—primarily their difficulty of access or their attachment to unusual natural features, such as grottoes, springs, ancient trees, or rock formations. Water from shrines attached to springs is usually considered to be endowed with the saint's *baraka* and is used by pilgrims for drinking or ablution purposes. Where trees or rocky protuberances are present, pilgrims may attach handkerchiefs or small strips of cloth to "remind" the saint of the need to "untie" their difficult problems.

Shrines of Conception

Shrines specializing in infertility can be found throughout Egypt (Biegman 1990), but three of those catering to Alexandrian women appear to be unique for a number of reasons. One of these shrines is a Muslim *shaikh*'s tomb, similar in some ways to those already described, but notable for its enclosure around an unusual rock thought to help "unbind" difficult physical problems, including the effects of *kabsa* and *khaḍḍa*. Another is a desert monastery dedicated to a miracle-making Coptic Christian saint whose mother bore him after many years of infertility and whose shrine is located on the site where camels deposited his dead body. The final pilgrimage "site," defunct as of mid-1989, was a secular one run by Bedouins of the Awlad 'Ali tribe; during the late 1980s, it served as a major pilgrimage center for Egyptian and other infertile Middle Eastern women and their husbands who came to drink the milk of a miraculous hermaphroditic goat.

Although differentiated along lines of sacredness versus secularity and Christianity versus Islam, these three pilgrimage sites are united by the fact that, as natural anomalies, they are believed capable of providing solutions to women *made anomalous* by virtue of their infertility. In all three of these sites, the "cures" offered for infertility are explained in religious terms, although the nature of the healing rituals taking place in them would be described as quite profane by orthodox Muslims.

While in Egypt in the late 1980s, I made my own *ziyārāt* to all three of these shrines of conception, in two cases with infertile women for the purpose of healing. The descriptions that follow reflect my own experiences at these pilgrimage centers and are based, in large part, on verbatim excerpts from my fieldnotes.

Tomb of Shaikh Il-Khibari

In a Muslim cemetery outside of the agricultural town of Kafr al-Dawwar, southeast of Alexandria, a small, domed building atop the cemetery hill contains the tomb of the community's most renowned *shaikh bil-baraka*, Shaikh Il-Khibari. Although the *shaikh*'s tomb itself—ensconced in a small, dimly lit room, with a brass grill enclosing the green-velvet-covered sarcophagus—is relatively nondescript, it is attached to a small chamber in which a powerful stone is located. According to sources at the pilgrimage site, this stone, which rises naturally out of the ground adjacent to the *shaikh*'s tomb, is considered to be geologically unlike any other in Egypt. It is phallic-shaped and, interestingly enough, is to be "licked" by the mostly female pilgrims to the point at which their tongues begin to bleed. If licked over three consecutive Fridays at the time of the Muslim noon prayer, the rock is thought to be extremely effective in causing the effects of *kabsa* to vanish, thereby curing *kabsa*-bound infertile women who want to become pregnant. According to sources at the rock-tomb, many women have unbound *kabsa* problems in this way; in fact, a woman in this study and the paternal aunt of another informant reported having successfully unbound their *kabsa* problems through such rock-licking rituals.

Because of the notoriety of this site as an infertility healing center, numerous women in this study noted their desires to visit the rock-tomb as pilgrims. This was difficult for most, however, because of the trouble involved in reaching this rather remote destination without a car. Because of my own desires to make this pilgrimage, I organized transportation for myself and two infertile women in the study who had shown particular interest in visiting this site. This excerpt from my fieldnotes depicts our journey:

"After driving through Kafr al-Dawwar and its Friday market, we found a back road that led to the *shaikh*'s tomb containing the rock. A large mosque stood on the way to the cemetery, and colorful horse-drawn carriages could be hired to ride from the mosque to the cemetery where the *shaikh*'s tomb stood. His small, single-domed tomb sat atop the open, hillside cemetery and could be seen from the road below, where we stopped and parked the car. All of us bailed out and began walking through the aboveground tombs to the *shaikh*'s tomb on high. It was a sunny day, and I felt as though I were on a hike, since I found us ascending on a small dirt path amidst boulders and tombs. Once we got to the top, we knew we had reached the proper destination. It was about 11:30 A.M. by this time, and soon the noon prayer would begin. Indeed, this ritual, as with most of the '*kabsa*-removing' rituals, was supposed to occur during the Friday noon prayer and was to be repeated by each participant over three consecutive Fridays.

"A number of people, mostly female but some males as well, had already congregated at the tomb. The tomb consisted of two rooms. To the right (facing it) was the dome under which was the *shaikh*'s tomb itself. It was an aboveground structure, about neck-high, and was covered with green velvet. On top of it was the Qur'an. The tomb was enclosed by a brass railing, but the gaps in the railing were large enough to allow insertion of a human hand and touching of the velvet—thereby procuring some of the *shaikh*'s *baraka*. Hadaya [one of the women accompanying me] asked me to join her in this *baraka*-procuring ritual, so I removed my shoes (mandatory) and walked around the *shaikh*'s tomb with her.

"As noon drew nearer, the licking ritual began in the small attached room to the left. This was the room housing the mysterious stone, which was not as I had imagined it at all. I was under the impression from informants' descriptions that the stone was pointed and that this 'point' caused the tongue to bleed when licked. Rather, the stone was dull and the consistency of sandpaper. It stood about two to three feet high and was large enough in diameter to allow two to three lickers at a time. The licking process was monitored by an old woman who stood at the door to the 'rock room' and allowed participants to enter and depart. She was piebald, having an advanced case of vitiligo. She was accompanied by a younger man who appeared to be mentally deficient or mentally ill. His role was undefined.

"Soon, the woman began ordering the participants in and out. Most of the women looked to be of the same [social] class as Hadaya and Madiha [the two women with me], and I noticed that one young peasant man and an adolescent boy also participated. The ritual began with a frenzy, and it was, for me, the most disturbing thing I had seen in a long time. Huge-buttocked women squatted aside the abrasive stone and began licking until

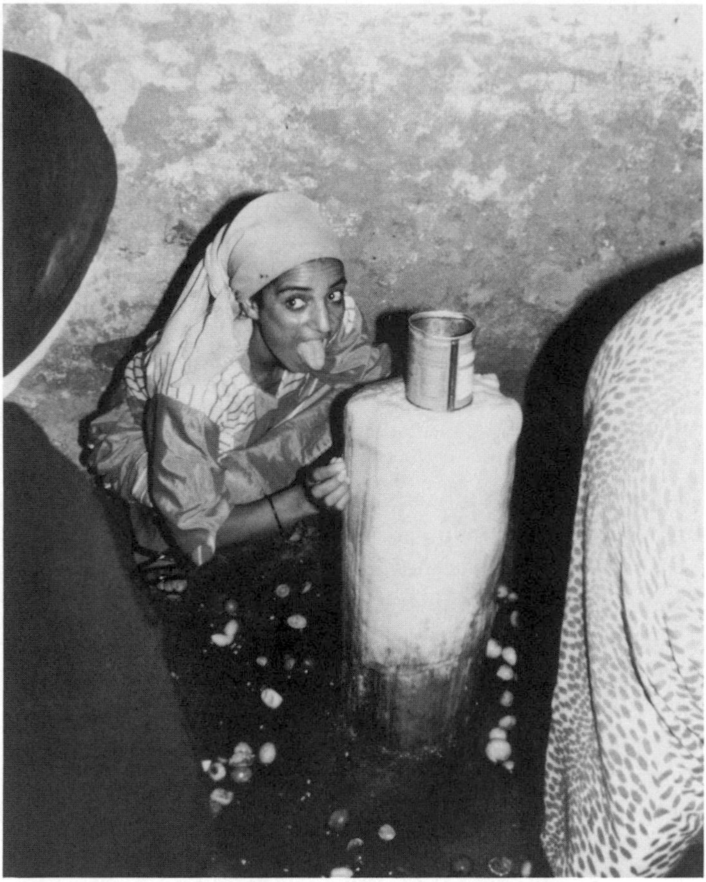

Photograph 7. A pilgrim licking the rock at Shaikh Il-Khibari's Tomb. (Photograph by Marcia Inhorn)

their tongues bled. Once blood was produced, they emerged from the room, squeezing lemons on their tongues and then spitting the blood and juice on the ground. Meanwhile, the piebald gatekeeper 'cleansed' the stone with water, which she poured over it from a small metal pitcher. The water trickled down to a 'moat' around the stone, and then out a drainage ditch that led downhill. I noticed that this thin ditch was filled with discarded lemons and coagulated blood. I almost passed out just looking at it.

"Apparently, Hadaya, too, was scared by the whole bloody event, because before her 'turn' had come, she went to the car, under the pretense of getting me my camera bag. [When she returned] I told her that she did not have to participate in it if she was scared and that I was scared, too.

Most of all, I could not imagine what one might contract from the licking, and I thought especially of blood-borne and -transmitted diseases such as hepatitis B and AIDS. However, Madiha was determined to undertake the licking, and Hadaya felt inclined to go with her. The two of them squatted against the rock, and Madiha was the first to bleed, despite her outbursts of laughter. Hadaya, on the other hand, was having a hard time producing any blood, and I believe this is what caused Madiha to laugh. After about five minutes, Madiha emerged with a completely bloodied tongue, which I photographed. Hadaya eventually followed and showed a little blood, but not as much as Madiha. Madiha had brought lemons to squeeze [on their tongues], and they completed the ritual in this way. I had never imagined such an episode, and, for me, the 'pilgrimage' was well worth it, although I felt rather unnerved by it."

Monastery and Church of Saint Mena

Although little has been said here about Coptic Christians in Egypt, Coptic women are just as likely as Muslim women to embark on an ethnogynecological quest for conception involving pilgrimages to sites associated with religious personages. In fact, although the Coptic Christian religion and its orthodoxy differ substantially from that of Islam, the nature of its local-level religious pilgrimages and pilgrimage centers does not. Essentially, both Christians and Muslims visit these pilgrimage sites because of the exalted character of the religious notables to whom the sites are dedicated and who are often entombed there. Both Christians and Muslims believe in the concept of the *baraka* of these religious figures, who, among Christians, are usually the purported descendants of the family of Jesus, Coptic saints, and notable priests or monks. Both Christians and Muslims accept the empowering prayers and *ḥugub* of living religious figures—priests and *shuyūkh*, respectively—at these sites. And both Christians and Muslims may attempt to obtain *baraka* through the ingestion of or anointment of their bodies with holy waters found at the pilgrimage site. Likewise, both Christians and Muslims accept the intermediary role of the religious figures to whom they pray, although this is considered to be orthodox in only one of these religions (namely, Coptic Christianity). And, although Muslims accept the notion of God's "miracles," Copts are much more likely to believe in and extol the miraculous powers of their once-human saints, such as the one to be described here.

Of the many pilgrimage sites visited by Coptic Christians in northern Egypt, the one frequented most often by infertile women is that dedicated to Saint Mena (also known as Menas), the "Miracle Worker."[7] According to legend, Mena was born in the second-century to Euoxius, governor of Pentapolis (to the west of Alexandria in eastern Libya) and his infertile Egyptian wife, whose prayers to God for a child were answered in the birth of her son, Mena. After his parents died, Mena entered the Roman army, where he was ordered to assist in the persecution of Christians. After deserting and then returning to the Roman army, declaring himself a Christian, and refusing to take part in the persecution, Mena was beheaded. Although his body was supposed to be cremated, it was rescued by the troops with whom he had fought, who were then transferred to Egypt. There, they were forced to abandon the heavy sarcophagus of their friend on their return to Phrygia when the camels bearing the exhumed coffin refused to carry it. They buried Mena where the camels stopped, at the small desert village called Est'. Many years later, villagers became aware of the healing powers of the tomb of Mena and built a small dome over it. Once discovered, the reputation of Saint Mena attracted other pilgrims, and a church was built. The relics of the martyr were transferred to the crypt of this church, which, within a few years, could no longer accommodate the throngs of pilgrims.

Thus, a major pilgrimage center, known for its healing powers, eventually developed, reaching its apex during the late fifth and early sixth centuries, when the emperor Zeno visited the site and built a palace and town for the pilgrims. Thousands of pilgrims coming from as far as Europe are thought to have visited the site to be healed by its sacred waters. (Flasks embossed with a relief of the saint have been found throughout the Middle East and medieval European sites.) However, by the twelfth century, the town was in ruins and was no longer a place of pilgrimage, having been ravaged by Bedouins. Centuries later, however, excavations of the site began, and the Shrine of Saint Mena was discovered in 1905. In 1959, the Coptic Monastery of Saint Mena was founded at the site, and the relics of Saint Mena were transferred there from Cairo. (The preparation and handling of relics, whether hairs or bones, is typically Christian.)

Today, the Monastery of Saint Mena, located in the desert west of Alexandria, is a thriving pilgrimage center, attracting nearly twenty thousand pilgrims on the saint's birthday alone. Pilgrims come largely for the healing powers of the martyr Saint Mena, who is said to perform many miracles in this respect. In addition, Pope Kyrillos VI, the former head of the Egyptian Coptic Church who oversaw the restoration of the Monastery of Saint Mena during his reign from 1959 to 1971, is buried there and is the best-known saint in the category of holy monks. According to Biegman (1990), "Father Kyrillos" may be the most actively venerated Coptic saint of this century, and he is said to work many miracles either by himself or with the aid of Saint Mena.

Because of the reputation of the Monastery of Saint Mena as a pilgrimage site specializing in infertility, I decided to visit the site with two American friends who, having been raised as Catholics, were interested in accompanying me. This excerpt from my fieldnotes depicts our "pilgrimage" to the site:

"I had been wanting to visit Saint Mena's monastery in the Amriya district and had been informally invited by a Christian family. Instead, I decided to make this excursion with Ellen and Bill [American friends], who, as Catholics, had been interested in this Christian pilgrimage center. I hired [a Muslim driver], who did his duty in getting us there, although I could tell that he was distressed at being so close to Christianity. The monastery was truly in the middle of nowhere, and when Ellen and Bill spotted what looked like a two-shafted mosque in the distance, I doubted that it was our destination. I was incredulous to discover that this was, indeed, the monastery, as apparent from the crosses atop the tall domes on the entrance.

"When we entered the monastery compound . . . a black-bearded Coptic monk appeared in a black robe and black hood with gold crosses [to greet us]. His job was to take us to the relics of Saint (Mary in Coptic) Mena, which had been found at the spot on which the monastery was built and which have been preserved in a gaudy shrine room. The small shrine room was full of aluminum-foil-type, sparkling religious pictures, and in the corner was a small 'tomb' filled with the relics of the saint. There, we stood (barefooted) with the monk as he explained to us the significance of Saint Mena, the 'Miracle Worker.'

"One of my Christian informants had told me that infertile Christian women visit this monastery to pray for fertility. Apparently, Saint Mena's mother had been infertile and had prayed to God to give her a child, and he blessed her with Mena. Thus, Christian women hope that such a 'miracle' will happen to them. When I asked the monk if this was true, he affirmed the story, and then proceeded to tell us of his own friend who had been infertile. After consulting physicians in Europe, the friend had returned to Egypt and to the monastery, where he visited the relics and took some of the sacred oil. (We were each given samples of this oil in small vials. The monk said that some people use it as a lotion, while others drink it.) Soon, the monk's friend's wife was pregnant, after being told that there was no chance of her ever having children. The monk told us of other miracle

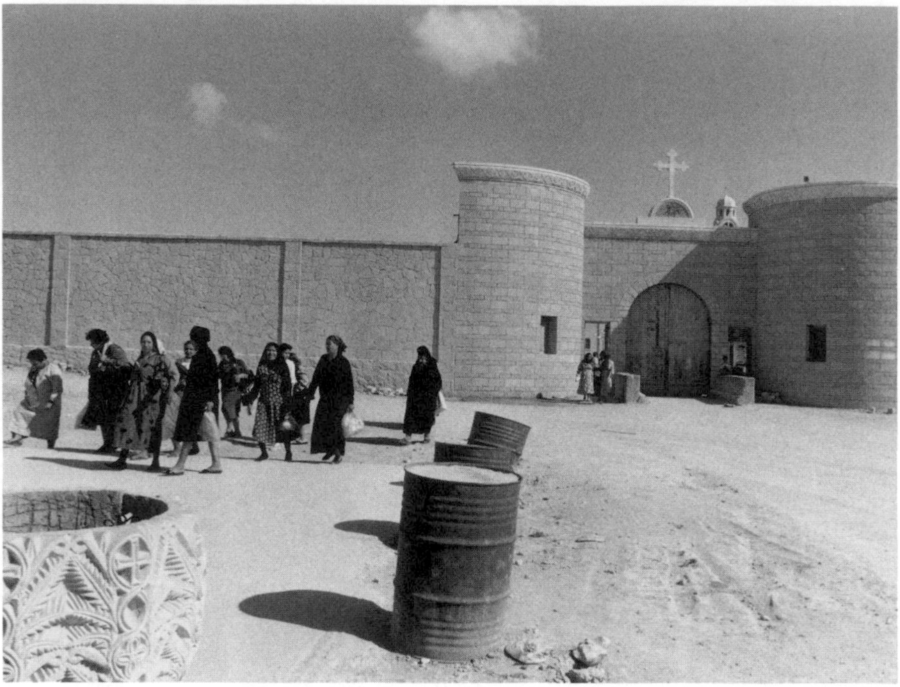

Photograph 8. Pilgrims leaving the Monastery of Saint Mena. (Photograph by Marcia Inhorn)

cures . . . and said that Christians throughout Egypt know Saint Mena not by his name, but by the title 'Miracle Worker.'"

The Hermaphroditic Goat

In Egypt, the sacred *baraka* and miracles associated with dead religious personages are the primary attractions for pilgrims, who seek the extraordinary powers of dead saints in an attempt to solve the problems of worldly living. Pilgrimage sites need not be sacred, however (Morinis 1992). Secular pilgrimage centers may take different forms, but may appeal to pilgrims for the same reason—namely, for their extraordinary ability to help human beings who are faced with seemingly insurmountable problems. Indeed, the anomalous nature of most secular pilgrimage sites is their main feature and is the one that imbues them with significance and power. Furthermore, as Preston (1992) has noted, unusual pilgrimage centers marked by their "spiritual magnetism" may achieve rapid notoriety and equally rapid decline. This should become abundantly apparent in the story of the hermaphroditic goat that follows.

During the period of this study, a secular pilgrimage center came to full fruition in Egypt—reaching over a period of ten months considerable notoriety throughout Egypt and neighboring nations for its hermaphroditic goat, a male whose anomalous ability to produce milk was believed to be therapeutically significant. The Awlad ʿAli Bedouin family who owned the ten-year-old, milk-producing *gidi*, or male goat, decided after some years of noticing the goat's aberrant behavior to tell tribal leaders of their unusual creature. News of the milk-producing male goat spread rapidly. Within months, hundreds of pilgrims made their way to the desert homestead of the Bedouin family, located outside of the seaside town of Marsa Matruh on the way to the Egyptian-Libyan border. There, as many as twenty-five to one hundred pilgrims per day waited from the period of the morning to evening milkings to obtain two drafts of the goat's fresh milk.

Some pilgrims, who had come from as far as central Libya and Saudi Arabia, remained overnight in one of the Bedouin family's houses, receiving the family's hospitality and utilizing the pit latrine that the family had constructed especially for the use of pilgrims. Although the Bedouin family did not charge for the goat's milk, pilgrims often volunteered donations to help offset the cost of foodstuffs and water provided by the family. Furthermore, pilgrims who were "cured" of their infertility, diabetes, or kidney ailments—the three conditions for which the goat's milk was considered particularly efficacious—often returned to the Bedouins' household to tell of their miraculous recoveries and to offer gifts and money as repayment for the *gidi*'s services.

As word of the hermaphroditic goat spread, the Egyptian news media picked up on the story and published several articles describing the goat, with its complete male and female reproductive systems and its purported ability to cure infertility. As soon as these infertility healing claims were published, women in this study began talking of the goat, seeking information on the location of the site, and debating among themselves as to whether the claims could be true. Eventually, one woman in the study obtained the "*gidi*'s address" and asked me to join her and her husband on this pilgrimage, knowing that I might be able to provide transportation. The story of our pilgrimage and our discovery at the pilgrimage site are described here in excerpts from my fieldnotes and interviews with the Bedouin family who owned the remarkable *gidi*.

"Halima [a woman in the study] remarkably obtained the address for the hermaphroditic male milk-producing goat about which I had heard so much all year. Its owner was a Bedouin man living outside Marsa Matruh, one of the beautiful summer beach resorts in the Western desert. I decided that I would take Halima to this goat, since I very much wanted to see it and Halima very much wanted to drink from it. . . . Before the day of our travels, Halima informed me that Farag [her husband] must accompany us, since husbands, too, were expected to drink the goat's milk. I assembled picnic supplies and we left at the ungodly hour of 5:30 A.M.

"At about 10:30 A.M., we arrived at the entrance to Marsa Matruh, where there was a small police station. Mustafa [the driver] asked the guards about the address, and this aroused their curiosity. Mustafa told them that I was a '*duktūra*' who had come to study the goat all the way from America, and they informed us that our trip was in vain because the goat had been killed. They told us that the owner had been accused of overcharging for the goat milk and that the goat had been confiscated some months earlier and slaughtered.

"The Egyptians in the car were convinced of the veracity of the story and told me that we might as well head for the beach. I, on the other hand, was not convinced, since one of the guards had mentioned that we might go to see the Bedouin owner if we promised not to drink. This, of course, suggested to me that the goat might still be alive, but that the milk business had been officially shut down. So I told them that I wanted to go anyway.

"Indeed, we went and found the Bedouin's compound, which was before the entrance to Matruh and only a few hundred feet from the highway. It consisted of a number of stucco-like, one or two-room structures over a small expanse of ground. Soon, a tall, extremely thin, late-middle-aged man appeared and asked who we were looking for. We read him the name on the address, and he said that he was the owner of the goat. He welcomed us, flashing what appeared to be a new pair of dentures, and soon procured for all of us small glasses of Bedouin tea, which we drank sitting against the wall of one of the houses. From him, the various women of his family (including two cowives), and his grandsons, we learned the story of the goat's demise as follows:

> An army officer from Ismailia came with his infertile wife to drink the goat's milk. Because of the publicity surrounding the goat by this time, numerous pilgrims were attending the milkings each day, and, as a result, the amount of milk to be dispensed to each person was quite small—a spoonful to be exact. After the officer's wife had taken her spoonful, the officer refused to take his share. He complained that the amount was too little and insisted on being given more. The Bedouin's grandsons, who were administering the milking and the allotment of milk to the long line of drinkers, told the officer that he could have no more, given that he was no different from the rest of the people

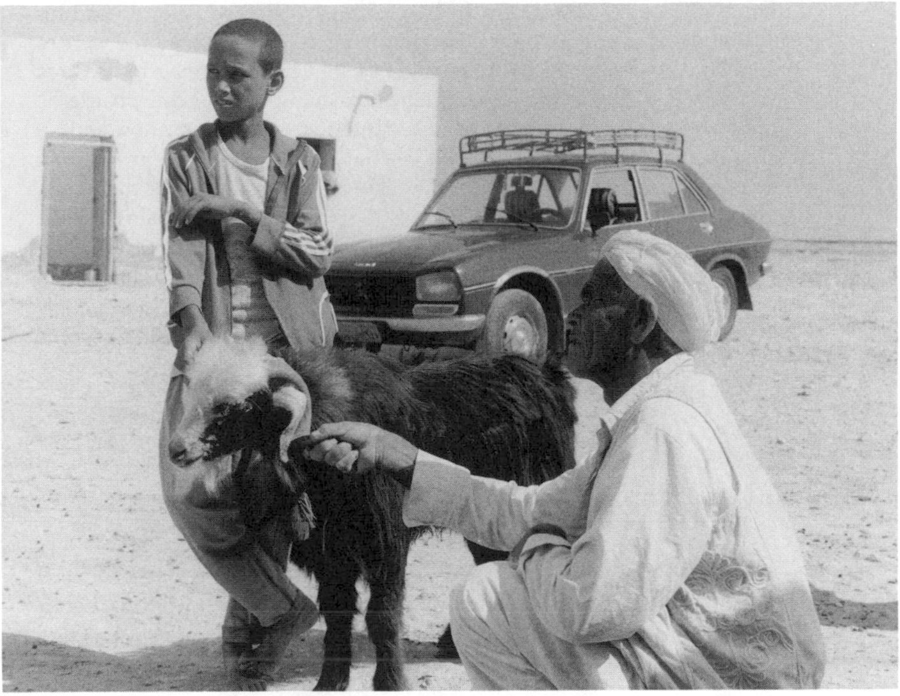

Photograph 9. The Bedouin owner and his grandson holding the hermaphroditic son of the hermaphroditic goat. (Photograph by Mia Fuller)

who had stood in line all day. The officer retorted by mocking them, saying, "You Bedouins need to learn manners. You are Bedouins with no blood." The adolescent boys were insulted, and one of them threw a can of cheese at the officer.

The enraged officer went to the police station, where he had "connections." He told his friends there that the Bedouins were operating a fraudulent business, giving people milk from a normal goat rather than from their *gidi*. As a result, the police came to carry out a search the next morning. The men and older women were gone at the time, and the police "ambushed" the young girls, which was sinful of them. When the Bedouin goat-owner returned, he was arrested along with his two grandsons, and the three of them were jailed for one week. During this time, the Bedouin told the police, "If this goat that did so much good for people led to my arrest, then go ahead and kill it. I don't care." That is, in fact, what the police did: they confiscated the *gidi* and slaughtered him.

Meanwhile, the disgruntled officer took his case to the governor and state security, claiming fraudulent misrepresentation of a product. Although the Bedouin and his grandsons were released from jail on bail and were then acquitted, the officer persisted with his case and won. The Bedouin and his grandsons received written notice that they were to be fined £E 50 and were to be sentenced to one year in jail. Terrified of this prospect, they hired three lawyers for £E 300, who will argue their case in an upcoming court battle.

As the Bedouin's senior wife lamented: "Infertile women come now and cry because the goat is dead. People used to come and see a miracle from God. Some people came and got cured; the milk was just an excuse for their cure, but the cure was a miracle from God. Every day, the goat had two kilos of milk, and it was heavy with extra hormones. But it was only two kilos; he was a *gidi* and not a buffalo! He was a male, and he had sex with other goats and had children by them, but he had two breasts in front of his testicles. Some people came to get children, and they got pregnant after drinking the milk. But some came just to mock us. The boys couldn't stand this, so now they're sentenced to one year in jail. All the good we did is paid for by one year in prison."

God and the Search for Children

As the Bedouin woman explained in this sorrowful tale of greed and treachery, the "cure" offered by her husband's hermaphroditic goat was actually a cure from God. According to her, many infertile women became pregnant after drinking the remarkable *gidi*'s milk, but these pregnancies were the result of divine intervention rather than the miraculous milk itself. If the *gidi*'s son—who is also a hermaphrodite—should begin to produce such milk in the future, she explained, his milk, too, will only cure the infertile "with the permission of God."

Thus, this woman expresses a widely held conviction among Egyptian women: namely, that the success or failure of any given remedy—and of the "search for children" itself—is "up to God," who determines if and when a woman will become pregnant. God's determinative role in the quest for therapy extends not only to ethnogynecological therapies, but to biogynecological ones as well. His desire for women to "search for children" is what motivates their pilgrimages for pregnancy—pilgrimages that take them to healers' and herbalists' back-alley practices and to the mosque-tombs and remarkable sites of *Ṣūfī*s and *gidi*s known for their healing powers. God's desire for his followers to "search" is also what motivates women's biogynecological quests for therapy—quests that are legitimated by powerful establishment forces in Egypt, but whose usefulness we will now consider.

Part 3

Biogynecology

8. Biomedical Bodies

The Stories of Ghada and Marwa

Born into a lower-middle-class Alexandrian family, Ghada was allowed by her parents to complete junior high school and to delay marriage until the age of nineteen—late by the standards of her *baladī* neighborhood. However, when Ghada married Saad, she was extremely sad, because, during the hasty month between her engagement and wedding, she had no opportunity to get to know the man who was to become her husband. As she explained, "I would have preferred to meet him first and know him—not directly like this. But his family wanted a quick marriage, and my family approved, and I agreed." Fortunately for Ghada, she found Saad to be an understanding husband, and, with time and the birth of their son during the first year of marriage, she grew to love him. However, within six months of his birth, the baby died of severe diarrhea and jaundice and, according to Ghada, "there was no medicine for that."

When Ghada was unable to become pregnant after her son's death, she began searching for biogynecological therapy—a search that has lasted fourteen years and has been aided by her emotionally and financially supportive husband. With her bit of education and her ability to read, Ghada has rejected ethnogynecological therapies altogether, despite her neighbors' attempts to bring her bloodied suppositories and other appurtenances of ethnogynecological therapy. Instead, Ghada and her husband are firm believers in biomedicine, the treatments of which she has tried repeatedly but, so far, have failed to help her.

Indeed, Ghada's search for a biogynecological remedy for her infertility has been truly valiant; it has taxed her body, her husband's financial resources, and, ultimately, her reproductive health. What this search has not called into question is Ghada's belief in biomedicine and its ability to provide an eventual cure—a cure that she hopes will come through a third attempt at making a "baby of the tubes" in Alexandria's Shatby Hospital. In fact, Ghada is one of the relatively few Egyptian women to have undergone in vitro fertilization—the making of a "test-tube baby"—an attempt that was extremely expensive for her and, despite two trials, ultimately unsuccessful. Likewise, Ghada has subjected her body to a dizzying array of other biogynecological diagnostic tests and therapies, including three hysterosalpingograms, two endometrial biopsies, four diagnostic laparoscopies, one hormonal blood analysis, one postcoital test, one cervical mucus analysis, twelve abdominal ultrasounds, seven or eight tubal insufflations, two cervical electrocauterizations, one dilatation and curettage of her uterus, one tubal surgery, two trials of artificial insemination with her husband's sperm, and fourteen years' worth of almost continuous, polydrug pharmaceutical therapy. Ghada estimates that Saad has spent more than five thousand Egyptian pounds (two thousand dollars) for all of her "medicines, tests, and operations," and she has sold every article of gold jewelry, as well as any presents she receives, in order to finance her biogynecological quest.

At least Ghada knows what is wrong with her, for several doctors have explained to her that "the way is blocked." As she understands it, "The tubes are blocked. That's the reason; there is no other reason. The tubes are blocked and the egg has no chance to come out, because the spermatic animals go to the tubes and an egg goes through the tubes. The spermatic animals and egg meet each other at a place in the uterus, like a warehouse, where they meet. The egg stays one week in the tubes then goes to the uterus and pregnancy occurs."

Ghada believes her fallopian tubes are blocked *because of biogynecological therapies themselves*—therapies she should have never tried. After her tubal surgery, several doctors that she visited "shouted" at her, saying, "This is the biggest mistake you did." As she explains, "When you do an operation, you normally get an infection. This helped the tubes to get blocked more." Likewise, she strongly suspects that the seven or eight tubal insufflations undertaken by various doctors contributed to further blockage of her tubes.

But Ghada feels no resentment toward the biogynecologists who have mishandled her case, because, as she realizes, it is God who "decides who gets and who doesn't." She feels she must try in vitro fertilization again, because "it's the last thing I can do." If several additional IVF trials fail, then her search will be "finished." As she says, "Is there anything else to do? If I don't get pregnant, that means God doesn't want me to have children. And maybe one day I can get pregnant without doing anything. Maybe it's blocked, but one day, in God's hands, it's not blocked anymore, and I can have a baby."

Marwa's case is a bit different from Ghada's, because, after eight years of searching exclusively in the biogynecological realm, Marwa has still not been given a definitive diagnosis by a physician, and, frankly, she has become "fed up," turning to the *wasfāt baladī* that she had previously rejected altogether. Because both Marwa and her husband, Amr, were divorced from previous spouses, because Amr and his ex-wife had a daughter who died, and because Marwa's ex-husband went on to have children by his second wife, Marwa believes that there must be something wrong with her, since she is the only one of the four who has not proven her fertility. Yet, having visited nearly fifteen physicians — all of them gynecologists — and having never been given a reasonable or consistent explanation for her infertility, Marwa is convinced that "it's something up to God, because I can't find any reason until now." According to Marwa, "I've looked for any problem wrong with my body. If there was anything wrong, all this treatment and all these operations would have worked. *Maybe* God is testing me — that I didn't give up. I still have hope in God's mercy."

Marwa, like Ghada, has endured a battery of diagnostic tests and therapies, including "drawing on the uterus" during her period (that is, tocography, an outdated test of uterine contractility for severe dysmenorrhea), one blood test, one cervical mucus analysis, three ultrasounds, one diagnostic laparoscopy (in which the doctor "scratched" her intestines, requiring therapy from another physician), one tubal insufflation, one dilatation and curettage, one cervical electrocauterization, and "lots of drugs," including almost continuous therapy with Clomid, a fertility drug that affected her adversely (with nausea and vomiting, blurred vision, dizziness, fatigue, and a "tired heart"). Furthermore, like Ghada, Marwa has sold all of her gold to finance these tests and treatments, and her husband, who is a driver, must work nights as well as days to pay for her therapeutic quest.

Reflecting on her experiences in the biogynecological realm, Marwa comments, "I believed everything I was told, and I took every treatment until I found no result and got very upset. I never stayed with a doctor for very long, because each one gave me many drugs at once and made me sick. Because each one said a different thing; they said, 'You have *ruṭūba* or pus on the ovaries or infections or fibroids.' This made me give up going to doctors. They're *exactly* like *munaggimīn*."

Although she has found a physician at Shatby Hospital with whom she feels comfortable, Marwa says that she has "lost faith" in biogynecologists and has turned in the past two years to ethnogynecological therapies, which she had never believed in before. Over the past two years, Marwa has made up for lost time in the ethnogynecological realm. She has undergone seven different *kabsa* healing rituals, including visiting the tomb of Shaikh Il-Khibari, where she licked his stone; two countershocking remedies for *khaḍḍa*; both *kasr* and *kawī* for *dahr maftūḥ*; and *tabwīkha* for uterine *ruṭūba*. In addition, Marwa visited one *munaggim*, who prescribed *ṣūwaf* and wrote *ḥugub*. But, because Marwa wasn't "convinced" of the *munaggim*'s methods, her mother has visited several *munaggimīn* on Marwa's behalf since then, and they have divined that Marwa's *ukht taḥt il-arḍ* is upset with her, because she poured hot water on the ground without saying, "In the name of God."

As for Marwa, she currently believes that she is infertile because her back is open and "slippery." "Yes, I feel it," she says. "I have lower back pain, and when I bend, I can't straighten up right away, maybe because I work hard and carry heavy things. If you carry heavy things on your head, it causes the back to open." Although she will continue seeking therapies for her open back and uterine *ruṭūba*, Marwa says that she will pursue simultaneous treatment by the university physician until, God willing, she becomes pregnant in a year or two. If this fails, she will go to no other doctors, but instead, will visit a man in Cairo who gets "things from Saudi Arabia" and makes *wasfāt baladī* from them. As she explains, "I'll continue to do *something*. One shouldn't give up on God's mercy. God says, 'You'll try, and I'll help you.'"

The Biogynecological Quest

Just as most infertile Egyptian women seek to understand and overcome their various ethnogynecological problems, the vast majority of Egyptian women, like Ghada and Marwa, search for ways to overcome their infertility in the biogynecological realm. As Egyptian women explain, "God created medicine," and, hence, therapeutically speaking, "God shows the way." Thus, it is incumbent upon all believers to continue to search for the proper remedy until therapeutic possibilities are exhausted. To cease this quest prematurely is, in effect, to admit doubt in God's wisdom and his ability to grant children to whom he wishes at times designated only by him.

For many women like Ghada and Marwa, this therapeutic quest in the biomedical realm begins early on—specifically, with visits to biogynecologists operating from either private clinics, private hospitals, or public clinics and hospitals specializing in maternity. Given the well-developed specialty of obstetrics and gynecology—*amrāḍ nisā'*, literally, "diseases of women"—in Egypt, most women restrict their biomedical searches to biogynecologists exclusively. However, as we shall see, very few biogynecologists restrict their practices to the problem of infertility. Hence, physicians visited by infertile women tend to be biogynecological generalists, whose knowledge of infertility diagnosis and management may be quite limited.

Yet, among most poor urban Egyptian women, belief in physicians and their treatments is quite high and is a reflection of the hegemonic penetration of the biomedical belief system in the Egyptian collective consciousness. However, as seen in the case of Marwa, the faith of some women in physicians and their remedies is undermined by years of endless therapy with "no results"—the expression used by women to represent their frustration over the failure of biomedicine to help them conceive. In fact, the "old school" of invasive, outdated biomedical procedures still employed widely in Egypt to treat infertile women is not only inefficacious in most cases, but may even lead to deleterious results, as seen in the case of Ghada. Yet, the "new school" of assisted reproductive technologies—namely, artificial insemination by husband (AIH) and in vitro fertilization (IVF), which have recently emerged in urban centers in Egypt—is largely unavailable to poor women without resources and probably offers false hope to many of those infertile women who are able to avail themselves of these technologies.

To understand this biogynecological "search for children," it is necessary to begin by exploring the nature of biomedicine in Egypt—first, how the colonial reproduction and historical expansion of British-style biomedicine throughout Egypt has led to a contemporary system of health care plagued by serious deficiencies, and second, how biomedicine's mechanistic, atomistic view of the reproductive body has come to inform not only Egyptians' theories of procreation, as seen in Chapter 3, but their theories of procreative failure as well.

Egyptian Biomedicine

Contemporary biomedicine in Egypt is, in many senses, a victim of its British colonial heritage. As described in Chapter 3, with the British takeover of Egypt and its health-care system in the late 1800s, many of the most important biomedical advances instigated under the reform-minded Egyptian ruler Muhammad Ali were effectively stultified (Sonbol 1991). Instead of encouraging the development of an indigenously appropriate system of medicine, which had been Muhammad Ali's major goal, the British debased all that was "Egyptian" about Egyptian biomedicine, and instead turned biomedicine in Egypt into a dependent, imported, and adulterated carbon copy of its own system.

The impact was, unfortunately, profound and, so far, has been difficult to reverse. Despite health-care reforms instituted under Nasser following the expulsion of the British from the country in the early 1950s, reforms have failed to transform the basic character of Egyptian biomedicine, which today bears the indelible mark of colonization and anglicization (Blizard 1991). Perhaps most discouraging, critics charge that the British colonial legacy has thwarted the potential excellence of Egyptian biomedicine as a system responsive to the *needs of its own citizens* (El-Mehairy 1984b; Kuhnke 1990; Sonbol 1991).

But what, exactly, are the colonially induced ills plaguing contemporary Egyptian biomedicine? Although numerous pitfalls have been pointed out by health-care analysts (Abu-Zeid and Dann 1985; Carney 1984; El-Mehairy 1984b; Institute of Medicine 1979; Kandela 1988), it seems worthwhile to highlight four problematic areas that are particularly germane to the discussion of Egyptian biogynecology, which, too, suffers from this inglorious legacy.

First and perhaps most important, the British privatized medicine, which was being made public and accessible under Muhammad Ali (Kuhnke 1990; Sonbol 1991). Instead of encouraging "health for all" in Egypt, the British exported their own brand of fee-for-service, private medicine, practiced by physicians as a trade for financial gain. Excessive entrepreneurialism in biomedical practice was the result, with Egyptian physicians, who were "second-class citizens" to the European doctors imported by the British, forced to compete in sometimes unseemly ways in order to make a living. Furthermore, biomedical services were no longer accessible to the Egyptian masses under this private, fee-for-service system, and, as shown by Kuhnke (1990), the health of the Egyptian populace suffered dramatically during this period of British domination.

Today, more than a century later, the foreign physicians are gone, and health-care reforms have again brought public-sector medicine to the masses. However, the effects of colonial privatization have been profound in Egypt and have resulted in a major chasm between public and private health-care services. According to Kandela (1988), Egyptian biomedicine has "three faces" — two public, one private — with quality care limited largely to the latter and to those who can afford it. The lowest tier of care is the purportedly "free" medical care available to all Egyptians through Egyptian Ministry of Health hospitals (including university teaching hospitals) and clinics constructed under Nasser's aegis. Yet, as apparent in the many complaints about public health care registered by poor Egyptians, this system of free clinics and hospitals is "crumbling under the weight of the huge demand and lack of resources" (Kandela 1988:34). Public hospitals are in disrepair, and many patients' stays are unnecessarily extended due to lack of physician manpower and crucial equipment and supplies (Institute of Medicine 1979). Similar problems plague Ministry of Health outpatient clinics, where the hours of operation are short, the waiting lines are long, and drugs and other materials are often in short supply. The result is serious underutilization of public, primary health-care services — underutilization that is fueled by the pervasive feeling among patients that it is wiser to spend one's hard-earned money on a visit to a private clinic (Abu-Zeid and Dann 1985; Institute of Medicine 1979). On the other hand, the second tier of care — namely, the public "health insurance" scheme, with its own system of government-run hospitals and ambulatory-care clinics — covers only about three million people in a nation of almost sixty million, with two million of the insured being government employees. Thus, not only is this "public" system exclusionary, but, according to Kandela (1988: 34), "the insured person's dependants are not covered and the low salaries of government employees means that this system cannot offer an acceptable level of medical care." The third tier of care is "private" care, for those who can bear the full cost of medical intervention without the help of insurance. A British colonial legacy, private medicine, which continued unabated during the period of Nasser's reforms, has proliferated in Egypt in recent years. The reasons are considered to be threefold: (1) the significant glut of un- and underemployed Egyptian medical school graduates who, upon completing their mandatory government service in often remote rural areas, cannot find substantial, well-reimbursed positions in "desirable" (that is, urban) areas of the public-sector system (El-Mehairy 1984b; Institute of Medicine 1979); (2) the significant numbers (75 to 80 percent) of active public-sector physicians, including university medical professors, who attempt to supplement their meager government salaries through afternoon and evening practice in their own private, fee-for-service clinics (El-Mehairy 1984b; Institute of Medicine 1979); and (3) Sadat's capitalist call for "open investment" in Egypt, including in private "investment" hospitals, which have been described as the "medical Hiltons and Sheratons" of Egypt, but which are considered by some critics to be one of the most prominent "diseases" of the free-market economy (Kandela 1988).

The result today is a schizophrenic medical landscape, with many Egyptian "biomedicines" being practiced according to patients' abilities to pay. For most Egyptians, who despise the quality of service and treatment in the overtaxed, underequipped public medical sector, private medical care is the first choice, pending sufficient out-of-pocket funds. But, for reasons to be detailed below, even private biomedicine is pluralistic, lacking uniform standards of quality. Thus, as it now stands, even patients who can afford to pay have no guarantee that they will receive appropriate care for what ails them.

Second, when the British took over medicine in Egypt, the quality of medical education deteriorated dramatically (Sonbol 1991). Medical school admissions of Egyptian students were cut drastically to make room for the European physicians who were soon allowed free reign in the country. Furthermore, medical school, which was free under Muhammad Ali and open to any bright (male) Egyptian student, became prohibitively expensive under the British, who thus restricted medical education to the wealthy elite. Language became an additional barrier; Arabic, the official language of biomedicine following Muhammad Ali's reforms, was replaced by English, which became a prerequisite for medical school admission. Finally, the British quashed critical, scientific inquiry and innovative medical research in Egyptian medical schools, encouraging instead traditionalism in education based on the rote learning of imported materials.

Today in Egypt, the state of medical education differs little from a century ago. Although Egyptian medical education has been opened up to the point of overextension, the quality of medical education is still seriously deficient (El-Mehairy 1984b; Institute of Medicine 1979). Classes are filled well beyond capacity, leading to a shortage of seats, textbooks, and opportunities for more individualized training, especially in critical clinical skills. Faculty members are often absent and, when they are present, encourage students to adulate them as "demigods" in a system that is blatantly paternalistic, hierarchical, and authoritarian (El-Mehairy 1984b). Furthermore, educators encourage medical traditionalism by often failing to take their own research mandate seriously, by relaying sometimes outdated knowledge and standards of practice to their students and expecting unquestioning acceptance of this material, and by failing to encourage the efforts of up-and-coming junior physicians who would like to engage in biomedical innovation. The result, according to El-Mehairy (1984b), is the graduation of thousands of poorly trained physicians, who forget much of what they were forced to memorize for exams, who are underspecialized, and who may never be forced to update their knowledge or standards of practice, due to the lack of continuing medical education (CME) requirements in the country. Moreover, because Egypt lacks a system of physician self-monitoring (for example, board exams or medical ethics review boards) as well as a system of medical malpractice, physician graduates are essentially free to do as they please once they enter community practice, with little surveillance or scrutiny of their capabilities or services.[1]

These deficiencies, according to critics, have led to poor quality care in many instances and the lack of a well-developed "medical morality" in Egypt, which, in fact, can be traced historically to the British, who scuttled ethical reforms begun under Muhammad Ali (Sonbol 1991). However, given the absence of health activist and consumer advocacy groups in Egypt today (Morsy 1985), individuals have little recourse when they feel their rights have been violated or their cases mishandled. Instead, the outcome is "lack of trust" in physicians (El-Mehairy 1984b), who, according, to Marwa's comments above, can be considered about as trustworthy as unscrupulous *munaggimīn*.

Lack of trust is also perpetuated by medical elitism of the worst kind, also a product of British medical domination. Not only did the British promote the idea that everything "European" was superior to everything Egyptian, but Egyptian physicians themselves were encouraged to look down upon the Egyptian masses, including the ethnomedical specialists who had practiced for centuries in their country and who had been incorporated into the biomedical system under Muhammad Ali (Gallagher 1990; Kuhnke 1990; Sonbol 1991). Efforts to train ethnomedical practitioners, such as *ḥallāqīn aṣ-ṣiḥḥa*, as ancillary medical personnel were entirely suspended under the British, and these healers were deemed "quacks" and "charlatans" and the poor folk who turned to them instead of physicians, "ignoramuses" (Sonbol 1991; Walker 1934). Furthermore, the new "language of biomedicine" in Egypt was English, which few Egyptians spoke; thus, increasing distance was often placed between physicians and patients, already separated by different class backgrounds.

Again, the situation in Egypt today is little improved from a century ago. Attempts to incorporate ethnomedical practitioners into the biomedical system have been feeble at best and limited to *dāyāt*, whose services remain officially illicit, as seen in Chapter 4. Furthermore, ancillary medical personnel of all kinds—including, among others, nurses, medical technicians, paramedics, medical social workers and psychologists—are undervalued, undertrained, and in chronically short supply (Carney 1984; Institute of Medicine 1979). Instead, only physicians are accorded professional prestige (although this prestige often outstrips their real contributions), and their attitudes toward other health-care personnel, including ethnomedical practitioners, remain supercilious at best (Pillsbury 1978). As a result, medical "teamwork" is lacking in Egypt, and such tasks as medical record-keeping, laboratory work, and basic primary-health-care services, which could be effectively delegated to trained paramedical personnel, are often handled, if at all, by physicians themselves (Institute of Medicine 1979). Furthermore, the patronizing attitudes and lack of cultural sensitivity of many Egyptian physicians regarding their patients—especially poor, uneducated patients presenting at public facilities—has been noted by a number of scholars, who have described the untoward effects of medical paternalism on doctor-patient communication (Assaad and El Katsha 1981; Early 1985; El-Mehairy 1984b; Lane and Millar 1987; Morsy 1980b, 1985, 1993).

Finally, the British, true to their heritage in industrializing Europe, exported to Egypt a brand of Western biomedicine enamored with technology for the "repair" of broken-down bodily "machines." Instead of developing prevention-oriented public health-care services, which were desperately needed throughout the disease-ravaged Egyptian countryside, the British promoted high-tech, curative, urban hospital-based health care, which was frankly unresponsive to the pressing medical needs of Egypt's largely rural populace (Kuhnke 1990; Sonbol 1991).

Today, the biomedical system in Egypt remains biased in similar directions. Namely, urban areas are favored over rural ones by health-care personnel, curative care is privileged over preventive services, and invasive "high-tech medicine" is often practiced at the expense of noninvasive "low-tech" medicine, even though the standards of technological medicine in Egypt often lag far behind developments in other parts of the (Western) world.

As we shall see in the chapters that follow, all of these problems are played out in the realm of biogynecology, which poses many difficulties for infertile patients. Yet, as El-Mehairy (1984b) points out, relatively little is understood about patients' responses as *consumers* of health care, and especially about women patients as they attempt to negotiate their ways through the often perplexing biogynecological treatment system. As she concludes, "More research is indicated for the consumer of the health delivery system, especially those women in childbearing years, so that services might be better tailored to their needs *as they perceive them*" (El-Mehairy 1984b:189–90; emphasis added).

In addition to understanding the perceived needs of Egyptian women as health-care consumers, it would be very interesting to know how the problems plaguing Egyptian biomedicine are similar to or different from problems confronting biomedicine in other postcolonial and especially anglicized societies. If it can be accepted that biomedicine is a social and cultural construction — a product, as it were, of particular social and cultural conditions, which are historically situated (Lock and Gordon 1988a) — then we must assume the local specificity of biomedicine in Egypt and the uniqueness of many of its problems and its contemporary character. Yet, the globalization of the Western medical model, based in many cases on the British medical education system, has resulted in the domination of neocolonial, urban-based, technologically oriented care in *many* postcolonial societies around the world (Blizard 1991; Bonair, Rosenfield, and Tengvald 1989). Thus, some of the problems facing contemporary Egyptian biomedicine, modeled as it is on the British system, are probably very similar to those found *wherever* a Western medical model has been transplanted, forcibly, into a non-Western, colonial setting.

Unfortunately, too little historically grounded, critically oriented, comparative research on biomedicine has been carried out in non-Western settings. Although medical anthropologists have been a major force in turning the "critical gaze" on biomedicine, the vast majority of this research has taken place *in the West*, despite the fact that most biomedicines around the world are also Western-based. This neglect of a comprehensive, international "cultural critique" of biomedicine is evident, for example, in the recent major volume *Biomedicine Examined* (Lock and Gordon 1988b), which pays little attention to biomedicine in the non-Western world. Furthermore, the call in that volume for "more comparative research among *western* contexts which not only grounds or challenges some commonly ascribed assumptions about western culture, but which also shows how medical practice reflects local culture" (Gordon 1988:22; emphasis added) seems, anthropologically speaking, too narrow.

Yet, Lock (1988) in that volume and Nichter (1991) in a recent commentary on ethnomedicine index, at least in part, the reason for this anthropological neglect. Lock (1988) points to the problem of the predominance of a symbolic-interpretive approach in medical anthropology, which has led, perhaps, to an excessive interest among medical anthropologists in nonbiomedical *ethnomedicines in other cultures*; this, in turn, may have led to the neglect of other important issues impinging upon both bio- and ethnomedicines wherever they are found — for example, in the control, distribution, and dynamics of the actual application of medical knowledge. Nichter (1991), furthermore, warns of the danger of "imperialist nostalgia" among medical anthropologists — namely, the juxtaposition of the positive aspects of traditional medicine / health culture with the negative aspects of biomedicine as it is practiced by doctors who rely on technological cures — leading to the potentially irresponsible portrayal of a reified biomedical hegemony.

With a few notable exceptions,[2] anthropologists have yet to turn their critical gaze to biomedicine in the Middle East, including Egypt. The result in Egypt, interestingly enough, is that the "cultural critique" of biomedicine comes from Egyptian physicians and patients themselves, who are often abundantly aware of the problems facing "modern" Egyptian health care. As we shall see in this chapter and especially the next, those involved in Egyptian infertility management, including both recipients and deliverers of care, are often incisive critics of current biomedical practice and feel free to offer censorious analyses of the host of problems plaguing biogynecology in general and infertility management in particular. Although the focus in this chapter is primarily on women's perspectives as patients, considerable attention is paid in the next chapter to physicians' frustrations over the current state of infertility care.

Indeed, Egyptian biogynecologists are not a monolithic force practicing medicine according to a uniform set of standards. It is, in fact, the variability of standards and the lack of a systematic, up-to-date approach to infertility management that bothers many Egyptian biogynecologists who treat infertile patients. Some biogynecologists — the minority, to be sure — take great interest in infertility and great pains to "keep current" in the field by following international journals and undertaking training and continuing medical education abroad (mostly in the West). This group — largely (although not exclusively) urban-based, university-affiliated, and part of the self-proclaimed "new generation" of younger physicians — tends to decry the poor quality of care being offered on a general level to infertile Egyptian women and the frank exploitation of this group of "desperate" patients.

Yet, infertile Egyptian women such as Ghada and Marwa have little recourse in a system which, as they too realize, exploits them. Although they can resist their exploitation by withdrawing their trust in physicians, most infertile Egyptian women continue to place their faith in "God and doctors," hoping that, together, they offer salvation.

Biomedical Bodies and Factor Fixation

Faith in biomedicine in Egypt on the part of most infertile women is evident in their faith in biomedical assumptions regarding the human reproductive body and its failure. Specifically, most infertile women who have participated to any extent in the biogynecological system in Egypt have adopted to a striking degree biomedical notions of infertility as a disease, caused by the machine-like bodily breakdown of specific reproductive parts.

This view of the body as "machine" is one of the dominant metaphors in biomedicine, according to Kirmayer (1988), and the accompanying belief in "atomism," the division of the body into parts or "factors," one of biomedicine's most tenacious assumptions (Gordon 1988). Together, machine metaphors and atomistic reductionism characterize biomedicine's understanding of the "infertile female body," which is viewed as affected by specific factors located in various reproductive organs. Because these factors can be localized so specifically, they are seen as being highly amenable to "costly and technologically specialized repair jobs"—or what Renaud (1978) has called "the engineering approach" to the human body.

But what, exactly, are these infertility factors? And how have they come to be viewed by infertile Egyptian women? As we shall see, "factor fixation" among biogynecologists in Egypt—and among biogynecologists wherever the Western model has been adopted (Becker and Nachtigall 1991)—has profoundly affected the infertile Egyptian public, which has also adopted the notion of localized, bodily pathology. Unfortunately for women, biomedical factors are predominantly "female" in nature; therefore, Egyptian women of all social classes are more likely to be assigned and to accept the blame for infertility by reference to their own "reproductive bodily breakdown" and to subject their bodies to costly, invasive, biogynecological "fixes."

To reiterate an important point made in Chapter 3, Egyptians today are exceptionally well apprised of the fact that both women *and* men may be infertile. Nevertheless, it is also true that infertility problems are thought to occur more commonly among women than among men, and women are more often assumed by others to be the infertile partner in a marriage. Although the advent of semen analysis in Egypt during the past two decades is probably more responsible than any other single factor in convincing Egyptians of the presence of male infertility, biomedicine has also shown that women may suffer from a host of infertility problems. The seeming multitude of "female factors" introduced by biomedicine has served to convince Egyptians that women are much more likely to be sources of infertility than men, even though, in any given population, the epidemiological distribution of male and female factors is thought to be roughly equal.[3] Yet, most Egyptians argue vehemently that "female problems" are much more common and more difficult to overcome, a belief that is grounded in their biomedically influenced views of men's and women's reproductive bodies. Whereas women are seen as having "many things that can go wrong" like "the parts of a junked car needing new equipment," men, on the other hand, have only one potential problem: their spermatic worms. Although "worm problems" are considered to be potentially serious, they are also thought by most Egyptians to be amenable to therapy and thus more easily overcome than many of the female factors of which they are aware.

The extent to which biomedicine has been successful in shaping Egyptians' asymmetrical views of men's and women's reproductive bodies is apparent in the litany of biomedical causes of infertility that most Egyptian women, both fertile and infertile, can list and describe in some detail (having been exposed, in many cases, to the discourse of doctors and patients in health-care settings, to discussions about infertility in the media, or to everyday conversations with other women). Furthermore, although Egyptian women demonstrate as much variability in their beliefs about reproductive failure as in their beliefs about procreative success, they tend to view the biomedical causes of infertility as falling neatly into the various categories of "infertility factors" promulgated by biomedicine.

Yet, as we shall see, the language of infertility factors used by these women is often quite different from that used by biogynecologists. Women transform foreign-sounding medical terms—translated into Arabic from the foreign language of Latin-based English medicalese—into a language of reproductive pathology that appeals to their commonsense models of the body. Thus, just as "spermatic animals" becomes "worms" in Egyptian popular parlance, "pelvic adhesions" become "sticky things around the tubes," and "tubes," when "blocked," are seen as requiring "plumbing."

Indeed, in attempting to understand the inner workings of their reproductive bodies, Egyptian women imagine the uterine *bait il-wilid*, or "house of the child," as a home with an intricate plumbing system, containing tubes that are easily clogged. Thus, women's representations of their reproductive "machinery" utilize creative imagery that transforms the intimidating jargon of biogynecological infertility factors into a colorful language of weak worms and jammed plumbing systems—notions that make greater sense in women's everyday worlds of experience.

Tubal Factor

According to the biomedical model, tubal-factor infertility (TFI) resulting from dysfunction of the fallopian tubes is one of the most common causes of infertility and is increasing in incidence among some populations, primarily due to rising rates of sexually transmitted infections and resultant pelvic inflammatory disease (PID) (Doyle and DeCherney 1993). TFI is a condition involving: (1) total or partial obstruction of the fallopian tubes; (2) distortion of the normal shape of the fallopian tubes, usually due to infection-induced adhesions forming on the external surface of the tubes or to endometriosis, a condition in which tissue from the interior surface of the uterus gains access to the pelvis, leading to marked distortion of the anatomy because of adhesion formation; or (3) denudation of the internal surface of the fallopian tubes, involving damage to the internal epithelium and cilia. Such tubal changes are usually the result of scarring due to infection, inflammation, or surgery. Infection leading to PID is thought to be the most common cause of tubal damage and is usually attributable to sexually transmitted diseases (gonorrhea or chlamydia) (Doyle and DeCherney 1993). However, in Third World countries such as Egypt, pelvic infections caused by tuberculosis may also be a significant problem (World Health Organization 1975), as well as iatrogenic infections caused by mixed aerobic/anaerobic organisms that gain access to the upper genital tract following various reproductive events (for example, childbirth, miscarriage, abortion, intrauterine device insertion, abdominal and reproductive surgery). Unfortunately, tubal-factor infertility, which is the most common cause of infertility in Egypt (Serour, El Ghar, and Mansour 1991), is one of the most difficult forms of infertility to treat and is one of the major indications for in vitro fertilization (IVF).

Among poor Egyptian women, tubal-factor infertility—which they know as *anābīb masdūd*, or "blocked tubes"—is the condition deemed most common and most serious. Tubes that are "blocked," "tight," or "twisted" are seen as needing "opening," "widening," or "plumbing." Furthermore, *iltiṣāqāt*, or "adhesions," that are viewed by women as either "sticky things," a "lining," or "leather" enveloping the tubes may need to be "peeled" or "cut away."

"Tube problems" of this nature are viewed as "the worst thing" to have by most infertile women and by many fertile women as well. This belief regarding the gravity of *anābīb masdūd* probably stems from several sources: (1) the widely recognized low success rate of tubal surgery among women who have undergone this procedure; (2) physicians who tell women with bilateral tubal obstruction that IVF represents their "only hope"; (3) occasional health programs on radio or television devoted to the serious problem of "blocked tubes" and ways to avoid them; and (4) the realization among many women that there are "no medicines" for blocked tubes, only "surgeries."

However, despite widespread knowledge of the problem of *anābīb masdūd*, poor urban Egyptian women display considerable confusion over the nature of the "tubes" inside their bodies. Whereas uteri and ovaries are organs whose location and functions are well-defined in ethnophysiological models of the reproductive tract, few women are certain about the location of their "tubes" (for example, between the vagina and uterus or between the uterus and ovaries); their number (one, two, or more); their size (as thin as "hairs" or as large as "pipes"); and their function in the "catching and carrying" of pregnancy. As we shall see in Chapter 11, such confusion is further confounded by the notion of "babies of the tubes" (test-tube babies), which are "made" for women with "tube problems" but in "test tubes" outside the body.

Furthermore, women with *anābīb masdūd* are often left to puzzle over why their tubes are "blocked." Many women assume this condition to be congenital, although others are informed by physicians of some probable infection in the past. But because many cases of PID are asymptomatic, women who are told they must have suffered from an infertility-producing infection are often hard-pressed to remember any occasion of pelvic pain, vaginal discharge, or other suspicious symptoms. On the other hand, women who underwent prior reproductive events or abdominal surgeries — including post-miscarriage D & Cs, vaginal and cesarean deliveries, appendectomies, splenectomies, fibroid tumor removals, and the like — are often quick to blame such events (and often themselves) for their past infections and current reproductive problems.

Ovarian Factor

According to the biomedical model, ovarian-factor infertility (OFI) involves a variety of problems leading to anovulation, or inability of a woman to ovulate. These problems are usually located in the ovaries themselves, but may also be associated with the thyroid gland or the central nervous system (the pituitary and hypothalamus), where hormones governing ovulation are largely regulated (Chang 1993; Liu 1993; Stradtman 1993). The most common ovarian cause of anovulation is the polycystic ovary syndrome (PCO), a condition of self-perpetuating, chronic anovulation (Seibel 1993). PCO, in fact, represents a complex ovulatory dysfunction involving the hypothalamus, pituitary, ovaries, adrenal glands, and peripheral adipose (fatty) tissues, all contributing to an endocrine imbalance usually associated with infrequent ovulation, hirsutism (excessive, male-pattern hair growth), the growth of multiple "follicles" (cysts) on the ovaries, and infertility (Seibel 1993). Because PCO is related to obesity, because obesity in and of itself is a risk factor for ovulatory problems (Azziz 1993), and because many poor urban infertile women are mildly to morbidly obese (as a result of carbohydrate-rich diets and excessive sedentariness), ovulatory problems are thought to be a common cause of infertility among women in Egypt (Serour, El Ghar, and Mansour 1991).[4]

Second only to "tube problems," ovarian problems are viewed by poor Egyptian women as a major cause of female infertility. *Mibāyiḍ daʿīf*, or "weak ovaries," are deemed the primary ovarian problem and are viewed as being amenable to medicines that "strengthen." As with weak worms, weak ovaries index the common cultural illness idiom of "weakness," which is viewed both as a general condition of ill health (DeClerque et al. 1986) and as a problem localized to specific parts of the body (for example, "weak heart," "weak lungs," and "weak blood"). In terms of ovaries, however, weakness is sometimes translated into functional but condemnatory terms, with ovaries often being referred to as "lazy" or "nonfunctioning" and in need of "activation."

Yet, according to Egyptian women, there are many other potential ovarian afflictions. *Iltihāb*, or inflammation, and *ʿadwā*, or infection, are seen as common problems of the ovaries, given the propensity of ovaries to develop *ruṭūba*, which is viewed by many women as synonymous with infection or inflammation. Thus, women speak of "inflamed ovaries," "swollen ovaries," and "infection in the ovaries," with such problems leading to "blocked ovaries" (as in "blocked tubes"). Furthermore, women are well apprised of ovarian growths and cysts of various kinds, which are sometimes referred to by these terms, but which are usually translated into a more familiar idiom. Thus, ovarian cysts are often referred to as "water around the ovaries," while other types of ovarian growths are referred to as "fat" or "leather" on the ovary. Likewise, given the popular procreative theory of ovaries that "catch" and sometimes "carry," many women refer to ovarian problems in these functional terms—for example, "ovaries that don't come out" and "ovaries that can't carry the baby." In addition, an absolute "lack" of ovaries or a "missing" ovary is sometimes mentioned as an infertility problem. Indeed, just as weakness and blockage are cross-cutting themes in illness discourse, the problems of "missing parts" and "lack of function" tend to cut across infertility categories, as we shall see.

In addition to problems of the ovaries themselves, problems of ovulation, or *tabwīḍ*, are frequently cited as causes of infertility by Egyptian women, especially by biomedically savvy infertile ones who hear this term used by physicians. In general, *tabwīḍ* is a term that is widely used by Egyptian women but one that is poorly understood. However, because of their considerable participation in the biogynecological system and their experience with matters pertaining to ovulation, infertile women are much more likely than fertile ones to: (1) understand (at least approximately) the biomedical meaning of ovulation; (2) associate ovulation with maximal fertility; and (3) assign this period of maximal fertility to the middle days of the menstrual cycle. Ironically, fertile women, whose ease of conception has allowed them to ignore such matters, are often uninformed about ovulation and are much more likely to: (1) attribute the so-called "fertile period" to the days immediately before or after the menstrual period, when the uterus is still "open" and receptive to "sperm-catching"; (2) believe that a woman can become pregnant on any day of the month; or (3) profess "no idea" about the period of maximal fertility.

Not surprisingly, ovulatory problems are usually seen as revolving around notions of weakness or lack of ovulation. Sometimes, however, women deem ovulatory problems to be related to the *buwaiḍāt*, or eggs, themselves. Among women who accept the egg-sperm theory of procreation, four types of "egg problems" are often mentioned: namely, "lack of eggs," "weak eggs," "blocked eggs," or "eggs that aren't released from the ovaries," again indexing the problems of missing parts, weakness, and blockage. However, among women who do not accept the egg-sperm theory, the equation of a woman's body with that of an egg-producing bird is simply impossible to accept. As one woman exclaimed following an ultrasound examination of her ovaries: "The doctor said I have three eggs! What am I? A chicken!"

Infrequently, problems of the *hormōnāt*, or hormones, are also mentioned in conjunction with ovulatory disturbances. Although very few women admit to understanding the function of these hormones, they hear about them from physicians, who relate them to ovulation. When hormonal problems are cited by women as a cause of infertility, the hormones are usually described as being "disturbed," "bad," or, in some cases, as a foreign agent that has mistakenly appeared "in the blood."

Given the high prevalence of menstrual irregularities among infertile Egyptian women, many women deem problems of the *daura*, or (menstrual) period as a cause of infertility. Inevitably, menstrual problems are viewed in terms of abnormality or irregularity, which can be overcome through regulation. Thus, "an abnormal period," "an irregular period," or "too many periods each month" are all deemed to be causes of infertility. The "lack of a period" is also considered a dire problem, one which is feared by women as a sign of premature menopause. As many women are apt to put it, "If you don't have a period, you can *never* get pregnant."

Uterine Factor

According to the biomedical model, various abnormalities of the uterus can lead to uterine-factor infertility (UFI), as well as a number of other reproductive problems, including recurrent miscarriage. The primary uterine cause of infertility involves uterine leiomyomas, commonly known as uterine "fibroids" or "fibroid tumors" (Winkel 1993). Although the mechanisms by which uterine leiomyomas cause infertility are largely hypothetical, it appears that they may mechanically obstruct conception, either by blocking the fallopian tubes or by distorting the relationship of the reproductive organs (Winkel 1993). In addition, some women suffer from congenital defects of the uterus that render them infertile or subfecund; these include Müllerian duct agenesis, in which the uterus and upper vagina are missing, and various congenital "divisions" of the uterus into unusual (even duplicated) configurations (Winkel 1993).

Although uterine-factor infertility is less common than both tubal and ovarian factors, poor urban Egyptian women deem "problems of the uterus," or *mashākil ir-raḥim* (alternatively, *mashākil il-bait il-wilid*, or "problems of the house of the child") to be the third major cause of female infertility. This notion that uterine-factor infertility is common has been forwarded by many Egyptian biogynecologists, who are responsible for promulgating among their patients two antiquated concepts:[5] (1) that a hypoplastic, or abnormally small, uterus is a cause of infertility, and (2) that uterine malpositioning, and especially retroversion, or "tipping back," of the uterus, is a major cause of infertility. Having learned this from biogynecologists, Egyptian women deem a "small" or "baby" uterus to be one of the most common infertility-related conditions. Likewise, many Egyptian women (and the *dāyāt* who sometimes claim to treat this problem) speak of uterine malpositioning, including "a folded uterus," "an upside-down uterus," "a backwards uterus," "a displaced uterus," "a tilted uterus," "a fallen uterus," and "a flattened uterus," as a major cause of infertility.

Furthermore, as with ovaries, uteri are seen as subject to various kinds of growths—not only fibroids, but cysts and tumors as well. Although these medical terms are occasionally used, women tend to transform them into the familiar language of "fat," "skin," "leather," and "meat," such that uterine growths become "fat around the uterus," "extra skin on the uterus," "leather around the uterus," and "a piece of meat in the uterus," which are thought by some women to lead to uterine "blockage."

Furthermore, uteri, like ovaries—both of which must function correctly in the catch-and-carry procreative process—are seen as suffering from "weakness" and "tiredness." As noted earlier, uteri may also become "disgusted"—a disgust stemming from the polluting menstrual blood with which it must constantly come into contact.

Finally, some women are aware of congenital uterine defects—defects "that a woman is born with." One such condition, being born "uterus-less," is referred to by women as being "born like a man."

Cervical Factor

According to the biomedical model, cervical-factor infertility (CFI) usually involves failure of the sperm to "penetrate" the cervical mucus because of poor mucus quality (Haas and Galle 1984). Normally, the cervical mucus provides the necessary chemical milieu for sperm transport to the upper genital tract; when its quality is deficient, due to, among other things, hormonal disturbances, trauma to the cervical-mucus-secreting glands, cervical tumors, or severe cervicitis (infection-induced inflammation), the cervical mucus acts as a barrier against, rather than as a medium for, sperm upon its entrance into the uterus (otherwise known as sperm/cervical mucus interaction problems) (Byrd 1993; McShane 1988; Rebar 1993).

In Egypt, this view of CFI is not the one most commonly adopted by biogynecologists. Rather, many biogynecologists promote to their infertile patients the atavistic notion that *iltihābāt*, or cervical inflammations, leading to subsequent "erosion" of the cervix, or *qarḥa*, are the primary cause of CFI. In this view—relegated long ago to the annals of gynecological history in the West (Child 1922)—the cervix, or *ʿunq ir-raḥim* (literally, "neck of the uterus"), requires treatment by *kayy*, or cervical electrocautery.

Unfortunately, many Egyptian women wholeheartedly accept this explanation of their infertility and are willing to subject their cervices to *kayy*, which is potentially iatrogenic. However, biogynecologists who are more familiar with currently accepted standards of infertility management and who thus adopt the current definition of CFI sometimes explain to women that "the husband's spermatic animals do not reach the uterus." Again, most infertile women who are told of this etiology wholeheartedly accept it—as well as the blame for their own "rejection" of their husbands' sperm, which, as they notice, "flows out" from the vagina shortly after sex. Although the discharge of seminal fluid from the vagina following intercourse is a normal occurrence and has nothing to do with CFI, Egyptian women, eager to consider all possible causes of their infertility, often fear that their postintercourse discharge is abnormal and then realize this fear when they are told by physicians of their husbands' "nonreaching sperm."

In addition, many Egyptian biogynecologists promote the outdated notion—as old as the "cervical erosion" theory cited above (Child 1922)—that the "stenosed cervix," or "pinhole os" (namely, severe cervical restriction) is a major cause of infertility. Unfortunately, many unknowing Egyptian women are led to believe that they suffer from such tightness—usually translated as *raḥim ḍayyi'*, or a "tight" or "narrow" uterus—requiring various invasive "widening" procedures to be described in the following chapter.

Immune Factor

In addition to all the infertility factors described above, it has come to be accepted in biogynecological circles in the West that some cases of so-called unexplained infertility are, in fact, due to immune factors of either female or male origin (Honea 1993). Female immune factors involve so-called antisperm antibodies, usually occurring at the site of the vagina, cervix, or uterus, which, as the phrase suggests, hinder or "kill" the sperm entering a woman's body. Male immune factors, on the other hand, involve the production of antisperm antibodies in a man's own body (calle autoantibodies), usually as the result of testicular injury.

Although antisperm antibody testing in Egypt is limited to only a few centers (primarily university hospitals in Cairo and Alexandria and selected private infertility clinics), women who have undergone such testing now speak of the problem of *agsām muḍādda*, literally "anti-bodies." They describe this problem in the following ways: "the ovaries and the sperm don't match," "the animals of rejection kill the sperm," or "something in the woman's body rejects the sperm."

Such a notion of antibodies accords well with a widespread, empirically grounded, popular belief among Egyptians that some husbands and wives are individually healthy, but do not match as fertile partners. In describing the causes of infertility, women often remark: "Both the husband and wife are okay, but they don't go together. If they split up and each remarries, they can both have children."

Miscellaneous Factors

Finally, in terms of female infertility, Egyptian women believe in a variety of other biomedical causes, the most common of which is *mashākil wirāthī*, or hereditary problems. With regard to hereditary infertility, there are two common views: (1) that having a first-degree female relative—for example, a mother, sister, aunt, or first cousin—with infertility problems is a sign of (or at least increases the likelihood of) familially based, hereditary infertility; and (2) that hereditary infertility is brought on by consanguineous marriage to cousins. This latter view is debated, however, with Egyptian women appearing to be about evenly divided between those who believe that marriage to a cousin decreases a couple's fertility (because "their blood, which is the same, doesn't mix") and those who believe that cousin-marriage has no effect (because "they have the same blood"). The belief in cousin-marriage causing infertility has *not* been promulgated by Egyptian biogynecologists, who appear to remain unconvinced of any connection.[6] However, biogynecologists do occasionally warn women married to cousins of the risks of congenital anomalies in offspring, as well as recurrent spontaneous abortion, ideas which have also been forwarded by the Egyptian media. Indeed, a nationally televised public service announcement (PSA) airing in the late 1980s warned Egyptians about the dangers of endogamy, pointing specifically to the increased risk of birth defects among the children of cousins. Although this PSA set fear into the hearts of many endogamously married (or about to be married) couples, many Egyptians dismissed the warning, given their own knowledge of many healthy children produced by married cousins.

In addition to hereditary diseases, some Egyptian women contend that major *amrāḍ*, or diseases, such as diabetes, heart conditions, and cancer—all of which, as "diseases of modernization," are becoming increasingly common in urban Egypt and are often related to the problems of female obesity described above—affect a woman's ability to become pregnant. Furthermore, psychological stress is widely acknowledged by Egyptian women as playing a causative role in infertility, a view that accords with biomedical knowledge of so-called psychogenic infertility (Mai 1978).

It is important to note here that *'aqm*, the "official" biomedical term for infertility, is a word that Egyptian women themselves rarely use. Rather, infertility, like fertility, is usually referred to by Egyptian women through use of the verb *khallafa*, which means to leave (someone) behind, have offspring, or have descendants (Cowan 1976). When a woman delivers a baby, she is said by others to have "had offspring." A woman who has never had any children, on the other hand, is referred to through verbal negation as "one who did not have offspring." Thus, infertile women rarely refer to themselves as suffering from *'aqm*, nor would the average Egyptian refer to a childless woman in this way. However, during the late 1980s, the term *'aqm* became popularized in Egypt by way of a series of clever, televised PSAs on the dangers of untreated schistosomiasis (also known as bilharziasis), a life-threatening, parasitic blood fluke infection affecting the majority of rural Egyptians. In one of these PSAs, the mayor of a village (played by a famous Egyptian actor) warns a fellow villager about the assorted serious health problems that may arise from the untreated infection. Of all of the problems mentioned, infertility is the one considered most fearful by the astonished villager, who repeats the word "*'aqm!*" with incredulity. Apparently, this message hit home with the Egyptian viewing public. Within weeks of the PSA's first airing, the term *'aqm* became part of the vocabulary of the Egyptian populace, whereas prior to this, most women admitted having never heard the term. Once *'aqm* became a household word, it also became an occasionally mentioned cause of infertility. But rather than viewing *'aqm* as the biomedical term for the generalized state of being infertile, most women deemed *'aqm* to be a separate, permanent, irreversible *form* of infertility. As they put it, "a woman who has *'aqm* can *never* get pregnant." Given the perceived gravity and intractability of this condition, few infertile women would admit to having such a problem.

Male Factors

Interestingly, this same PSA caused Egyptians to rethink their ideas about the causes of male infertility. Soon after the PSA first aired, Egyptian women began to report that the schistosomiasis parasite, also known as a *dūda*, or "worm," causes male infertility by "eating the husband's worms"! However, given the pervasive tendency for women to be blamed for infertility, others reported that infertility results when the "worm" of a woman with schistosomiasis "eats her husband's worms."

In areas of the world where schistosomiasis is endemic, this disease may, in fact, lead to infertility in the male, through destruction of the urinary tract and blockage of the vessels necessary for the passage of sperm-containing seminal fluid (McFalls and McFalls 1984). Thus, schistosomiasis must be viewed as a risk factor for male-factor infertility (MFI) in Egypt, although its causal role has been poorly investigated (Inhorn and Buss 1994).

Typically, male-factor infertility is due to one or more of the following problems (McConnell 1993): (1) low ejaculate volume; (2) poor sperm density or count, including azoospermia (lack of spermatozoa in the semen) and oligospermia (deficiency in the number of spermatozoa in the semen); (3) poor sperm motility and/or problems with forward progression; (4) abnormalities of sperm morphology, or shape; (5) hyperviscosity of the seminal fluid and pyospermia (presence of pus in the seminal fluid); and (6) autoantibody formation against sperm, a problem described above.

Among poor urban Egyptians, *mashākil id-dīdān*, or "problems of the worms," is the generic term for all of these factors. Within this category of worm problems, however, a number of more specific conditions are widely recognized. The primary cause of male infertility is considered to be "weak worms," which is not surprising, given the aforementioned idiom of "weakness" which pervades reproductive imagery. In addition, because men's worms are considered to be *living spermatic animals*—animals with the important job of carrying men's fetuses to women's wombs—they are seen as suffering the problems of other animals, including excessive somnolence, natural death, and even murder. Thus, many Egyptian women speak of "sleeping worms," "dead worms," "worms that die quickly," "an infection that kills the worms," "discharge from the woman that kills the worms," "bacteria [or pus or a microbe] that kills the worms," or "suffocated worms." Furthermore, the problem of not having enough worms—namely, the problem of low sperm count—is one that is recognized as important. Some men are seen as having "no worms at all," "a low percentage of worms," "too few worms," or, in a fusion of popular and biomedical language, "a low worm count"!

Men are also seen as having problems of *sā'il*, or seminal fluid, which is deemed necessary as the medium for spermatic worm transport to the woman's reproductive body. Thus, "pus in the fluid," "weak fluid," "bad fluid," "watery fluid," and "fluid like liquid" are all considered to be prob-

TABLE 5. Biomedical Causes of Infertility in the Study Sample of One Hundred Infertile Women and Their Husbands.

FACTOR/ PROBLEM	NUMBER SUFFERING FROM FACTOR (OF TOTAL NUMBER TESTED)	PERCENTAGE
Male factors	40/87	46
Female factors	82/100	82
Ovarian	49/87	56
Tubal	41/89	46
Cervical	25/56	45
Uterine	19/100	19
Miscellaneous	10/100	10
Unknown factors	6/100	6
Sexual problems	13/100	13

lems associated with male infertility. Furthermore, the "tubes" transporting the fluid may suffer from blockage, or, as one woman put it, "one of the veins may be weak." In addition, the term *brūstata* is occasionally used to refer to prostatitis, or an infection-induced inflammation of the prostate leading to pus in the seminal fluid. Unfortunately, the problem of pus—in semen or urine—is a major problem for poor urban Egyptian men, who, in many cases, probably suffer from sexually transmitted infections of which their wives are unaware.

Many poor urban Egyptian women view their husbands' sexual problems as another major cause of infertility. Although sexual problems are rarely addressed by Egyptian biogynecologists, even when conferring with their infertile patients, Egyptian women themselves are often very concerned about the effects of their husbands' sexual performance problems on their own fertility. Impotence, which is often attributed to sorcery, is usually described by women in terms of the husband being "tired," "sick," or "weak" in the genital region (or "from down," as Egyptian women usually refer to this area). Other male sexual problems also revolve around the idioms of weakness and blockage—namely, "weak ejaculation," "blocked ejaculation," or "a weak testicle." A few women also believe a "small penis" to be a male problem, but it is unclear whether this problem is seen as related to male infertility per se or to sexual performance alone.

Given these various understandings of male and female infertility, the

TABLE 6. Multifactorial Etiology of Infertility Problems in the Study Sample of One Hundred Infertile Women and Their Husbands.

NUMBER OF BIOLOGICAL FACTORS DIAGNOSED	PERCENTAGE OF COUPLES
None (unexplained)	6
One	36
Two	29
Three	18
Four	10
More than four	1
Total	100

MALE OR FEMALE FACTORS DIAGNOSED	PERCENTAGE OF COUPLES
Female only	42
Male only	11
Female and male	31
Unknown	6
Total	100

important question remains: Are infertile Egyptian women aware of which of these assorted problems affects them and their husbands? For the most part, the answer is "no," for reasons to be described shortly. However, to demonstrate this, one need only consider the "distribution of understanding" among the one hundred infertile women in this study. As shown in Tables 5 and 6, these women and their husbands suffered from a variety of infertility factors, including many cases with so-called multifactorial etiology. However, the degree of disparity between the known biomedical causes of these couples' infertility problems, as diagnosed at the time of this study, and women's knowledge of these diagnosed causes was quite profound. Specifically, fifty-seven of one hundred women, or more than half, were unaware of one or more of the biomedical factors relating to their infertility. In addition, seventeen of these women were entirely unaware of the biomedical nature of their infertility problems. Moreover, twenty-seven of the one hundred women believed they were suffering from biomedical causes that, in fact, had never been diagnosed. Among this population of poor urban Egyptian women, only twenty-two, or less than one quarter, were accurately apprised of all of the diagnosed causes of their infertility, and, in most of these cases, this was probably due to the single-factor nature of their problems.

But why do poor infertile Egyptian women, so well informed about biomedical causes in general, remain so strikingly *uninformed* about the particular facts of their own cases? The reasons for this disturbing disjunction are the subject to which we now turn.

The Dilatory Reproduction of Biomedical Knowledge

It is important to state from the outset that infertile Egyptian women's critical knowledge gap with regard to the nature of their infertility problems is a direct reflection of the knowledge gap of most Egyptian biogynecologists with regard to recent advancements in infertility diagnosis and management. In plain terms, biomedical knowledge about the mechanisms underlying infertility causation and the ways in which specific etiological factors can be satisfactorily diagnosed and treated is constantly being updated and, in fact, has been transformed dramatically over the past two decades; yet, the reproduction of such metamorphosing knowledge has lagged far behind in Egyptian biogynecological circles. This dilatory reproduction of new knowledge, and the resultant knowledge gap among many Egyptian biogynecologists, has created critical problems for the infertile women who must seek treatment from these physicians. Although some Egyptian biogynecologists manage to stay well-informed, many display an understanding of infertility diagnosis and therapy that is abysmally outdated. Moreover, those who are able to diagnose women's problems correctly are often reluctant to convey this "sacred knowledge" to their female patients for reasons to be examined shortly.

To understand what goes wrong in women's biogynecological searches for children—including the lack of conveyance of information to them about the nature of their own infertility problems—it is necessary to address a number of critical features of Egyptian biogynecological infertility practice, beginning with issues of diagnosis and proceeding in the following chapters through issues of therapy.

The first problem is that, in Egypt, formal subspecialization within the larger specialty of obstetrics and gynecology is largely absent; thus, there is no official mechanism by which motivated biogynecologists can become experts in infertility. In the West, infertility subspecialization has been viewed as a necessity, particularly since the advent of IVF in the last two decades and the veritable explosion of infertility-related biomedical knowledge. In the United States, for example, board certification in reproductive endocrinology and infertility was established twenty years ago in 1974, and, since that time, membership in the American Fertility Society has risen dramatically (Aral and Cates 1983). Biomedical residency training and postresidency fellowship programs in reproductive endocrinology and infertility have also proliferated in recent years, and treatment centers and physicians specializing in infertility can be found in most urban centers in the United States (U.S. Congress, Office of Technology Assessment 1988). Furthermore, among this group of infertility subspecialists, widespread consensus exists regarding the major etiological factors in infertility, although differences of opinion may occur over the best diagnostic and therapeutic regimens, particularly with regard to the so-called assisted reproductive technologies (including artificial insemination and IVF).

In Egypt, on the other hand, biomedical subspecialization of this sort—gynecological or otherwise—has essentially not taken place. Thus, as it now stands, most Egyptian biogynecologists, even those who claim to have primary interests in infertility, are obstetric and gynecological generalists, who deliver babies, provide prenatal care and contraception, treat miscellaneous gynecological complaints, and perform gynecological surgery, among other things. Because of their needs to survive economically in a poor country with an overabundance of physicians and a lack of specialized biomedical technology, most biogynecologists are unwilling to turn away any potential patient; thus, they effectively reduce their chances of gaining expertise in any one area of biogynecological practice.

The untoward consequences of biogynecological practitioner competition in an economically depressed environment cannot be underestimated. In Egypt, biogynecologists—the vast majority of whom hold assigned government posts but who earn their livings through after-hours, private, fee-for-service practice—are eager to gain patients, especially in urban areas, where biogynecologists are in oversupply. Thus, as we shall see in the following chapter, biogynecologists, spurred by the profit motive, are willing to offer purportedly therapeutic infertility procedures that are guaranteed to generate income for them, but that may lead to destructive rather than curative changes in patients' reproductive tracts. Furthermore, much of this infertility "therapy" is undertaken with minimal diagnosis, since diagnostic procedures may be unavailable, are less lucrative than most therapies, are time-consuming, and may cause patients to become bored and lost to other physicians.

In other words, biogynecologists who are pressured to make money may, in fact, perform procedures for this reason, rather than to help patients overcome their problems. In addition, because most biogynecologists struggle to meet the overhead of their private practices, they are unwilling to invest the time or money in continuing medical education (CME), available mostly abroad. Frankly, recent periodicals containing specialized biomedical literature on topics such as infertility are extremely expensive to obtain in Egypt, and computers providing up-to-date information on medical literature are largely absent, even in urban centers. Coupled with the lack of CME requirements, physicians of all types lack incentives to update their biomedical knowledge.

As one Egyptian biogynecologist viewed the situation,

> We need more specialized physicians. They need to get exposure to the rest of the world to update themselves on the modern treatment of infertility. I think associations of gynecologists and obstetricians should be more active in this respect. They need a good budget to bring people, to get doctors to take a course for one week to update their knowledge. And they should make it cheap so they [doctors] can sacrifice their [private] clinics for one week, and this would help our community. . . . Actually, for me, you may have noticed, I paid £E 13,000 [$5,200] for this trip to Australia, and I go to conferences in Berlin, Singapore. It is my duty, my patients are paying me. I reward them by helping them to know more. The only teaching that was done in Shatby was laparoscopy, because this was financed by international aid. I hope some international aid promotes more activity in this respect, because many physicians, their information stopped at some point.

Thus, as suggested by this physician, the reproduction of contemporary biomedical knowledge regarding infertility has occurred in a haphazard fashion in Egypt and, on a general level, has lagged far behind in many areas. Consequently, it would not be overstating the case to claim that, in Egypt, biogynecologists demonstrate a striking lack of uniformity in their understanding of the biomedical model of infertility causation and accompanying diagnostic methods. Generally speaking, those physicians who are most well informed are university-based biogynecologists, or, in a few cases, exceptionally motivated private practitioners who, at their own expense, have sought specialized training in infertility outside the country. However, the majority of Egyptian biogynecologists appear to base their practice of infertility diagnosis and management on information gained as medical students from textbooks, written, in some cases, decades ago by Egyptian biogynecologists who were then deemed authority figures in the field.

Herein lies another problem, one that is rooted in the history of biomedical colonialism in Egypt and is raised as critical by some Egyptian biogynecologists themselves. According to them, the widespread practice in Egypt of following the traditions set down by earlier biomedical authority figures is culturally grounded in the nature of Egyptian society itself and the tendency of Egyptians to follow patriarchal authority figures—what El-Mehairy (1984b) calls "demigods"—of all kinds, including, for example, charismatic rulers or religious leaders. According to these physician critics, this tenacious pursuit of biomedical tradition has thwarted biomedical innovation in Egypt and has led to biogynecological practices based on outdated and, in some cases, clearly erroneous beliefs about the nature of disease causation and treatment.

As one such physician critic noted in condemning the practice of cervical electrocautery,

> If you open a book written by [a professor] thirty years ago, you will find it. But things change. If this was a good treatment thirty years ago, it doesn't have to be kept because a professor mentioned it in a book. People here are sensitive about this; they say, "We are insulting our professor." Because here there is no democracy at any level. . . . In places like the U.S. and England, these are democratic countries, and any young doctor will question anything which is not logical. . . . There is no monopoly on scientific thinking, but this is a problem we have here. A professor will be very much offended if you tell him something against his opinion. This helps to propagate the wrong things. They're doing it, and no one is talking to them. The juniors are stuck to them in the beginning, and they keep on doing it. And if you start criticizing, you end up having some problems.

The issue of cervical-factor infertility to which this physician refers provides a case in point of the problem of medical traditionalism. As described above, in current biogynecological thinking, cervical-factor infertility refers primarily to poor cervical mucus quality, leading to a failure of sperm transport to the upper genital tract. Initial diagnosis of cervical-factor infertility generally requires only one of two simple tests—namely, microscopic examination of the cervical mucus itself, or, ideally, a postcoital test (PCT), in which a sample of cervical mucus is taken several hours after intercourse to assess the success of sperm penetration and transport in the mucus (Bradshaw and Carr 1993). The PCT is also an effective initial test (although not a definitive one) of immunological problems between infertile partners (Honea 1993).

Some biogynecologists point to the practical difficulties in Egypt of undertaking the PCT, which, among Egyptian women, is known as *ʿayyina min il-mahbal baʿd il-iktimāʿ*, or "a specimen from the vagina after sexual intercourse." Indeed, of all of the procedures employed in the diagnosis of infertility in Egypt, the PCT is the most problematic on cultural grounds. Because it involves taking a sample of cervical mucus from the woman's vagina several hours (from zero to twenty-four) after intercourse, it violates two important sexual norms found in Egypt.

First, Egyptian women maintain rather rigorous standards regarding genital purity, and the PCT violates these standards. Most poor urban women practice frequent manual vaginal douching, sometimes once or twice daily, sometimes before prayer, and usually immediately following sexual intercourse.[7] As women explain, immediate internal washing of the vagina with warm water, using the first and second fingers, is imperative as a purifying method within the first half-hour or so after the sex act is completed. Given this behavioral norm, the PCT essentially requires that a woman remain "unpurified" for up to twenty-four hours after sex—a condition that many women find defiling and even repugnant. Physicians are often forced to insist that patients refrain from genital washing until after the PCT is performed (and in general when their patients are trying to become pregnant). When a PCT is performed and spermatozoa are absent in the cervical mucus, physicians often suspect that the patient has douched in this way.

Second, the PCT also requires that a husband and wife perform sexual intercourse "on demand." In most cases, a woman is told by her physician to ask her husband to have sex during a given evening and to return the following morning for the PCT. Thus, female patients are compelled to ask their husbands to have sex with them, which is contrary to gender expectations. As women explain, it is men—not women—who initiate sex. For a woman to do so would be both abnormal and even shameful. Thus, for yet another reason, the PCT is problematic for women, some of whom are forced to ask their physicians the humiliating question, "But how can I go home and ask my husband to have sex with me?"

Yet, given these cultural barriers to the PCT, it is extremely important to note that they do not represent the major obstacle to the effective diagnosis of cervical-factor infertility in Egypt. Rather, relatively few Egyptian biogynecologists understand the contemporary biomedical meaning of cervical-factor infertility, nor do they attempt to diagnose it through such biomedically accepted techniques. Instead, among most biogynecologists in Egypt, cervical-factor infertility is essentially synonymous with cervicitis, or inflammation of the cervix, which is diagnosed through standard speculum examination. Indeed, *qarḥa*, or cervical erosion, resulting from the breakdown of the cervical epithelium presumably caused by severe, chronic cervicitis, is one of the most often cited (by both physicians and patients) biogynecological conditions in Egypt. As we shall see in the following chapter, infertile patients are often told by their physicians that their problem lies in a cervical erosion, which must be treated by electrocautery of the cervix. Yet, as some Egyptian critics of the "erosion myth" explain, cervical erosions (1) are diagnosed in Egypt far more often than they actually occur, (2) are probably not a major cause—if at all—of infertility, and (3) are treated in ways that probably *produce* true iatrogenic cervical-factor infertility, through the destruction of cervical-mucus-producing glands and subsequent fibrosis and stenosis of the cervix.

As one Egyptian biogynecologist lamented,

> Did you hear about the "honey month [honeymoon] erosion"? A woman doesn't get pregnant after one or two months, so she goes to a physician. He examines her and tells her, "You have a honey month erosion. You *must* have cautery." This is the time he must teach her about the fertile period and things that may benefit her, instead of doing cautery. She has no indication for cautery. But many doctors don't know how to investigate cervical factor. This is not due to its difficulty, but due to ignorance, and few doctors consider it important. *Very few* can investigate it properly, can do the PCT.

Dismal Diagnostics

The lack of Egyptian biogynecologists' common understandings of what cervical-factor infertility means, as well as their lack of up-to-date understanding of other important infertility factors, has produced two important effects. The first has to do with diagnosis itself and the second with the disclosure of diagnostic information.

With respect to the first point, the diagnosis of infertility in Egypt frankly lacks standardization, because of the lack of uniformity in etiological understandings among Egyptian biogynecologists. Depending upon the physician's state of knowledge, resources, and enthusiasm, the biomedical diagnosis of an Egyptian woman's infertility problems can proceed in any one of four ways.

No Diagnosis

Many biogynecologists treat infertile women without recourse to diagnostic techniques of any kind. After taking a brief medical history, they may prescribe "empiric therapy," or therapy given without specific diagnostic tests. In the case of infertility, biogynecologists tend to prescribe an ovulation-induction regimen, usually the drug clomiphene citrate, or Clomid, which will be described in greater detail in the following chapter. However, in some cases, biogynecologists may proceed to more invasive therapeutic procedures. Although biomedical treatment of infertility without specific diagnosis appears to be a common practice in Egypt, it is condemned by many Egyptian biogynecologist critics as being unwarranted, potentially harmful, and a reflection of a lack of knowledge about infertility etiology, diagnosis, and management.

As one biogynecologist stated,

> This is what you call "drug abuse." Some physicians, when they see an infertile patient, they start to give her Clomid, and this is wrong, as you know. First, you must do investigations and decide which factor is responsible for the infertility, whether tubal, ovarian, and so on. After an accurate diagnosis, then you can start to treat. I don't believe in empiric therapy, only in a very, very few cases in which the patient cannot afford to do investigations, or she is in a hurry for some reason, and I do it with shame. It's very rare that I do this.

Minimal Diagnosis

Perhaps the most common diagnostic course undertaken by Egyptian biogynecologists is one of minimal diagnosis. This usually involves a history and pelvic examination (by speculum) of the infertile woman and a request that her husband undergo semen analysis, which is called *taḥlīl l-guz*, or "analysis of the husband." To their credit, most Egyptian biogynecologists are adamant that semen analysis must be the initial diagnostic step and must be undertaken before the wife undergoes further diagnostic evaluation or treatment. But, as many Egyptian biogynecologists acknowledge, semen analysis in Egypt is fraught with difficulty and may provide little in the way of accurate etiological assessment.

First, truly accurate semen analysis requires sophisticated technology and is difficult to perform and interpret in any setting, despite the efforts by the World Health Organization to implement worldwide standards for quality control among laboratories undertaking this procedure (World Health Organization 1987b). Second, problems of performance and interpretation are exacerbated in Egypt, where laboratories vary considerably in their equipment, personnel, and quality control. Egyptian biogynecologists sometimes complain that semen analyses are considered by Egyptian laboratory staff to be unimportant and unpleasant and are left to the most junior personnel, who lack knowledge about this procedure. As a result, many semen analyses are replete with obvious errors. Third, semen samples are often produced through masturbation at home, sometimes with contaminating lubricants, and then are brought to laboratories for analysis (often by men's wives) after they are no longer of optimal quality. Fourth, many husbands are simply unwilling or reluctant to undergo semen analysis, for reasons having to do with pride and social embarrassment. Thus, some husbands may refuse to undergo semen analysis altogether, or they may undergo it secretely and hide poor results from their wives and families. Fifth, even when husbands agree to go to a laboratory for semen analysis, it is said that they may bribe the technicians to write "a really good report." Thus, semen analysis reports may be inauthentic in addition to objectively unreliable. Finally, some men refuse to turn over the results of their semen analyses to their wives and their wives' treating physicians. Men who can read may tell their wives, who are often illiterate: "My semen analysis says that I'm okay, and the problem is with you."

Nonetheless, given these inherent difficulties, it appears that most Egyptian biogynecologists attempt to enforce this diagnostic measure in order to relieve the burden of responsibility from women whose husbands happen to be infertile, and most Egyptian husbands comply with physicians' requests, sometimes repeatedly. When husbands can be shown to be suffering from a male factor, women are often told by their physicians to wait to undergo further evaluation and treatment until their husbands receive therapy. Unfortunately, however, male-factor infertility is often not remediable by current drug therapies, and few Egyptian urologists or andrologists are specialized in treating this difficult problem.

Specific Diagnosis

Although specific diagnostic measures other than semen analysis are often ignored, some Egyptian biogynecologists do make an attempt to diagnose the biomedical causes of infertility in their female patients, utilizing available diagnostic resources. In Egypt, the most common diagnostic procedures, other than semen analysis, include: (1) premenstrual endometrial biopsies (*'ayyina min ir-raḥim*, or "a specimen from the uterus") to detect the presence of ovulation; and (2) hysterosalpingography (HSG) (*ṣūra ashi"a bi ṣibghā*, or "an X ray by dye"), an X ray of the pelvis in which dye is injected to determine uterine abnormalities and blockage of the fallopian tubes. Less common diagnostic procedures include: (1) diagnostic laparoscopy (*il-manẓar*, or "the view"), a surgical procedure in which a scoping instrument is inserted through the abdominal wall to assess tubal blockage and the presence of fibrous adhesions around the fallopian tubes and uterus; (2) serum hormonal assays (*taḥlīl id-dam*, or "analysis of the blood") and/or ultrasound monitoring (*it-taṣwīr*, or "the photography") of the ovarian follicles to assess ovulation; (3) PCTs (as described above), cervical mucus studies (*'ayyina min il-mahbal*, or "a specimen from the vagina"), and other sperm-penetration tests to detect cervical and cervical-immunological factors and various sperm abnormalities; and (4) specific immunological, or antisperm antibody tests (*taḥlīl agsām muḍādda*, or "analysis of antibodies").

Yet, as with semen analysis, many of these available diagnostic procedures are fraught with difficulty in Egypt. Diagnostic laparoscopy, one of the most powerful tools for assessing the status of a woman's reproductive tract, is one such problematic procedure. Currently, diagnostic laparoscopes are available in most major hospitals in the urban centers of Egypt, thanks to international agencies that have donated this equipment. As a result, a number of hospitals, including the University of Alexandria's Shatby Hospital, have offered diagnostic laparoscopy training programs for Egyptian biogynecologists. These programs have been popular with physicians. However, because of the large number of biogynecologists attending these courses and the limited number of laparoscopes and educated instructors, many biogynecologists have left these programs with limited experience—only to practice diagnostic laparoscopy in their home communities. According to some university-based infertility specialists, this lack of expertise has led to problems, because laparoscopy is relatively easy to perform but difficult to interpret. The occasional result is that major interpretive errors are made. For example, a woman who had undergone laparoscopy by an inexperienced physician was told that both of her fallopian tubes were blocked and that she would never be able to conceive without undergoing IVF. However, when her laparoscopy was repeated by a competent, university-based biogynecologist who suspected the error in reading the first laparoscopy report, it was revealed that both of her tubes were, in fact, unobstructed.

In addition, as with men and semen analysis, some women may refuse to undergo diagnostic laparoscopy, which they view as a nontherapeutic surgical procedure.[8] As will be apparent in the following chapter, Egyptian women are usually willing to undergo surgery if they believe it is potentially curative. But surgery for the sake of diagnosis alone is viewed by some as posing an unreasonable risk. In fact, because of problems of hygiene and sepsis in most Egyptian hospitals (especially public ones), postlaparoscopy infections may lead to further tubal-factor infertility problems.

Thus, in most cases, decisions about if, when, and how these various diagnostic tests and procedures are performed on a given patient often have less to do with the patient's history and the clinical suspicion of the physician than with a number of other intervening variables, including: (1) the infertility factors the physician views as most common in his/her practice and therefore most likely in a given patient; (2) the infertility factors the physician considers easiest to diagnose; (3) the availability of diagnostic equipment and materials to the physician; (4) the ability of the physician to perform the diagnostic procedure himself/herself, thereby generating additional income; (5) the patient's ability to pay for the test or procedure; and (6) the patient's willingness to undergo the test or procedure.

The case of the premenstrual endometrial biopsy provides an excellent example of the power of many of these factors in determining diagnostic decision-making. To wit, more Egyptian women undergo premenstrual endometrial biopsies for the evaluation of ovulation than less invasive and more diagnostically specific serum hormonal assays, which only require that a sample of blood be drawn. Why? First, Egyptian biogynecologists view the premenstrual endometrial biopsy as a technically easy, income-generating procedure that they can perform by themselves, usually on an outpatient basis. Second, hormonal assays, unlike premenstrual endometrial biopsies, require the services of one of the few Egyptian laboratories able to provide this type of testing, and these laboratories are notoriously slow and are viewed as taking business away from the physician (even though they are deemed as excellent by specialized biogynecologists who use them). Third, patients are usually willing to undergo a painless biopsy, which is performed under anesthesia. And, finally, premenstrual endometrial biopsies are often accompanied by dilatation and curettage (D & C) of the uterus, which many Egyptian physicians tell patients is curative for infertility.

Given these types of intervening factors, diagnostic regimens in Egypt tend to vary from patient to patient and from physician to physician.

TABLE 7. Diagnostic Histories of Ninety-five Infertile Women in the Study Sample and Their Husbands.

DIAGNOSTIC TEST	PERCENTAGE OF WOMEN / MEN TESTED
Male factor:	
Semen analysis (*taḥlīl l-guz*)	92
Sperm penetration assay	6
Hormonal assay (*taḥlīl l-hormōnāt*)	3
Ovarian factor:	
Hormonal assay (*taḥlīl id-dam*)	49
Endometrial biopsy (*'ayyina min ir-raḥim*)	44
Ultrasound (*it-taṣwīr*)	83
Tubal factor:	
Hysterosalpingography (*ṣūra ashi''a bi ṣibghā*)	74
Diagnostic laparoscopy (*il-manẓar*)	63
Cervical factor:	
Postcoital test (*'ayyina min il-mahbal ba'd il-iktimā'*)	55
Cervical mucus study (*'ayyina min il-mahbal*)	21
Immune factor:	
Antisperm antibody study (*taḥlīl agsām muḍādda*)	11

Furthermore, when patients switch physicians, which is commonplace in Egypt, diagnostic procedures may be randomly repeated, often with little attention to previous tests the patient may have undergone. Because most infertile Egyptian women "doctor shop" in this way—visiting as many as twenty physicians during their careers as patients—they are likely to undergo a variety of diagnostic tests, even though the majority of Egyptian physicians may treat them empirically. For example, most of the women in this study had already been subjected to an array of diagnostic tests before coming to the university teaching hospital, where they often underwent additional, more sophisticated procedures, including diagnostic laparoscopy, ultrasound follicular scanning, and, in a few cases, antisperm antibody studies. A review of the diagnostic histories of these women is presented in Tables 7 and 8. However, it is important to bear in mind that these

TABLE 8. Total Number of Types of Diagnostic Tests Undertaken by Ninety-five Infertile Women in the Study Sample.

NUMBER OF TYPES OF TESTS	PERCENTAGE OF WOMEN TESTED
None	1
One	13
Two	9
Three	15
Four	21
Five	16
Six	14
Seven	8
Eight	3
Total	100

women are diagnostically atypical, in that they had undergone many additional tests by virtue of their participation as patients at the university infertility clinic.

Systematic Diagnosis

Given this rather complicated state of diagnostic affairs, it is not surprising that few infertile Egyptian women are systematically diagnosed, despite repeated visits to physicians. Certainly, biogynecologists who maintain an up-to-date, systematic approach to the evaluation of infertile patients exist in Egypt, in both public and private practice settings in urban areas. For example, in terms of diagnostic capabilities and knowledgeable personnel, the University of Alexandria's Shatby Hospital offers exceptional diagnostic services, undertaken by a number of qualified staff members who have devoted their primary energies to the problems of infertile patients. Yet, it is important to reiterate that this public hospital, which has made a major commitment to infertility services, is exceptional by the standards described above. Although knowledgeable and competent private practitioners of infertility care do exist in Alexandria, they are not particularly common. Thus, outside of the hospital, infertile Alexandrian women encounter varying experiences in diagnosis, as well as generalized frustration in their own quests for diagnostic information and etiological understanding.

Summing up the situation, one physician critic commented,

> There is a major problem in Egypt in that obstetrics and gynecology [are] practiced by many nonspecialists. They just had the usual training in medical education. This is not at all enough to manage especially infertile patients. They misunderstand many things, and they abuse many things, and people will never have a result with such doctors. And I find many of the specialists, if they are not interested in infertility, they do not have a logical way of how to deal with a case. They do not know what to do first, what's the next step. They cannot pinpoint the problem, because infertility is a little more complicated. One who is dealing with [infertility] should be interested in infertility, should have good knowledge, and should be trained and have some experience.

Disclosure of Sacred Knowledge

This brings us to the second main effect of the variability in Egyptian biogynecologists' understandings of infertility etiology—one that involves disclosure of etiological and diagnostic information to infertile patients. In short, physicians who are not adept at assessing etiological possibilities through diagnostic methods are less likely to find an actual biomedical cause of a patient's infertility, and are therefore also less likely to provide the patient with information about causation.

Despite most infertile women's eager participation in the biomedical system, despite their ardent desires to understand the reasons for their failures to conceive, and despite their constant speculation about the possible causes of their infertility (and their tendency to blame themselves for multiple possible causes), relatively few women understand their own biomedical profiles, as described earlier. In fact, many poor urban Egyptian women are at an almost total loss to explain their infertility problems from a biomedical perspective, despite, in many cases, years of participation as consumers of biomedical care. Many women state flatly that they have "no idea" what is wrong with them, having never been informed by a single physician of the cause(s) of their infertility.

Furthermore, when physician-to-patient disclosure does occur, it tends to take one of the following forms: (1) the physician tells the patient, "There is nothing wrong with you," when, in fact, later diagnoses reveal a biomedical problem; (2) the physician offers an explanation, such as "an infection," "an erosion," or "a hypoplastic [small] uterus," which is not the actual causative factor of the infertility; (3) the physician accurately identifies a causative factor but misrepresents it to the patient through superficial explanation or gross oversimplification; or (4) the physician identifies a causative factor and attempts to explain it to the patient, but the patient misunderstands the physician's complicated language or partial representation of the problem.

Thus, disclosure of etiological as well as other biomedical information from physicians to patients in this setting can only be described as suboptimal, especially considering patients' desires to comprehend causation. As with the problems of diagnosis described above, some Egyptian biogynecologists decry the current state of affairs, blaming physicians for a reprehensible lack of patient education.

As one critic stated,

> It's very easy to tell most patients. With only very few do you find it impossible. The patient should be informed, should know everything, even if you find that they are illiterate, they are ignorant. They have some sort of reasoning, they can imagine what you're telling them, they can understand what's the problem. I think the only problem is that you have to get their confidence first of all; if you get that, they will do everything.
>
> Another problem is that patients try to ask, but doctors give imprecise information. He puts the thing in his own words in Arabic. He may tell her anything. Probably she has some sort of disease and can't say it in Arabic, and he wants to make it clear in Arabic, so he tells her something else. So we have to use precise and exact terms to explain what's wrong.
>
> Because many of the doctors do not inform the patients, this is the problem [leading to "doctor shopping"]. They don't tell them what's the problem, what's to be done, what's the program, and when to begin therapy, what are the results, what are all the therapies available, what are those available somewhere else. If the patient is so informed, she will be aware that the best doctor is *that* doctor, that he knows what's the problem, and he is efficient to treat and that he will tell her to go elsewhere if he can't treat her. So the problem is from the doctor mainly, because we do not inform. I, myself, I inform the patient, and I tell her what I've told you. But many of them just say, "Come to do that. Don't ask! Don't ask!" This is a problem with medical education, which doesn't emphasize informing patients. Because of the law, you have no responsibility if you don't inform, if you don't have consent, because the patient doesn't know what are her rights. Medical behavior—the behavior of the medical class itself—has to be changed.

Unfortunately, such enlightened attitudes are relatively hard to find in the Egyptian biogynecological community. Most Egyptian biogynecologists support a minimal disclosure position, justifying it on three grounds: (1) the lack of time for such discussion with patients; (2) the belief that patients actually fear knowledge about causation and will fail to return to the physician who has made them afraid by providing such information;

and (3) the belief that most patients are ignorant, especially in matters of reproduction, and are therefore incapable of understanding sophisticated biomedical information even after considerable effort to educate them.

Given the pervasiveness of such attitudes in the Egyptian biomedical community, critical examination and demystification of these various rationales for lack of disclosure are required, as well as an attempt to provide alternative explanations for what may be viewed as a significant problem of doctor-patient miscommunication.[9]

First, it is true that some physicians lack time to provide adequate patient education and counseling. Because of the lack of qualified paramedical personnel, every task—from drawing blood to counseling patients to cleaning instruments—may be left in the hands of physicians, who are overburdened with responsibilities that could best be handled by others. As a result, many physicians rightfully feel pressured for time. But whether this effectively prevents most physicians from talking to patients is doubtful.

For example, in the busiest and most successful private infertility practice in the Alexandria vicinity, the practicing biogynecologist routinely spends up to an hour with the woman—and ideally her husband if he is present—explaining basic reproductive physiology and what the husband and wife can expect to take place, both diagnostically and therapeutically, in the coming weeks. Although this "interview," as the physician calls it, requires valuable time, it leads to greater compliance, a sense of empowerment for the infertile husband and wife, and a relationship of trust between patients and the physician, which he believes is requisite for success in what may be a long-term diagnostic and treatment regimen. From the experience of this physician and others like him, motivation to spend such "downtime" with patients has been a crucial variable in the development of a highly successful practice.

Second, although few physicians are motivated to tell patients about the cause of their infertility problems, most patients are highly motivated to find out. Yet, this is a fact not widely perceived by physicians, who say they do not want to lose patients by worrying them with their biomedical problems.[10] Furthermore, because medical examinations are often rushed, allowing little time for discussion, many women are reluctant to ask physicians—by whom they are generally intimidated and who do not give them "the chance to speak"[11]—the simple question: "What is wrong with me?" Because most women do not ask this question directly, most physicians assume incorrectly that their patients do not want to know. Consequently, physicians may be reluctant to volunteer information that may be upsetting and that they suspect may cause the patient to "escape" to another physician. Furthermore, and very significantly, most physicians appear to be quite sympathetic to the social plight of infertile women; thus, they fear that providing an actual diagnosis of female-factor infertility may be used against the woman by her husband and his family. This is perhaps the major reason why infertile women are repeatedly told by physicians the reportable statement, "There's nothing wrong with you," even in the face of convincing countervailing evidence. Thus, *not* telling women the cause of their infertility may be viewed by physicians as the most socially sensitive measure—one that is even perceived as preventive against divorce.

Infertile women, on the other hand, are already upset, for a variety of social relational reasons (Inhorn n.d.), and not knowing the cause of their reproductive failure tends to make them suffer even more. In reality, women spend considerable time pondering the possible biomedical causes of their infertility and asking themselves questions such as: "Is the problem from him or from me?" "Is it incurable?" "Will it require surgery?" "Did I do something to cause the problem?" Most women are, in fact, desperate for biomedical explanations to such questions, and this is especially true in cases in which women suspect infertility on the part of their husbands, but are unable to verify this possibility.[12]

Third, it is true that many Egyptian patients are uneducated and illiterate. But this is not synonymous with uneducable or ignorant, the latter being the pejorative term often used by Egyptian physicians to describe their lower-class patients. As already seen, many infertile Egyptian women who have never been schooled in biology, reproductive physiology, or sex education manage to absorb, on their own, a tremendous amount of biomedical information, which they piece together as best they can in an attempt to make sense of their cases. In fact, infertile women often pick up most of this information during their many hours spent sitting with other infertile patients in the waiting areas of physicians' offices, hospitals, and clinics. There, they overhear information from doctors and from other women, and they may become involved in active exchanges of such information, some of it accurate and some of it not.

Given the seemingly indefensible nature of physicians' arguments for minimal disclosure, this lack of doctor-patient communication may be more usefully viewed from the perspective of social control and the monopolization of power in the biomedical encounter (Becker and Nachtigall 1991). As Oakley (1987) has argued in her examination of infertility practice in the West, physicians' retention of absolute control over expert knowledge and procedures is intrinsic to their claims of professionalization. Similarly, for Egypt, it can be argued that the minimal disclosure of crucial information to patients is a direct reflection of what Ehrenreich (1978) has called "the problem of professionalism":

> In our system, professionalism is primarily a defense of status and privilege. Although doctors and other health professionals have defended professionalism as a bulwark of quality, it has functioned more effectively as a mechanism to protect professionals from scrutiny, to limit access to the occupation and to medical knowledge, and to preserve doctors' control over the health system. To change the health system at all, much less to create a medical system which maximally utilizes self-help and mutual help and which encourages an active rather than a passive role for the patient, will require radical deprofessionalization. We will have to expand radically the use of community health aids; to spread medical knowledge to patients and to nonphysician health workers; to minimize the social distance between doctors and patients. . . . It is the privileges, the power, and the monopolization of medical knowledge that I am speaking of removing when I speak of deprofessionalization. (Ehrenreich 1978:28–29)

In Egypt, it is certainly in the best interests of physicians as a professional group—consisting of individuals drawn mainly from the upper and upper-middle classes—to maintain the privileges of elite status through the social distancing of largely lower-class patients and through the monopolization of quasi-sacred, specialized knowledge, available to only the chosen few. Although Egyptian biogynecologists tend to rationalize their control of etiological and diagnostic information through the three aforementioned arguments, it is equally plausible that physicians' failure to "reveal themselves" is primarily an attempt to maintain their privileges—especially exclusive rights to esoteric information, authority to label and legitimate sickness, and the acquisition of social prestige and economic reward for the monopolization of authoritative knowledge (Jordan 1993).

The major clue that such controlling processes are operative in Egypt lies in most physicians' insistence that all medical records, which are usually revealed to patients, be written in English, which remains the official, postcolonial language of biomedicine in Egypt and serves as an effective language of social control. Because only a small, educated minority of the Egyptian populace reads English, the consistent use of the English language in the biomedical setting serves as an effective barrier to the dissemination of biomedical knowledge. The records that patients are given to carry from physician to physician—and which, in the case of infertile patients, tend to become voluminous over time—can only be read and comprehended easily by other physicians. As a result, even educated individuals who are literate in their rather difficult native language, classical Arabic, are unable to decipher the mysterious contents of their written biomedical records.

Again, Egyptian physicians argue that they employ English because (1) it is the standardized language of biomedicine in Egypt, (2) it is used worldwide, and (3) it is the language in which they are trained. Yet, most Egyptian physicians do not *speak to each other* in this language—using instead their more familiar Arabic, sometimes interspersed with English terms that do not have direct Arabic translations. But even English-language biomedical terms are often replaced in physicians' verbal parlance with Arabic equivalents—equivalents that, as we have seen, are often picked up by patients and transformed into a more comprehensible idiom. Thus, as it now stands, English is the language of *written* records—records that are not kept by physicians, many of whom lack any system of medical record-keeping, but rather are given to uncomprehending patients, who literally carry them with them on their quests for therapy.

Overall, it can be argued that the way in which biomedical information is *not* disclosed to infertile patients has more to do with physicians' maintenance of professional boundaries than with patients' ability to fathom biomedical information. This argument gains credence in the memorable comment of one Egyptian infertility specialist, who stated firmly: "No patient should know even 10 percent of what I know!" In the case of nonspecialist biogynecologists—who, as shown, often know less about infertility than they should, given their treatment of infertile patients—*not* disclosing etiological information may be a way of preventing patients from knowing just how little they *do* know about infertility!

In either case, no system exists in Egypt to encourage—or to demand—disclosure. Legislation mandating disclosure of biomedical information as a right of all patients, as well as an accompanying system of malpractice to make physicians accountable for their professional performance, is entirely absent in Egypt. Thus, physicians are able to proceed as they do now with only their professional reputations to consider and without threat of legal challenge from disgruntled patients.

Despite the willingness of patients to participate in the biomedical system, which most view as their best chance for help, many infertile patients are, in fact, dissatisfied with physician caretakers who repeatedly fail to inform them of pertinent information—including, most significantly, the biomedical problems from which they suffer—and, ultimately, who fail to cure them of their infertility. Despite biogynecologists' statements otherwise, infertile women *do* desire detailed biomedical information regarding the causes of their infertility and are grateful when they receive it—even from a foreign anthropologist speaking, at times, garbled colloquial Arabic (see Appendix 1).

As one poor infertile woman lamented, "Of course, if you understand more, you're more comfortable when you know rather than when you're blind. Here [in Egypt], the doctors don't tell you anything. They *must* tell the patients everything, and I don't know why they don't. But most don't."

The power of physicians to keep their infertile patients in the dark is summed up in the poignant story of a middle-aged Nubian woman, whose valiant "search for children" ended at Shatby Hospital in Alexandria in the late 1980s. Nine years earlier, the woman had undergone a postmiscarriage operation in a public hospital in Cairo. Although this woman realized that her "tummy" had been "opened," her menstrual period had subsequently waned, and a postoperative problem had developed "from down" (for which she came to Shatby Hospital seeking care and which turned out to be a prolapsed vagina), she was still under the impression that she could have a child and had continued her quest for therapy over the postoperative decade. Little did the woman realize, however, that the scars crisscrossing her abdomen like a set of railroad tracks were the result of a hysterectomy—the total removal of her *bait il-wilid*—of which the doctors in the Cairo hospital had never informed her. Although the physicians at Shatby Hospital would ultimately tell her the truth about her missing uterus and repair her vagina to its prehysterectomy configuration, what they would never be able to restore was her faith in physicians, who, in her eyes, had robbed her of her fecundity, femininity, and desperate hopes of becoming a mother.

9. Untherapeutic Therapeutics

Maisara's Story

When Maisara did not become pregnant during the first three months of marriage to Munir, and Munir's stepmother told him he should divorce Maisara and remarry a fertile woman, Maisara became worried. Although she did not tell Munir or his family, Maisara, too, blamed herself for her inability to conceive, because while still a virgin, she had experienced very irregular menstrual periods, which only came when doctors gave her injections. Now, as a married woman, Maisara surmised that her previous menstrual problems might be related to what Munir and his family perceived to be her infertility problem. So, eschewing ethnogynecological therapies as being *ḥarām,* or improper, and borrowing money from her parents, Maisara began her biogynecological quest for therapy—a quest that has lasted eleven years.

In the first year of her marriage, Maisara's physicians prescribed "medicines only," all of them to "strengthen the ovaries." However, when drug therapy failed to make Maisara pregnant, Maisara went to a physician who examined her and told her that she had *qarḥa,* or an erosion of her cervix, which was preventing pregnancy. For this, the physician undertook *makwa,* or "ironing" of Maisara's cervix—a painful procedure that he called *kayy* (electrocautery) and which involved the insertion of an instrument to heat her cervix like an iron. Maisara waited several months following the "ironing" procedure to see whether she would become pregnant. But, there were "no results."

Therefore, she went to another physician who told her that she needed an operation called *nafq* (tubal insufflation), which Maisara understood as an operation to "widen either the ovary or uterus." Maisara was neither hospitalized nor anesthetized for this operation, because she was required to tell the physician whether she experienced any pain, especially in her shoulders. Although the operation was extremely uncomfortable "from down" (that is, in the genital region), Maisara did not experience any shoulder pain, and the physician did not tell her whether this was good or bad.

Again, Maisara waited for pregnancy results after this torturous operation, but none were forthcoming. So, she decided to "rest" from painful operations and to take only drugs as prescribed by physicians. For a period of four years, Maisara visited *many* different doctors, all specialists in *amrāḍ nisā'* (diseases of women), and all of them prescribed many different medicines. Some were pills of different colors, shapes, sizes, and dosages. Some were suppositories for the vagina. Some were vaginal douches. And some were injections. Maisara took these medicines in whatever form they were prescribed to her, and, after time, began to feel like "a pharmacy inside." In order to pay for these medicines, some of which were very expensive, she sold all of her gold jewelry, including her bracelets and her *dibla,* or wedding ring, and eventually had to begin to borrow money from her father. Munir's salary as an army driver was simply not enough to cover the costs of living, as well as Maisara's treatments, which during this four-year period exceeded one thousand Egyptian pounds (four hundred dollars) in cost. Yet, despite the expense and numerous unpleasant side effects of these drugs, none of them caused Maisara's ovaries to become "strong" enough for pregnancy. As Maisara explains, "I don't know why they didn't work. I used to take all the drugs they gave me regularly. I thought it might be from my husband, because most of this time, he was away, and we didn't have normal intercourse every time. But, they told me my ovaries were weak, and it wasn't from my husband."

Thus, Maisara decided to visit Shatby Hospital, which she heard specialized in infertility. At Shatby, they told her she needed *il-manẓar,* a diagnostic laparoscopy, for which she was hospitalized overnight. Maisara was told by the doctors that she had "something like leather on the ovary," and, following the laparoscopy, she received drug treatment for another year.

However, failing to become pregnant, she visited another women's hospital, where a doctor prescribed the drug Clomid and a vaginal douche for a period of nine months. Having experienced only minor side effects before, Maisara found Clomid therapy to be particularly "severe," given that it caused strong headaches, pain in her eyes, blurred vision, and engorged breasts. Thus, after nine months, she discontinued taking Clomid and stopped seeing this physician.

The next "outside" (private) physician Maisara visited told her that she had a cyst on her ovary that needed to be removed through surgery.

Although Maisara had undergone "little operations" before—including the electrocautery, the tubal insufflation, and an appendectomy when she was seventeen—she was unprepared for the magnitude of the ovarian operation. After it was over, she discovered that they had "opened my whole belly." Later, she would come to "curse this doctor, because he did the wrong operation." Namely, when she visited another physician following the operation, she was told that her tubes had become "closed *from the operation* itself"! To "open" her tubes, the physician prescribed a series of tubal insufflations—one every month for three months following her menstrual period. After this series of insufflations was completed, Maisara underwent *ṣūra ashi"a bi ṣibghā* (hysterosalpingography) to see if the insufflations had opened her tubes, but she was given her X ray to take home and was never informed of the results.

Thus, after some recuperative time had passed, Maisara went to another physician, who told her that she needed thirty sessions of *makwa,* but this time on her abdomen, "through the stitches of her operation." Maisara underwent the *galsāt kahraba,* or "sessions of electricity" (shortwave, or infrared, therapy), in which heat was applied to her abdomen. However, Maisara found "no results" with this therapy either, which was extremely expensive and time-consuming.

Finally, ten years into her therapeutic search, Maisara's friend encouraged her to return to Shatby Hospital, where her infertile sister had gone seeking treatment and had become pregnant. Maisara consented and was taken by her friend to Shatby, where she underwent her second diagnostic laparoscopy. Unfortunately, the doctors "saw nothing at all." As they explained to Maisara, the ovarian operation she had undertaken had not been successful and, in fact, had increased the "leather" (pelvic adhesions), enclosing both of her ovaries beyond the point of diagnostic visualization. While in her hospital bed, Maisara confronted a passing physician, asking "Oh, doctor, can you *please* tell me what's wrong with me?" He examined her chart and said to her, "You will never be pregnant. The only chance that you might have is a 'tubes baby.'" When Maisara told him that she didn't have the money for that, he encouraged her by saying that in Shatby, the public hospital, making a tubes baby would be "cheap."

Since then, Maisara has been a patient of an infertility specialist at Shatby Hospital, who has taken two samples of "water" from her vagina (cervical mucus samples) and has performed fifteen to twenty abdominal ultrasounds on her. Although the doctor has not told her specifically what is in store for her, Maisara believes that she is a candidate for *il-ḥu'an,* or "the injections," using her husband's sperm (namely, artificial insemination by husband, or AIH). Maisara has heard from women in the Shatby clinic waiting area that, "to do the injection, they take liquid from the man, put it in a machine, and inject it in the uterus, for up to three times, and then it's in God's hands." Although she has also heard women talking about *ṭifl l-anābīb,* or a "baby of the tubes," she has no idea what this really means or whether she will be scheduled to "make" one. But, whatever her future holds at Shatby, Maisara says she will try "*anything,* just to get pregnant." And, if this does not work, her pilgrimage for pregnancy will continue—or, as she puts it, "I will *never* give up."

Features of the Biogynecological Quest for Therapy

For many infertile Egyptian women like Maisara, the quest for biogynecological therapy for infertility begins early—some as early as the first month of marriage[1]—and may last many years, involving scores of physicians, the expenditure of thousands of Egyptian pounds, and the production of irreparable scars to women's minds, bodies, and souls. Yet, in most cases, women's visits to biogynecologists, especially during the early months of marriage, are volitional and are often discouraged by husbands, who, while enjoying their honeymoon period, attempt to reassure their new wives that the timing of pregnancy is something in "God's hands." However, as in the case of Maisara, women's mothers-in-law are less sanguine, prompting, through their running commentary, their daughters-in-law's trips to physicians and supplying them with the names of "good doctors."

For women like Maisara who do not become pregnant after several years of marriage, their quests for biogynecological therapy often become engrossing endeavors, totally absorbing their thoughts, time, energy, daily bodily regimens, and financial resources. The consuming nature of this quest is evident in several primary features of women's pilgrimages to physicians—pilgrimages that are especially difficult for women such as Maisara with seemingly intractable infertility problems.

Spending and Selling

First, being infertile is an impoverishing experience for many Egyptian women, especially those who are already poor and subsisting on limited financial resources. Despite the official rhetoric of "free" health care in Egypt, very little health care, even in public facilities, is without some cost to the patient. In public facilities such as Shatby Hospital, patients may end up paying for many nonsubsidized items, including supplies, drugs, and certain diagnostic and therapeutic procedures. For example, patients undergoing "free" infertility-related surgeries in public Ministry of Health hospitals are required to pay for all "extras," including blood for transfusions, syringes for the injection of anesthetics and painkillers, pre- and postoperative analyses, and usually their own food, given the poor quality of the meals offered. The inability of poor women to readily pay for these pre- and postoperative expenses keeps many of them in the hospital for extended periods, until the necessary funds can be obtained by their husbands and families. Likewise, in the fee-for-service world of private medicine in Egypt, patients are required to subsidize everything from needles to hospital beds with their own financial resources—and to meet the high fees of the physicians who treat them as well.[2] Because of the absence of a private health-care insurance industry in Egypt, expenditures for health care—private or public—are made by patients in cash, with no expectation of any reimbursement. The costs of actual health-care services are compounded by the costs of the therapeutic quest itself, including bus, train, tram, and taxi transportation, food and accommodations when physicians are visited in distant cities (such as Cairo), *baqāshīsh,* or tips, that must be paid to various minor functionaries, such as hospital guards and technicians, and various, other unplanned expenses that tend to arise on the therapeutic journey.

Given this situation, many infertile Egyptian women end up spending vast amounts of money in the biogynecological realm—quantities far exceeding the average expenditures of other patients utilizing public and private health-care facilities in the country (Abu-Zeid and Dann 1985). Among women who have sought biogynecological therapy for any extended period of time (say, longer than two years), expenditures for the types of infertility services listed in Table 9 begin to add up, with total expenditures ranging anywhere from £E 100 to £E 10,000 ($40–4,000), depending on the length of therapeutic involvement, the intensity of the biogynecological quest, and the severity of the infertility problem.[3] Although these costs may seem reasonable by Western standards, among poor Egyptians, whose monthly incomes are usually less than one hundred pounds (see Appendix 2), this represents a substantial investment, one that is deemed to be lost when a woman fails to become pregnant.

Because few poor urban women work, women's husbands are the major financiers of their therapeutic quests, and, perhaps contrary to expec-

TABLE 9. Costs of Infertility Diagnostic and Treatment Services as Reported by One Hundred Infertile Women in the Study Sample.

SERVICE	COST IN EGYPTIAN POUNDS	COST IN U.S. DOLLARS*
Examination in a private physician's office	10–50	4–20
Hysterosalpingogram	25–50	10–20
Serum hormonal assay	15–40	6–16
Ultrasound	25–40	10–16
Artificial insemination	40–100	16–40
Invasive infertility procedures (e.g., D & C, electrocautery, tubal insufflation)	40–100	16–40
One packet of ovulation-induction therapy	6–400	2.40–160
Diagnostic laparoscopy in a private facility	100–600	40–240
Infertility surgery in a private facility	1,000–3,000	400–1,200

*The average 1989 exchange rate of £E2.5 = $1 is used here.

tation, are often very generous with their wives if the money is to be spent purposefully on therapy. Yet, given poor men's insubstantial earnings, very few women are able to rely on their husbands' wages alone, resorting to borrowing from parents, parents-in-law, and siblings in most cases, or, rarely, obtaining small loans from employers, neighbors, or savings clubs.

The most common strategy women use when they have "spent down" existing cash resources is to begin to sell their possessions—typically their gold jewelry, which is usually given to them as a bridewealth payment and which represents their most valuable and easily salable item. Although some women refuse to part with their gold (which may be their only form of economic "security"), preferring to wait for therapy if they are too poor to afford it, many women, like Maisara, are willing to sell back to jewelers some or all of their gold, including occasionally their gold wedding bands. Women may also sell off other precious bridewealth items, including sewing machines, china dishware, copper kettles, and their best dresses. Women who live in rural or peri-urban areas may deal in small livestock, such as goats, geese, and other fowl, in order to subsidize their therapeutic quests. Occasionally, women who are truly destitute are forced to limit their searches to "charity" clinics, such as the Islamic clinics that offer treatment to the poor for nominal fees (Morsy 1988), or to plead their cases to the

Ministry of Health in order to obtain special letters labeling them as "charity cases" and entitling them to completely free treatment in Ministry of Health facilities.

One woman, infertile for fourteen years and heavily engaged in the biogynecological system for the last ten years, described her financial situation in the following way: "I sold all of my gold—six bracelets, three rings, a necklace, and four pairs of earrings. There is none; I have only silver now. And I used all of our savings—six thousand pounds [$2,400]—plus any money my husband gets. Everything is very expensive. Now, I'm paying every month forty pounds [$16] for ultrasounds, six pounds [$2.40] for injections, and thirteen pounds [$5.20] for Clomid. And our income is just one hundred pounds [$40] a month. So sixty pounds [$24] is most of it."

Most women are adamant that they would not have begrudged this expenditure of money had it "brought results." Many of them say they are willing to spend "every piaster" (equivalent of a penny) that their husbands earn if it would bring them a child. But many women who do not achieve results in the biogynecological system believe they are "spending their money for nothing." Eventually they begin to condemn physicians who they believe are less interested in treating infertile women than in "gaining money" from them.

Doctor Shopping

This is largely why so many infertile Egyptian women "doctor shop"[4]—moving from one physician to the next in the hope of finding a doctor who "takes money" only to cure. Women who feel tricked by physicians who prescribe expensive but fruitless therapies are unlikely to remain with them or to follow their prescriptions, and they often end up moving quickly from doctor to doctor, even when courses of therapy have not been completed.

However, doctor shopping, one of the major features of poor urban infertile women's therapeutic quests, also stems from a number of other sources.[5] First, infertile women often feel compelled to visit any physician whose name has been volunteered to them by an acquaintance—particularly by overzealous mothers-in-law, but also by other family members, neighbors, and friends. Furthermore, when a mother-in-law insists on dragging an infertile daughter-in-law from physician to physician, the daughter-in-law is rarely in a position to refuse. This is even the case when a woman's *husband* is the confirmed infertile partner, but her mother-in-law denies this reality and seeks to blame the childlessness on her son's healthy wife.

Second, women are occasionally referred from one physician to another. Some Egyptian biogynecologists are honest about their limited abilities to treat infertility, especially more difficult cases, and refer patients to more qualified colleagues or to specialized facilities. Others refer patients for specific diagnostic procedures, such as diagnostic laparoscopy, which they do not offer in their practices. Thus, some doctor shopping on the part of infertile women actually comprises interphysician referral of patients. This is particularly true of women who end up seeking treatment at Shatby Hospital, a place of frequent referral by doctors in the Alexandria vicinity.[6] Because of its status as a university hospital, a tertiary care facility, and an institution specializing in infertility, physicians throughout the Nile Delta region and from as far away as Cairo sometimes refer infertile patients there, particularly poor women who cannot afford private treatment services. As one such poor woman who was referred to Shatby explained, "I went to a *duktūra* outside. She told me, 'I can't prescribe anything because you already took all the drugs.' After she saw all my X rays and analyses, she prescribed that I go to Shatby to have diagnostic laparoscopy. 'This is the only way we can know anything,' she said."

Thus, for many poor infertile women, Shatby Hospital serves as a place of last resort—a place that women can go before "giving themselves up to God." However, some infertile women deemed "beyond hope" at Shatby or elsewhere continue to doctor shop in their sheer determination not to give up—even after physicians tell them to "go home and leave your case up to God." Granted, such "prescriptions to do nothing" are made more often than they should be, given many Egyptian biogynecologists' lack of ability to diagnose and treat infertility appropriately. Nevertheless, some women with infertility problems are truly beyond medical "repair"—for example, those with severe endometriosis or tubal blockage/pelvic adhesions who require but cannot afford IVF, those with irreparable congenital malformations of the reproductive tract, those with irreversible premature ovarian failure (premature menopause), and those whose husbands have severe male-factor infertility. Indeed, it is quite common to find Egyptian women whose husbands are infertile moving from biogynecologist to biogynecologist hoping to discover that the infertility problem really lies with them and not their husbands. Because husbands are sometimes reluctant to admit male infertility or, more commonly, are noncompliant with their expensive therapy, their wives attempt to assume responsibility for the situation by "shifting the blame" to themselves. Thus, for these women, as well as for women with intractable female infertility problems, doctor shopping provides a means of taking charge of a situation essentially beyond their control. As they often say, they will "*never* stop searching," so that, when they reach menopause, they will feel "no regrets."

Finally, many infertile women admit to doctor shopping because of impatience with physicians or, as they put it, of becoming "fed up" quickly with any physician who does not offer a rapid cure or, minimally, a therapy different from that offered by other physicians already visited. Therapeutic redundancy is a major complaint of many women, who are asked to repeat trials of the same drugs or undergo repetitive invasive procedures by biogynecologists who ignore their colleagues' previous prescriptions or who have nothing better to offer. On the other hand, many women also complain of the seeming randomness of physicians' therapies, which are often provided with little diagnostic verification, as described in Chapter 8. As one woman put it, "Each doctor does something different. Each doctor says something different. It made me give up going to them."

For their part, many biogynecologists acknowledge doctor shopping as a serious problem in Egypt and complain when their patients "escape" to another physician. Yet, they explain this habit variously, sometimes blaming the infertile women they treat and sometimes blaming physicians themselves.

As one physician who had worked in Saudi Arabia commented, "You know, this is our main problem. The patient comes to you and takes medicine for one month, and if no pregnancy, she escapes and throws away all the medicine and all the prescriptions and goes to another doctor and starts all over again. The main reason is because she is desperate to get a quick result and also because it's a habit here. I didn't find this in Arabia."

Another physician who viewed doctor shopping as a problem of "impatient patients" explained,

> This is a problem, especially with infertility. Infertility requires a very long time to diagnose and treat. So this patience is lacking in patients. Some will spend some time with one physician, and if, in their opinion, there is no progress, they will start to go to another one. This will do harmful effects to the patient, because the next one will start new investigations and a second wrong line. One patient I met a few weeks ago, I did an exam and found some bleeding points from the cervix. When I asked her, "When is the last time you were examined?," she said, "One hour [ago]." I didn't believe this—a patient would go from one doctor to another in just one hour! The problem is related to the education of patients. They go from small doctors to bigger ones, then to professors.

However, other biogynecologists say that physicians must assume at least part of the responsibility for doctor shopping. As one such critic argued,

> The main difficulty here in treatment is follow-up, because most patients escape after the first appointment. Many patients, if I start with Clomid again and they've received it for years, I'll never see her again. I must tell them about a new line for maintenance. It's a problem because the lines of treatment are common and most of them have received the common lines of treatment, such as induction of ovulation, insufflation, and so on. . . . But I tell them about all these new lines of treatment, so they stick to me.

As another physician concluded, doctor shopping

> is a problem of patients *and* doctors. It's a problem of doctors, because there are no subspecialties in ob-gyn. For example, if we had specialists in endocrinology, endoscopy, or operative endoscopy, someone in insemination, IVF, then, honestly, we could tell the patient, "Your problem is so-and-so, and you should go to that doctor." To cut short her search and get her the right treatment. From her side, the problem is from lack of confidence [in physicians]. But if she is confident, she will really stick to that physician.

Ambivalence Toward Physicians

As suggested by this final comment, many infertile women do, in fact, openly admit that they lack confidence in most physicians, viewing them with as much suspicion as they view *munaggimīn*. A common complaint heard among poor infertile Egyptian women is that there are "no good, conscientious doctors anymore." Rather, many Egyptian women, as angry consumers of biogynecological care, criticize the incompetence, ineffectiveness, and avarice of biogynecologists, especially private ones. And, as suggested by Becker and Nachtigall (1991), both doctor shopping and the withholding of trust and respect are ways for them to reassert their nebulous power as self-determining actors in the therapeutic quest.

However, as also noted by Becker and Nachtigall (1991), infertile women's feelings of hostility toward physicians are often mixed with desires to be viewed by physicians as "good patients," who do the routine work of infertility therapy in an exacting manner. Generally speaking, infertile Egyptian women proudly view themselves as being obedient to physicians' authority—of "following doctors' orders" religiously—even if the result for them is a loss of power, as well as increasing dependence and passivity.

Furthermore, despite the widespread perception that Egypt is plagued with many bad doctors, doctors who have gained good reputations in infertility management are often deemed by desperate patients to have *baraka* — similar to dead *shuyūkh* — and these highly sought after physicians may find it relatively easy to obtain their patients' complete submission. For example, women's faith in what they perceive to be the particularly knowledgeable and gifted "professor-doctors" at university hospitals such as Shatby is quite high,[7] and, for this reason, they may entrust them with their bodies and dreams in ways that they might not otherwise.

Drugs and Delirium

For the vast majority of infertile women in Egypt, part of being seen as a dutiful patient is taking the drugs prescribed by physicians. Drugs are an integral part of the therapeutic quest — the feature of therapy that is most characteristic of infertile women's careers as patients.[8] The taking of fertility drugs — more properly known as ovulation-inducing agents — is part of the routine work of the biogynecological quest (Becker and Nachtigall 1991), and, for many women, it is a task that continues indefinitely. When an infertile Egyptian woman is asked if she has ever taken fertility drugs, the most common immediate response is "*katīr*!," meaning "a lot!" Many women explain that their bodies are "full of drugs" — including pills, tablets, injections, suppositories, and medicated douches — or, as Maisara put it, "it's like a pharmacy inside of me."

To a large extent, infertility therapy in Egypt has been subject to the forces of pharmaceuticalization and commodification, namely, the notion that fertility can be "purchased" through medicine taking. This belief is promulgated by Egyptian physicians, who are quick (often too quick) to write prescriptions for fertility drugs, and it is accepted wholeheartedly by many infertile patients, who say that they would take "*any* drug, even one with side effects" just to get pregnant.

Yet, most poor infertile women who have accepted this philosophy do not know the names of the medicines prescribed to them, or the specific reasons why they are taking them. Although most women understand that they are taking fertility drugs, designed to "get them pregnant," their specific understandings of the mechanism of action of these agents on their reproductive systems are not well developed. Occasionally, women who are able to read Arabic examine the package inserts of these drugs in an attempt to derive such understanding. Likewise, husbands may read these inserts for their illiterate wives. However, for most of these minimally schooled men and women, the medical language of package inserts is obfuscating, despite its translation into Arabic, leaving readers with only vague impressions of a drug's intended use and benefits.

Given their understandings of the reproductive body (and occasional explanatory comments made by taciturn physicians), most women connect these agents to the uterus, ovaries, ovulation, or eggs, which are seen as being weak and in need of strengthening, activating, or increasing. Sometimes, drugs are seen as "regulating the menstrual period," especially among women who suffer from amenorrhea. In fact, one of the most popular self-prescribed infertility remedies in Egypt is a one-month regimen of oral contraceptives, which are widely perceived to regulate the period in this way.[9] Given the importance of "blockage" in women's ethnophysiological models, it is not surprising that infertile women also view drugs as being like drain openers, which, when poured in, are capable of unplugging clogged tubes or ovaries.

Despite the ambiguity surrounding how fertility drugs work, one thing is certain: most infertile women know that they have received clomiphene citrate (Clomid, Clostilbegyt), an ovulation-inducing agent that is widely prescribed in Egypt and the rest of the world. Because many Egyptian women have received repeated trials of clomiphene citrate, they are more aware of this drug than any other agent, identifying it by name and on sight as "the one in the blue box."

Clomiphene citrate is considered to be the drug of choice for ovulation induction in anovulatory patients with intact pituitary function (Hammond 1984; Steinkampf and Blackwell 1993). As a fertility drug, clomiphene citrate has several advantages: (1) it is relatively inexpensive, costing approximately six Egyptian pounds ($2.40) for a box of ten fifty-milligram tablets, with the normal initial dosage being fifty milligrams daily for five days; (2) it is readily available in pharmacies throughout Egypt; (3) it is relatively safe; (4) it is easy to prescribe and administer in tablet form; and (5) it is quite effective as a first-line therapy in patients with simple ovulatory failure (officially known as WHO group II amenorrhea) (Steinkampf and Blackwell 1993).

In addition, because clomiphene citrate was one of the first drugs to be described for use in ovulation-inducing therapy nearly thirty years ago (Hammond 1984), it is widely known to Egyptian gynecologists, many of whom are less familiar with the new generation of ovulation-inducing agents introduced into the biogynecological world during the past decade. In Egypt, ovulation induction with clomiphene citrate is taught to medical students, whereas ovulation induction with new-generation drugs is not. Furthermore, the scientific literature on ovulation induction is vast and growing rapidly, ensuring that most Egyptian biogynecologists, as generalists, lack up-to-date information concerning this rapidly evolving field.[10]

Given clomiphene citrate's tried-and-true reputation among Egyptian physicians, it is one of their first-line therapies for the treatment of infertile women. But, herein lies the problem. Because most biogynecologists consider clomiphene citrate to be safe and effective, they prescribe it empirically—without first determining whether the patient is anovulatory. In patients who ovulate normally but who have other infertility factors, such as blocked fallopian tubes, the drug is absolutely useless and should not be prescribed. Nevertheless, many biogynecologists write a three- or six-month clomiphene citrate prescription figuring that it "can't hurt," especially when patients are poor and are unwilling (if offered) to undergo expensive diagnostic tests. If the treatment regimen fails, patients are told to return to the physician's office, at which time the patient may be diagnostically evaluated for ovulatory or other factors *or* given another course of clomiphene citrate—this time at a higher dosage.

Unfortunately, clomiphene citrate *can* hurt, causing serious side effects that are clearly described on the package insert but are often ignored by physicians when they occur. Visual problems, and especially blurred vision indicative of pituitary enlargement, are among the most common (Steinkampf and Blackwell 1993). As stated on the package insert (in both English and Arabic), "a feeling of blurred vision or other visual symptoms may sometimes occur in the course of treatment with [clomiphene citrate]. If they occur treatment must be immediately and *permanently* discontinued; a complete ophthalmological examination is recommended" (emphasis added). Many infertile women who have taken clomiphene citrate say they have suffered from *zaghlala,* or blurred vision;[11] yet, in most cases, clomiphene citrate therapy is repeatedly prescribed by biogynecologists, who fail to ask about previous side effects. Furthermore, Egyptian biogynecologists who are not specialized in infertility rarely monitor clomiphene citrate's reproductive side effects; these include decreased cervical mucus quality and the much more serious complication of ovarian hyperstimulation, which occurs in about 10 percent of patients and which is associated with abdominal fullness, weight gain, and pain followed by nausea and vomiting (Steinkampf and Blackwell 1993).

Drug side effects, including, most commonly, dizziness, nausea and vomiting, weakness, fainting, enervation, depression, headaches, breast enlargement, and loss of appetite, are part and parcel of most infertile women's experiences. For example, bromocriptine mesylate (Parlodel), another ovulation-inducing drug often prescribed empirically with clomiphene citrate, is associated with many of these side effects, primarily nausea and vomiting, headache, fatigue, and lightheadedness (Hammond 1984). Furthermore, bromocriptine is intended for use in a particular type of anovulatory patient—namely, those with hyperprolactinemia, manifested as milk in the breasts (Hammond 1984). Yet, bromocriptine is one of the major drugs prescribed empirically to infertile Egyptian women, probably because it is actively promoted by the manufacturer (Sandoz Pharmaceuticals) to Egyptian biogynecologists.

Other types of ovulation-inducing agents present different problems for infertile patients, the primary ones being cost and availability. Women who are prescribed "new-age" fertility drugs—including human menopausal gonadotropin (hMG), follicle-stimulating hormone (FSH), or gonadotropin-releasing hormone (GnRH) analogs—are often faced with insurmountable difficulties in obtaining these drugs, either because of the exorbitant cost of the agents (up to one thousand Egyptian pounds [four hundred dollars] for one cycle of therapy, plus an additional one thousand pounds for costs of monitoring) or because few, if any, pharmacies stock these imported agents. For example, in one pharmacy in an upper-class Alexandrian neighborhood known for specializing in fertility drugs, the pharmacist explained that imported ovulation-inducing agents, such as the drugs Pergonal (hMG) and Metrodin (FSH), are obtained *in Europe* by pharmacy staff making trips there. Furthermore, although the Italian division of Serono Laboratories was engaged in importing gonadotropins into Egypt by the late 1980s, some infertility specialists speculated that these agents, which were relatively inexpensive in Egypt by worldwide standards, were being manufactured by subcontractors in the Middle East. Thus, the quality of these agents, some of which are manufactured from human products (for example, postmenopausal women's urine), could not be ensured.

For poor infertile women, attempting to obtain these agents is often a nightmare. Pharmacies stocking these expensive medications tend to be located in wealthier neighborhoods. As a result, poor women or their husbands must often travel the length of Alexandria scouring pharmacies in an attempt to fill their prescriptions. In addition, women who are able to locate and pay for these expensive agents often face another problem: lack of refrigeration. To ensure the biological viability of these agents, continuous refrigeration is necessary; but because many poor women expend all of their economic resources on biogynecological therapy, they lack such luxury items as refrigerators.

Given these difficulties, it is not surprising that many women fail to become pregnant with ovulation-inducing therapy. For example, only four women in this study had become pregnant on fertility drugs. In one case, a woman became pregnant (although she later miscarried) after taking, by mistake, three fifty-milligram clomiphene citrate tablets per day rather than two, as ordered by a university-based biogynecologist. In another case—the only one of one hundred women who actually conceived and delivered a living child during the course of this study—ovulation-inducing therapy that was given and carefully monitored by the same university-based biogynecologist succeeded in causing the woman to become pregnant after only three months. However, as she explained, she had spent the first fourteen years of her marriage taking one drug after another, sometimes simultaneously, as prescribed by private physicians who had offered neither diagnostic evaluation nor therapeutic monitoring. Thus, she attributed her pregnancy to the "clever" university-based physician, whom she "could not thank enough," and to the university's ultrasound machine, which she called *ḥulw,* or sweet, and believed to be largely responsible for her successful treatment. (This woman's success story—pregnancy after fourteen years—became so widely disseminated in her community that fifteen infertile women sought her out to learn about where and how she had been treated.)

Women who are unable to become pregnant with ovulation-inducing drugs often puzzle over why these drugs have not worked for them. In general, women believe in the efficacy of these agents, pointing to other cases in which women have become pregnant. Thus, treatment failures are often attributed by women to: (1) some other infertility factor not amenable to drug treatment (for example, blocked tubes); (2) lack of knowledge on the part of the treating physician, who prescribed "the wrong medication"; (3) the need for some other type of biomedical therapy (for example, "an operation"); or, ultimately, (4) God's decision to wait before granting them a child. As one woman philosophized, "God knows, because not all bodies are similar and not all diseases are similar. So if one medicine works with one woman, it doesn't necessarily work with another."

Yet, despite their lack of success with drug therapy, many women emphasize that they would "take *anything,* no matter how strong" in order to become pregnant. Some women point to the Arabic proverb "What made you stick to the bitter thing? The more bitter thing" to explain why they are willing to subject their bodies to powerful drugs that make them suffer delirious side effects. In fact, dizziness and delirium are often less worrisome to women than the cost of the drugs themselves, which many women consider to be their major obstacle. This willingness to "try anything" no matter how dangerous or expensive—or, as one woman put it, "to even take poison"—is also evident in women's attitudes toward "operations," the subject to which we now turn.

The Technological Obsession

Very few infertile women in Egypt complete their biomedical quest for therapy without undergoing one or more invasive procedures. Although women call these procedures *'amalīyāt,* or operations, surgery comprises only one aspect of the procedure-oriented old school of infertility therapy in Egypt. Other invasive technological measures, primarily electrocautery of the cervix, dilatation and curettage of the uterus, and tubal insufflation, are frequently undertaken as outpatient procedures in biogynecologists' offices throughout the country. Their prevalence, which is strikingly high, is apparent in infertile patients' biogynecological histories (see Tables 10 and 11).

That Egyptian biogynecologists favor technologically oriented procedures in the treatment of infertility is a reflection of a number of forces.

The Technological Imperative

First, it is a reflection of the "technological imperative" in postcolonial Egyptian biomedicine—namely, the pressure to perform technological procedures simply because they are there and can be done (Barger-Lux and Heaney 1986). Certainly, Egypt's love affair with what Alubo (1987) has called "white elephant" medical technology—namely, imported, curatively oriented technology that does not meet the most pressing health needs of Egypt's masses (Carney 1984; Institute of Medicine 1979; Kuhnke 1990)—is not unique and is found in many neocolonial settings where massive technology transfer has occurred, including in other parts of the Middle East (Alubo 1990; Bolton et al. 1990; Bonair, Rosenfield, and Tengvald 1989; Gallagher and Searle 1984, 1985; Haddad 1988; MacCormack 1989;

TABLE 10. The Old Reproductive Technologies (ORTs) for the Treatment of Infertility: Histories of Ninety-four Infertile Women in the Study Sample.

PROCEDURE	PERCENTAGE OF WOMEN UNDERGOING THE PROCEDURE	
	Once	*More than once*
Procedure		
Electrocautery (*kayy*)	29	9
Dilatation and curettage (*tausīʿ wi kaḥt*)	37	20
Tubal insufflation (*nafq*)	39	18
Hydrotubation (*ḥu'an fir-raḥim*)	2	3
Shortwave (infrared) therapy (*galsāt kahraba*)	1	10
Surgeries (*ʿamalīyāt*)		
Ovarian (cystectomy/wedge resection)	11	—
Tubal	10	1
Uterine (myomectomy/ventral suspension)	13	—

Turshen 1991). Nonetheless, the "smothering dominance" of technology in Egypt is certainly felt in infertility practice (Barger-Lux and Heaney 1986), where most of the "cures" offered to infertile female patients are technological and invasive in nature.

Critics of biomedicine have pointed to various problems promoted by the technological imperative—problems that are profoundly apparent in Egypt. Barger-Lux and Heaney (1986), for example, have argued that the technological imperative leads to the valuing of things over people, leading to impaired communication between givers and receivers of health care via technological barriers. In addition, they note that the technological imperative leads to insurmountable conflicts of interest for physicians, who (1) feel compelled to "do something" in the face of uncertainty, (2) experience significant opportunities for financial gain through the use of technologies, and (3) begin to see solutions to health problems in terms of their technological power.

In Egypt, profit-oriented biogynecologists view infertility procedures as relatively easy to perform and more lucrative than other lines of therapy (including drug therapy). And, because infertile patients have been led to consider these invasive procedures to be maximally effective, they are willing to subject their bodies to this technological invasion. In fact, biogynecologists who prey on the bodies and pocketbooks of Egyptian women

TABLE 11. Number of Types of Old Reproductive Technologies (ORTs) Administered to Ninety-four Infertile Women in the Study Sample.

NUMBER OF TYPES	PERCENTAGE OF WOMEN
Zero	12
One	27
Two	21
Three	27
Four	10
Five	3
Total	100

often point to the enthusiasm of their patients for these invasive technologies, especially if undertaken *bil bang* (under anesthesia). Physicians sometimes justify their use of invasive technologies by arguing that, if they do not use them, patients will plead for them to perform such procedures or they will go elsewhere. Because most physicians view these procedures as benign if not always therapeutic, they believe that they are demonstrating their commitment to patient care by performing "mercy treatment" for desperate patients who need *some kind of help,* if only a placebo.

Unfortunately, many of these procedures reduce physicians' own feelings of uncertainty and impotence, but produce iatrogenic, rather than placebo, effects in their patients.[12] Many of the most commonly employed invasive procedures in Egypt are actually iatrogenic causes of further infertility problems in female patients (Inhorn and Buss 1993; Inhorn and Buss 1994). However, the problem of gynecological iatrogenesis is too easily dismissed by many Egyptian physicians.

As one Egyptian biogynecologist lamented, "Permanent infertility is induced by procedures which are not indicated. Any infertile patient here, if you ask her about tubal insufflation and D & C and cauterization of a cervical erosion, this is the dominant finding in all cases. These three factors may induce infertility itself. . . . They are mainly used by physicians for getting money."

In addition to these problems promoted by the technological imperative, Koenig (1988) describes how technology becomes "routinized" in biomedicine—how physicians come to define "standard therapy" as being technological in nature—and how, once entrenched, such "technological rituals" become difficult to eliminate. In Egypt, the routinization of questionable technological procedures is a significant problem, one made all the more compelling because of the lack of bioethics and technology assessment fields in the country. Routinization of technology in Egyptian infertility practice is most blatantly manifest in the fact that the majority of therapies are *old:* outmoded, antiquated, primitive, obsolete, and in every other way "premodern." Most of these technological procedures were in vogue in Egypt decades ago and are used routinely today as they were then. Some of these procedures, such as tubal insufflation and uterine suspensions, can be traced to the early part of the twentieth century in the annals of Western biogynecological history (Speert 1958, 1973, 1980), but have long since been abandoned in infertility practice in the West. Furthermore, some of these procedures were never intended as *therapies* for infertility, but are employed as such by Egyptian biogynecologists. In other words, Egyptian infertility practice today can be characterized as both "unprogressive" and "irrational"—terms used by Egyptian biogynecologist critics themselves—and these problems have much to do with the routinization of biomedical tradition in a cultural setting where "tradition" is extremely important.

In criticizing the unevolved nature of Egyptian infertility practice, the intent here is not to uphold Western biomedicine and its technologies as some sort of state-of-the-art, progressive, "gold standard," against which Third World biomedical practices should be judged. Rather, the point is that biomedical progress—including technological progress—is not a cross-cultural universal, in part because "progress" as an ideal is not as dearly held in many countries as it is in the Enlightenment-influenced West. Thus, what represents progress in one country where biomedicine is practiced may never be reproduced in another—either because of lack of technology transfer, which is not the main problem in Egypt, or because of lack of transfer of the associated values necessary for "progressive" biomedical technologies to be adequately instated and integrated. Thus, in Egypt, Western-based biomedicine and its technologies have been reproduced, but without concomitant ideologies of progress and modernity, including the idealization of science as an objective and value-free body of knowledge (Lock 1988), which are deemed necessary for biomedicine to adapt and transform itself.

As one Western-educated Egyptian biogynecology professor and proponent of science complained,

> We have a major difference between what people believe here and in the West: that medicine is a science and not an art. . . . People here don't really believe in

> science on all levels, from the highest place in government to the lowest place. You will find very famous professors and they will not work in a scientific way. I think this is very important and if I just succeed in teaching my students this, I think I will have done a very big thing. So this is a big problem you will find in this country.

Biopower and Technopatriarchy

The obsession with technology in Egyptian infertility practice is also related to what Foucault (1977) has called "biopower," in which the human body itself becomes the site of surveillance and control and is manipulated through biomedical "technologies of the body" designed to discipline and subdue docile subjects, most often for political ends. Thus, the body itself becomes a text upon which a society's dominant ideologies—of biomedicine itself or of the state—are encoded and from which they can be read.

It can be argued that, in Egypt, infertile women's bodies serve as the site of biomedical, "technopatriarchal" control (Mies 1987; Rowland 1987). Infertility, the failure of women's bodily machines to nurture men's fetuses, is never a tenable option in Egypt and is one that must be overcome through the bodily invasive repair jobs of mostly male biogynecologists. Indeed, in Egypt, male biogynecologists—who symbolically intervene in intercourse by surgically and vaginally "penetrating" the bodies of other men's infertile wives—are applauded for their efforts to overcome a difficult "problem." This problem is a social one and is at the heart of the patriarchal value system in Egypt: namely, by virtue of their "defective" bodies, infertile women thwart the creation of men's most important product, children, and, in so doing, thwart the reproduction of society at large. Thus, by correcting female bodily defects through increasingly invasive and manipulative procedures that "plunder women's inner space" (Baruch 1988), male biogynecologists, as technopatriarchs, facilitate *other men's patriarchal powers* to bring life into this world.

Although numerous feminist scholars have described the transfer of procreative control to biomedicine and, hence, to mostly male experts,[13] the analysis offered here of the Egyptian case diverges somewhat from that of Western feminists, who point to Western men's "disconnectedness" from procreation and consequent "womb envy" (Baruch 1988) as the reason for their desires to assert such penetrating, biogynecological control. As one such author argues:

> It is suggested that men's alienation from reproduction—men's sense of disconnectedness from their seed during the process of conception, pregnancy,

> and birth—has underpinned through the ages a relentless male desire to master nature, and to construct social institutions and cultural patterns that will not only subdue the waywardness of women but also give men an illusion of procreative continuity and power. New reproductive technologies are the vehicle that will turn men's illusions of reproductive power into a reality. By manipulating eggs and embryos, scientists will determine the sort of children who are born—will make themselves the fathers of humankind. (Stanworth 1987b:16)

In Egypt, men experience none of this alienation from procreation. Rather, they experience *frustration* when women prevent the demonstration of their virile procreative powers. For this reason, many men in Egypt, even poor men, encourage their wives to seek the technological intervention of male biogynecologists—as opposed to female ethnogynecologists—and, after some time, may themselves be encouraged by their patrilineal extended-family members to dispose of their defective wives whose faulty bodies cannot be repaired.

The question, of course, is whether women are major benefactors or major victims of this patriarchal "technocratic pressure" (Ruddick 1988). In the substantial Western discourse on the new reproductive technologies (NRTs), feminist scholars find little to praise and much to fear about the increasing medicalization and subjectification of women's bodies under regimes of "assisted conception." Yet, in this almost exclusively Western discourse, little attention is paid to the precursors of the NRTs—to the invasive interventions that continue to be practiced on infertile women's bodies worldwide and that were often in place long before the arrival of test-tube babies and the other NRTs in the West. As we shall see here, in a place like Egypt, it is the old reproductive technologies (ORTs) that currently pose the greatest cause for concern.

The Old Reproductive Technologies

In Egypt, desperate infertile women living in an emphatically patriarchal society are often willing to subject their bodies to painful, costly, invasive procedures that are widely touted by Egyptian biogynecologists as therapeutic when, in fact, most of these procedures are outdated, unindicated in the treatment of infertility, and the probable cause of further iatrogenic infertility problems. Although the new reproductive technologies have recently arrived in Egypt and are the subject of Chapters 10 and 11, it is necessary first to examine the old reproductive technologies, which, as the normative standard of current Egyptian infertility practice, are the therapies that most infertile Egyptian women will experience during their careers as patients.

Ironing the Cervix

In Egypt, one of the most common treatments for infertility is the invasive procedure called *kayy* (electrocautery), which is deemed useful by many Egyptian biogynecologists for the treatment of *qarḥa* (cervical erosion), the purported major cause of cervical-factor infertility. With *kayy,* the endocervix is cauterized with an electrocautery device, consisting of a platinum wire in a holder which is heated to a red or white heat when the instrument is activated by an electric current.[14] In other words, with *kayy,* cervical tissue—including the purported erosion—is cauterized by the application of heat, which many patients understand as "ironing" or "burning" the cervix.

Although electrocautery *may* have a limited role in the treatment of severe endocervicitis that is unresponsive to antibiotic therapy, it is overused and abused in the treatment of infertility in Egypt for a number of reasons.

First, cervical erosions themselves are not a sufficient cause of infertility and, in fact, are not even mentioned in contemporary textbooks of reproductive medicine (e.g., Carr and Blackwell 1993). Although chronic infections causing cervical erosions may lead to inadequate cervical mucus production, thereby leading to cervical-factor infertility, many patients with so-called erosions become pregnant without treatment. According to Singer and Jordan (1976), the changes usually labeled as cervical erosion are probably a result of squamous metaplasia (namely, the replacement of columnar epithelium by squamous cells) that occurs continuously and *normally* at the transition zone of the cervix. Therefore, it is quite probable that chronic cervicitis and so-called cervical erosion are overdiagnosed and are usually *not* manifestations of an active cervical infection (Haas and Galle 1984).

Second, if endocervicitis can be proven—following cytological study or cervical biopsy to exclude a cervical malignancy, and cervical culture to identify the causative organism (all of which are rarely performed in Egypt)—then antibiotic therapy to eliminate the infection is indicated. Cautery is required *only* in intractable cases of cervicitis, unresponsive to antibiotic therapy. Such cases are, in fact, rare (Haas and Galle 1984).

Third, if performed aggressively or repeatedly, electrocautery can lead to permanent damage and destruction of the cervical-mucus-secreting glands, *leading* to subsequent cervical-factor infertility that can never be corrected.[15] Other complications include fibrosis (scarring) and stenosis (narrowing) of the cervix and cervical incompetence, all of which may affect pregnancy prognosis. Cryocautery is safer than electrocautery, but, because the former is not widely available in Egypt due to the expense of the equipment—that is, two thousand Egyptian pounds (eight hundred dollars) for a cryocautery apparatus versus thirty pounds (twelve dollars) for an electrocautery device—it is rarely used in outpatient practice.

The abuse of electrocautery in the treatment of infertility in Egypt is decried by numerous biogynecologists, even those who do not view themselves as specializing in infertility.

As one such physician stated, electrocautery "is used for the treatment of *every* case of infertility in Egypt—the first thing. They [physicians] misdiagnose about 80 percent of cases as having erosions, and their improper technique in doing cauterization can cause cervical stenosis."

Another biogynecologist noted,

> Especially now, a lot of doctors are doing electrocauterization for money. The lady goes to the doctor, he examines her and says she's in need of cauterization, and he does it. Because it's easy to do, it can even be done in these Islamic clinics. It's being abused very much. They do it once, twice, or thrice, either correctly or wrongly, causing cervical stenosis and difficult labor. The doctor must be honest. If she's not in need of cauterization, he shouldn't do it, because you harm the patient more than benefit her. He needs more money, and the infertile lady wants to do anything.

Cleaning the Uterus

Dilatation and curettage (D & C) of the uterus, or *tausīʿ wi kaḥt*—literally, "widening and scraping"—is another common invasive procedure that is unindicated and abused in the treatment of infertility in Egypt. Unfortunately, many infertile Egyptian women are told by their physicians that they can be cured of their infertility through simultaneous "cleaning" of their uteri (D & C) and "blowing" of their tubes (tubal insufflation, to be described below).

Cleaning—or *tanẓīf* as Egyptian women call it—refers to removal of the endometrial lining of the uterine cavity through dilatation (widening) of the cervix and subsequent curettage (scraping) of the uterine contents. D & C has absolutely no therapeutic role in infertility and is not included in contemporary textbooks of reproductive medicine (e.g., Carr and Blackwell 1993). Currently, its major therapeutic role is in postabortive bleeding (Bates and Wiser 1984), and, although it was once recommended for dysfunctional uterine bleeding, ablation of the endometrium by laser is now the treatment of choice (Winkel 1993). During the 1960s and 1970s, D & C was also recommended for treatment of intrauterine adhesions (Asherman syndrome), an uncommon but infertility-related, iatrogenic condition *caused* by overly vigorous endometrial curettage. By 1978, however, the recommended treatment for intrauterine adhesions had changed to hysteroscopic lysis (Bates and Wiser 1984; Winkel 1993), meaning that, by the late 1970s, D & C no longer had any biomedically recognized role in the treatment of infertility.

However, in Egypt, the use of D & C in infertility management continues unabated. Some of those biogynecologists who perform D & Cs on infertile women justify their practice through the simultaneous performance of diagnostic endometrial biopsies. However, many Egyptian biogynecologists disagree with this rationale.

As one such physician commented,

> D & C became now a tradition among physicians and many patients. This is completely wrong. It has no place in the treatment of infertility. It has a place in diagnosis: in the premenstrual biopsy to detect ovulation, which is an outpatient procedure without anesthesia. But this is different than D & C. Many physicians do D & C, telling the patients that it's diagnostic *and* therapeutic. So patients believe it is a sort of treatment. Patients tell their neighbors, so you find patients coming and asking to do D & C. Many physicians will do it for two reasons: One, money; and, two, ignorance. Some doctors practice their job not from true knowledge, from textbooks or reading, but just from hearing from their friends. Young physicians hear this from older physicians, so they start to go along this line, the lines of their bosses, without thinking.

Another physician added,

> [D & C] is nonsense. The bad thing is that the nonobstetricians are doing D & Cs, and they believe they are doing something. I don't know, probably it is a very, very old method, and it became obsolete a decade ago. Even, unfortunately, some highly trained gynecologists do it for money, but they know it will not do anything. But many [physicians] do not know that they should not use it to diagnose ovulation or for removing the unhealthy endometrium, which is removed monthly by menstruation!

Blowing Open the Tubes

Along with *kayy* and *tausīʿ wi kaḥt,* tubal insufflation, or *nafq,* is the third component of the traditional triad of most commonly performed infertility procedures in Egypt, which, according to one Alexandrian infertility specialist, came to be touted as the best line of treatment for infertility by one of the major Alexandrian maternity hospitals literally decades ago. Since then, these three procedures have been rendered obsolete, but continue to play a major role in the contemporary treatment of female infertility in Egypt.

Tubal insufflation, also known as the Rubin test because of its introduction by Isidor Rubin in 1919, has been relegated to the annals of gynecological history in the West (Speert 1958, 1973, 1980) and is represented that way in modern gynecological textbooks (e.g., Aiman 1984). In the earlier part of this century, however, tubal insufflation was used as the main diagnostic procedure to ascertain obstruction of the fallopian tubes. With an instrument called a tubal insufflator, carbon dioxide was to be insufflated into the uterine cavity at sixty to ninety millimeters per minute for a maximum of two minutes. If the tubes were open, the gas entered the peritoneal cavity, as demonstrated by X ray (showing gas under the diaphragm), by referred pain in one or both of the patient's shoulders, and by a drop in pressure as the gas passed into the peritoneal cavity. However, the test was not error proof, with both false-positive and false-negative results reported.

Commenting on the procedure's continuing use in Egypt, Sallam (1989) notes, "The test is potentially dangerous and should be conducted carefully. The following complications may be encountered: (i) Gas embolism which may be fatal; a soluble gas is therefore preferred (e.g., CO_2) to air or nitrogen. The pressure should not exceed 200 mm Hg or the volume 200 ml; (ii) Exacerbation or introduction of infection; (iii) Uterine or tubal perforation; (iv) Severe pain and vasovagal block" (Sallam 1989:130).

Given these dangers and the fact that both hysterosalpingography and diagnostic laparoscopy provide superior information, tubal insufflation has been superseded by these newer methods of diagnosis. Furthermore, tubal insufflation was *never* intended for therapeutic use and, as suggested by Sallam (1989), is likely responsible for *causing* tubal-factor infertility in some patients, by forcing pathogenic bacteria from the lower into the upper genital tract, leading to tubal infection.[16] Yet, in Egypt, the many biogynecologists who perform this procedure tell patients that "blowing" will open or widen the fallopian tubes, particularly if the tubes are mildly obstructed. For this reason, many patients willingly undergo the painful procedure—often more than once, as demonstrated in Table 10.

Unfortunately, many Egyptian biogynecologists defend their use of tubal insufflation as a diagnostic and therapeutic procedure. However, many critics also exist.

As one such critic argued,

> The old gynecologists do tubal insufflation in their private clinics, because they think it opens the tubes. But the new generation doesn't believe this, because there may be many factors other than obstruction causing tubal infertility—for example, tubal function only or pathology of the tube. But if the doctor has the apparatus and she [the patient] wants insufflation, he will do it for her. I heard about one [physician] who did insufflation in his private clinic and the patient died from anaphylactic shock. Although its use decreased over the last ten years, some still do it.

Another physician remarked,

> I tell patients when they say that "Mrs. So-and-So got pregnant after *nafq* and *tausīʿ wi kaḥt*" that "She would have become pregnant after she had eaten watermelon!" I'm not angry because these things are perpetrated among patients, but because they're perpetrated among doctors. They say, "I've done this before and she became pregnant." I say, "This doesn't prove anything; there's something called a controlled study." Of course, it's stupidity. Insufflation, some people do it to check the tubes, clear the tubes. I don't do it; I don't believe in it. . . . Of course, if there is an infection in the cervix, tubal insufflation can cause it to ascend. There was also a death several years ago because the doctor was injecting air; he didn't have carbon dioxide, so he injected air and produced an air embolism.

Yet another physician concluded,

> When first introduced, insufflation was a diagnostic test, before the era of diagnostic laparoscopy. Then it became abused as a therapeutic modality. Actually, the problem is that we [Egyptian physicians] don't have a systematic approach to studying problems. Some people get pregnant after diagnostic laparoscopy, some after insufflation. So, when working on your own and depending on your clinical impression, yes, it happens. If you don't have a systematic approach to treating infertility even in your mind, let alone some written protocol, then you say, "I want to do something for the patient." A lot [of physicians] have tubal insufflators, and they think this is the most benign approach.

Injecting "Cocktails"

A much rarer but occasionally employed procedure is hydrotubation (also known as hydroinsufflation or pertubation), or what is known to Egyptian patients as *ḥu'an fir-raḥim,* meaning "injections in the uterus." In hydrotubation, saline solution with a "cocktail" of antibiotics, corticosteroids, and anti-inflammatories (usually alpha-chemotrypsin) is injected by a cannula through the cervix into the uterus. Purportedly, such injections, if repeated over three to six months, dissolve mild tubal adhesions, thereby opening partially blocked fallopian tubes or maintaining openness following tubal surgery. In most cases, physicians charge approximately three hundred pounds ($120) for a series of these injections—an exorbitant price for most poor Egyptian women.

As with tubal insufflation, hydrotubation has no proven role in the treatment of tubal-factor infertility and is not mentioned in contemporary textbooks of reproductive medicine (e.g., Aiman 1984; Carr and Blackwell 1993). According to an Egyptian infertility specialist and critic of the procedure, "Repeated hydrotubation using antibiotics, corticosteroids is also of little value, and unless carried out under sterile conditions, may in itself spread any localised infection" (Sallam 1989:140). Other Egyptian biogynecologists agree. One commented that hydrotubation is "the same as insufflation but less common. Some doctors may consider it somewhat 'sophisticated.' But it has no therapeutic role for tubal infertility patients with adhesions."

Another critic argued that hydrotubation is "useless. You are not going to remove adhesions at all. It's been advocated with tubal surgery, but nowadays they do not use it. Sometimes some surgeons say they do it to keep the tube patent and to keep anastomoses corrected. But this is useless and may be even harmful."

Another physician agreed, saying, "[Hydrotubation has] been condemned in many centers. They say it doesn't benefit the patient, and, contrary, may even worsen the problem. Now, because of laparoscopy, we can determine the site of obstruction and can deal with it either surgically or send [the patient] to a specialist of IVF."

Sessions of Electricity

Like hydrotubation, shortwave (infrared) therapy—known as *galsāt kahraba,* or "sessions of electricity," to Egyptian patients—is an uncommon but occasionally employed therapy for tubal adhesions. Although most biogynecologists themselves do not perform this procedure (which may explain why it is not used more often), they may send tubal-factor infertility patients to radiologists or physiotherapists, who administer thermal radiation to the patient's external abdominal wall to supposedly increase circulation to the internal, adhesion-congested pelvic region. Unlike hydrotubation, which is usually administered in less than ten sessions, suggested courses of shortwave therapy are long and tedious for patients, who are often asked to come for as many as twenty to fifty "sittings."

As with the other procedures described above, many Egyptian biogynecological critics argue that shortwave therapy is of little value in the treatment of tubal-factor infertility.

As one such critic stated,

> This is a sort of therapy to supposedly reduce the effects of inflammation by inducing more blood supply to the area of inflammation. But, in established PID [pelvic inflammatory disease] with adhesions and tubal destruction, it will do nothing. It may be used in the acute phase or in patients with some pelvic pain, but in infertile patients, it will do nothing. In many cases diagnosed as tubal factor, her doctor may tell her to have this. [Short-wave therapy is] common, but not like D & C and insufflation, because the [gynecologist] doesn't do it by himself. If he did, it would be common.

Another critic of the procedure added, "Actually, [shortwave therapy] is not *kahraba* [electricity]; it is infrared, or heat. Radiologists and maybe physiotherapists do it, but I don't know why. If the gynecologist himself had this machine, he would do it for the same reason—money. It has no merit."

Opening the Belly

In addition to the "minor" outpatient procedures described above, many infertile Egyptian women are admitted to hospitals for major reproductive surgeries, or *ʿamalīyāt,* to correct various ovarian-, tubal-, and uterine-factor infertility problems. The primary infertility surgeries performed in Egypt are listed in Table 10 and are as follows: cystectomies and wedge resections of the ovaries; myomectomies for the removal of uterine leiomyomas (fibroids) and uterine suspension surgeries for uterine displacements; and tubal surgeries to remove adhesions and unblock obstructed fallopian tubes.

So commonly are such surgeries performed that nearly one-quarter of all infertile women in this study had undergone one or more major surgeries. Yet, surgery had failed to correct the infertility problem in every case.

As in the case of Maisara, surgery probably *leads* to further infertility problems for some women, through postoperative scarring and infection-induced pelvic adhesions. Furthermore, most poor women who are scheduled for surgery are never clearly told about therapeutic rationales or success rates of these operations. In other words, with the exception of most tubal surgery cases, few poor Egyptian women who undergo reproductive surgery understand exactly why their "bellies are being opened"—the Egyptian colloquial expression for all abdominal surgeries. Rather, most are simply told by a biogynecologist that they are "in need of an operation" in order to become pregnant.

Driven by their desires to conceive and by the low cost of surgery if performed in a public hospital, many poor infertile women agree immediately to surgery, although sometimes without the initial consent of their husbands or other concerned family members. Occasionally, women are told of the low success rates of various surgeries or of possible iatrogenic complications, but decide to proceed with the surgery anyway out of sheer desperation for a child. Furthermore, because such operations are undertaken under general anesthesia, infertile women do not fear the pain that is known to accompany most of the other procedures described above.

Although a detailed description of the various surgical methods employed for infertility in Egypt is beyond the scope of this discussion, a number of salient points about the practice of infertility surgery in Egypt must be made.

First, because most Egyptian biogynecologists are generalists, they do not specialize in biogynecological surgery, including infertility surgery. However, because gynecology, by definition, is a surgical specialty (Becker and Nachtigall 1991), most biogynecologists receive some surgical training in medical school and continue to perform such surgeries, for better or for worse, once they are established in practice.

Second, the major problem with surgery in general and reproductive surgery in particular is postoperative sepsis due to the lack of sterile operative conditions in biomedical settings throughout Egypt (Inhorn and Buss 1993). In addition to normal, postoperative, adhesion-producing scarring, pathogenic microorganisms introduced into the pelvic region during surgery lead to pelvic infections in many patients; these, in turn, lead to further adhesions and subsequent tubal-factor infertility. Thus, much of the reproductive surgery carried out in Egypt—even that undertaken to "cure" patients of infertility—is iatrogenic, causing in some cases irreparable infertility problems. Occasionally, these iatrogenic surgeries are carried out in unmarried women (for example, for ovarian cysts), thereby permanently destroying their future reproductive potential.

Third, many of the infertility surgeries performed in Egypt are truly unindicated. For example, as we have seen, some women are told that their uteri are malpositioned—a situation reflected in women's beliefs about infertility-producing "upside-down," "tilted," and "reversed" uteri. Infertile women who are diagnosed as having retroflexed uteri are often encouraged by gynecologists to undergo uterine-suspension surgeries to correct the purported infertility-causing displacement. However, as noted by Bates and Wiser, "Uterine retroversion, of itself, rarely causes infertility. Occasionally, a cervix that is positioned sharply anterior may be unable to receive the ejaculate. In an earlier era, the finding of a retroflexed uterus was indication (even in young women who had not tested their reproductive potential) for a uterine suspension. In modern infertility practice, this is not warranted" (1984:154).

Likewise, wedge-resection surgery for women with polycystic ovary syndrome (PCO) is frequently performed in Egypt, where PCO is a common finding. A history of wedge-resection surgery is, in fact, a common finding in women with *both* ovarian- and tubal-factor infertility, the latter probably resulting from the ovarian operation itself. However, with the advent of powerful ovulation-inducing therapies, especially during the past decade, wedge-resection surgery has become obsolete. As noted in a recent textbook:

> The use of wedge resection to treat the ovulatory problems associated with PCO resulted from a clinical observation. PCO patients with bilaterally enlarged ovaries initially thought to be pathological often begin to ovulate following wedge resection performed to establish a diagnosis. However, the significant incidence of postoperative adhesions and the increased number of ovulatory-inducing agents have resulted in wedge resection falling into disfavor. (Seibel 1993)

Myomectomies—which are more difficult than hysterectomies and are associated with greater complications (Winkel 1993)—are also frequently performed in Egypt, even when the benign uterine fibroids removed in these operations are small, asymptomatic, and unrelated to infertility. In fact, the relationship between fibroids and infertility has been questioned (Winkel 1993). As noted by Bates and Wiser, "If the endometrial cavity is normal in size, shape, and configuration, it is unlikely that leiomyomata are the cause of infertility" (1984:154).

Finally, laparotomies (abdominal surgeries) for the treatment of tubal-factor infertility are commonly performed in Egypt, given that newer alternatives, including laparoscopic surgical techniques and assisted reproductive technologies such as IVF, are not widely available. Unfortunately, because surgical microscopes are rarely used,[17] virtually every patient who undergoes tubal surgery, especially in public hospitals, is actually undergoing gross (macroscopic) surgery. Because the fallopian tubes are such delicate and complex structures—actively participating in transport of sperm, fertilization, and embryo migration—their functional integrity is easily impaired by what Eddy (1984) calls "injudicious surgical techniques," such as those performed on most tubal-factor infertility patients in Egypt.

In fact, many Egyptian biogynecologists feel strongly that tubal surgery, as practiced in their country at this time, harms patients more than it benefits them. Some of these physicians argue that, until the new reproductive technologies such as IVF become more widely available in Egypt, women should not be subjected to tubal surgery at all, because of the untoward consequences of this most invasive form of therapy.

As one such physician stated, "I don't recommend tubal surgery here, because there are no facilities for microsurgery. What's done here is not tubal surgery. They remove adhesions in a way that is not suitable for the fallopian tube, and the manipulations done will induce more adhesions after closing up. It needs microsurgery and experience and training. They do it now in private hospitals without microscopy. [Tubal surgery] is common but useless."

Another commented,

> Tubal surgery may play a role in causation [of tubal-factor infertility]. Sometimes, we get a patient with just adhesions or tubal obstruction, and a surgeon, not well trained, may try [tubal surgery] and do so much harm to the tube. The patient will become worse. [The physician] will add something to previous adhesions. I've seen so many cases of this. [Physicians here] have no experience in this. They do tubal surgery on their own basis: cut the tubes and try to resuture, cut again and suture again, without using the microscope or microsurgical techniques. The result will be shortening of the tube, many more adhesions, iatrogenic stenosis, and obstruction. The patient becomes much worse.

Speaking of his own experience, an Alexandrian infertility specialist concluded, "Actually, I don't do tubal surgery. Although I've been working in infertility for many years, I can't get myself to do surgery, because I believe someone better than me in surgery should be doing it. There should be two or three people who are specialized and do nothing but microsurgery. You can't be a jack of all trades, master of none. Some people here say they do microsurgery, but I think they are actually harming patients."

But, if not these "untherapeutic therapeutics"—including surgery, drugs, and the wide array of old reproductive technologies to which infertile Egyptian women are currently subjected—then where can these women turn to overcome, *safely,* their infertility in the biogynecological realm? This brings us to the topic of the NRTs—both artificial insemination and in vitro fertilization—and to the complexities of "assisted" conception in Egypt.

10. The Injection of Spermatic Animals

The Stories of Lubna and Nermin

Of very different backgrounds and social classes, Lubna and Nermin became fast friends—a friendship forged while waiting in a hospital clinic to undergo *il-ḥu'an,* or "the injections" of their husbands' "spermatic animals" into their barren wombs. In fact, artificial insemination—and the shared misery of their infertile lives—is the only thing that brought Lubna and Nermin together, Egyptian women who, under different circumstances, would never have associated with one another.

Lubna is a Bedouin woman, born in Burg al-'Arab in the "Bedouin" section of the Western Desert of Egypt. Since moving to Alexandria a decade ago, Lubna has become more Alexandrian than Bedouin and no longer identifies herself with her Bedouin past. Likewise, Lubna's husband, Ahmed, one of her cousins, comes from a sedentarized Bedouin family and works as a driver in Alexandria.

Having been married for nine years, Lubna and Ahmed began experiencing significant marital problems "only because of not having babies." As Lubna explains, "Every year that passes and I'm still not pregnant, he becomes more severe. He is cold; with words, he hurts me. He doesn't hit me, but he makes me *feel* that I'm not a complete women, although he doesn't say it. He *always* tells me he wishes to have a child. He doesn't push me to get treated, but if it's my time to come [to the hospital], he tells me to go."

After many attempts at different biogynecological and ethnogynecological therapies, including *ṭibb il-'arabī,* or Bedouin medicine, Lubna became a patient in the artificial-insemination-by-husband, or AIH, program at Shatby Hospital. This is where she met Nermin, a college-educated, middle-class woman who was also experiencing severe marital problems as a result of her secondary infertility.

Although Nermin had a seven-year-old daughter, Hala, by a previous marriage, Sharif, her second husband of four years, was under considerable family pressure to divorce Nermin and replace her with a "fertile" wife. As

Nermin saw it, her in-laws never liked her because she was a divorcée with a child and because her family was of a slightly higher social class, making her in-laws jealous. Thus, Nermin considered her marriage to Sharif to be extremely unstable because of the interference of his family, particularly his mother.

Both Lubna and Nermin, when they met, were desperate for a cure for their infertility, and thus both of them were willing to undergo several cycles of artificial insemination using their husbands' sperm. Lubna never became pregnant, despite her healthy fallopian tubes and her husband's excellent semen quality; therefore, the doctors suspected that Lubna and Ahmed had an immunological incompatibility, perhaps because of being cousins. Nermin, on the other hand, became pregnant on only her second attempt at AIH, and, ecstatic, she immediately told Sharif and his family of her AIH pregnancy. Thus, it came as a shock to her when she miscarried only two months later. Realizing that her in-laws' knowledge of her miscarriage would have a devastating impact on her marriage, she decided not to tell either Sharif or his family of the miscarriage and to attempt to become pregnant again. When she asked Sharif for additional samples of his semen in the second month of her "pregnancy," she told him that these samples were needed for "genetic analyses." Meanwhile, Nermin was working on an alternate plan to obtain an abandoned baby from an orphanage without Sharif's knowledge—a baby that would be born at the approximate time that she was "due."

Although Lubna warned Nermin that her plan to fake a pregnancy for the next six months and to obtain an illegitimate child was risky, Nermin saw no other way out of her predicament. Wanting to hold onto her husband, Nermin knew that the only way to keep him was to have a baby *soon,* and, since she could not seem to produce a living child by him, she felt that deception was the only answer.

Thus, over the ensuing months, Nermin took to wearing pillows under her clothing and staying at her mother's home, so as to avoid intimate contact with Sharif. She told him that the doctors said that she could not have sex with him and, therefore, that she needed to stay away from him for the duration of the pregnancy.

Unfortunately for Nermin, Sharif became suspicious about her story, did some checking on his own, and discovered that his wife had, indeed, become pregnant through AIH, but had miscarried soon thereafter. Incensed by her deception, Sharif divorced Nermin immediately.

As a result, Nermin no longer comes to the AIH clinic for the "injection." And, Lubna, who is no longer considered a good candidate for AIH but who is still holding onto her marriage, has not seen her friend Nermin since the calamitous discovery.

Technico-Moral Pioneers

Lubna and Nermin are both Egyptian "pioneer" women (Rapp 1988)—pioneers in a biotechnical revolution of the body that promises pregnancy at the expense of moral certitude. Among the first group of Egyptian women to subject themselves to the new reproductive technologies (NRTs), Lubna and Nermin have ventured into uncharted technical-ethical-legal territory in their pilgrimage for pregnancy. That this environment is murky is seen in the stories of both women, one of whom fails to become pregnant through artificial insemination and the other of whom becomes pregnant but fails to deliver a child, resulting in a panicked act of deception followed by divorce. In both cases, artificial insemination raises more questions than it answers and brings more suffering than salvation.

Within the past decade, the assisted conceptive technologies of artificial insemination (AI) and in vitro fertilization (IVF) have come to Egypt and have created new options—as well as new dilemmas and new disappointments—for women like Lubna and Nermin, who were under the assumption that their therapeutic quests had ended for want of other possibilities. Hungry for finality in their therapeutic quests, women like Lubna and Nermin are often overjoyed to hear of new procedures being introduced into Egypt that hold the promise of overcoming women's infertility problems for good.

Indeed, it would seem that Egypt is on the verge of a therapeutic revolution—one that will eventually lead to the eradication, or at least the reduction in prevalence, of the less-than-therapeutic procedures described in the previous chapter. On the other hand, this therapeutic transformation can never be total. With the NRTs, Egyptian women still undergo painful, invasive procedures by mostly male biogynecologists—procedures with low therapeutic efficacy rates and high price tags. And, as with the ORTs, the NRTs involve attempts by male "technopatriarchs" to facilitate the patriarchal agenda through the creation of other men's babies in women's wombs.

However, with the NRTs, male biogynecologists not only repair women's bodies using specula, scalpels, scopes, syringes, and the other tools of the biogynecological trade, but they actually place other men's fetus-carrying worms—liquified, spun, and washed—inside the bodies of men's wives, bypassing the need for the original male "tool," the penis. In other words, the NRTs represent the ultimate technology of the reproductive body in a patriarchal society, allowing a few, select, biomedical father figures to facilitate other men's fathering through extrasomatic control over men's worms and the invasion of women's reproductive receptacles.

For women in Egypt, the introduction of the NRTs—extremely masculinist technologies in which women (and, to a lesser extent, men) must submit to the will of male biogynecological authorities—is a mixed blessing. As in the cases of Lubna and Nermin, it is clear that participating in a collective therapeutic revolution—and a male-dominated revolution at that—is no guarantee of individual women's therapeutic victories. Furthermore, with the NRTs, the moral burden of responsibility placed on women is tremendous. They must convince their husbands—and themselves—that procedures such as artificial insemination and in vitro fertilization are *ḥalāl* (permitted) by Islam and by the mores of the communities in which they live. As we shall see, with the NRTs, moral concerns often outweigh practical-logistical ones, and the "local moral worlds" (Kleinman 1992) in which women like Lubna and Nermin live become places fraught with anguish over sometimes insoluble moral conflicts. As noted by Rapp (1988:114), "Until we locate and listen to the discourses of those women who encounter and interpret a new reproductive technology in their own lives, we cannot evaluate it beyond the medical model."

To understand the troubled moral worlds of infertile Egyptian women, it is necessary to examine the eventful introduction of the NRTs into Egypt, the participation of both men and women in this event, and the response of the infertile and fertile Egyptian publics to new technologies of the body that manipulate not only the soma but the soul, not only the reproductive organs of women but the conceptive substances of men. In this chapter, we will examine artificial insemination alone—or what infertile Egyptian women have come to understand as the "injection of spermatic animals" into their empty wombs. In the following chapter, we will examine the creation of "babies of the tubes"—babies much awaited by the infertile women of Alexandria.

Arrival of the NRTs

In March 1986, the new school of assisted reproductive technologies was formally introduced into Egypt with the establishment in Cairo of a private in vitro fertilization and embryo transfer center (Serour, El Ghar, and Mansour 1990, 1991). The following year, the first Egyptian test-tube baby was delivered in Cairo (in July 1987) (Serour, El Ghar, and Mansour 1991), and technology transfer within Egypt began, with the announcement of both public and private AI and IVF programs in Alexandria, the second largest city.

By 1988, a full-scale artificial-insemination-by-husband (AIH) program was in place at the University of Alexandria's Shatby Hospital. In addition, by that time, plans were also well underway at the hospital for the establishment of Egypt's first public-sector IVF program, which had been widely publicized in the mass media and for which patients at the hospital were being selected and prepared.

Because of the publicity about the introduction of the NRTs at Shatby Hospital, physicians in the Alexandria vicinity began referring their intractable infertility cases, especially those with bilateral tubal obstruction, to the hospital. Such women were usually told by their physicians that Shatby Hospital—with its "new machines from abroad" and its "free test-tube baby program"—was their best hope. In addition, many patients began coming on their own or with their husbands, often at the urging of other family members, after exposure to media publicity about the hospital's AIH/IVF program.

By the fall of 1988, the artificial insemination (*talqīḥ iṣṭināʿī*) program at the hospital claimed many participants, as well as many pregnancies. The program was strictly AIH—or artificial insemination *by husband*—because of religious prohibitions in Egypt against AID, or artificial insemination *by donor*. Given the necessity of using only husbands' sperm, the primary indications for insemination developed by the physicians administering the program included: (1) cervical-factor infertility, in which intrauterine AIH allowed for the safe passage of sperm beyond the cervical mucus barrier; (2) immunological infertility problems also at the level of the cervix and for the same reason as (1); and (3) "unexplained" infertility problems, many of which were suspected of being problems of (1) and (2). In addition, some women were chosen for AIH if their husbands had moderate to mild male-factor infertility problems, amenable to the sperm-washing techniques used in AIH, and their own difficult ovulatory problems required careful ultrasound follicular monitoring and precisely timed intercourse more easily controlled through AIH. To a much lesser extent, women with tubal-factor infertility were also chosen for AIH *if* their tubal obstruction was not bilateral; however, the pregnancy prognosis for many

TABLE 12. New Reproductive Technologies (NRTs) Administered to Ninety-four Infertile Women in the Study Sample.

TIMES PROCEDURE WAS ADMINISTERED	PERCENTAGE OF WOMEN
Artificial Insemination by Husband (AIH) (talqīḥ iṣṭinā'ī)	
One	17
Two	9
Three	5
Four or more	4
Scheduled (but not yet administered)	5
In Vitro Fertilization (IVF) (ṭifl l-anābīb)	
One	1
Scheduled (but not yet administered)	15

of these women was poor, and some of them were encouraged to undergo IVF, particularly following failed AIH attempts.

Given the many indications for AIH, 35 percent of the infertile women in this study underwent AIH at least once, while others were viewed as future candidates for this procedure, as shown in Table 12. In fact, so many of the infertile women attending Shatby Hospital as outpatients had either undergone or were being scheduled to undergo AIH that *il-ḥu'an,* or "the injections" as women called them, were the subject of significant discourse and eager anticipation on the part of women who had yet to be "injected" with their husbands' sperm.

Wombs with a View

According to the practice at the hospital, women who were scheduled to undergo AIH were first evaluated diagnostically, to assess their candidacy for the procedure according to the aforementioned indications and to establish the exact timing of their ovulation and, hence, insemination, through ultrasound follicular monitoring. Women who were deemed candidates for the procedure were asked to come regularly—and even daily—to the hospital for *it-taṣwīr,* or abdominal ultrasound (literally, "the photography"), used to chart their ovulatory cycles through measurement of ovum-containing follicles in the ovaries. Women whose follicular measure-

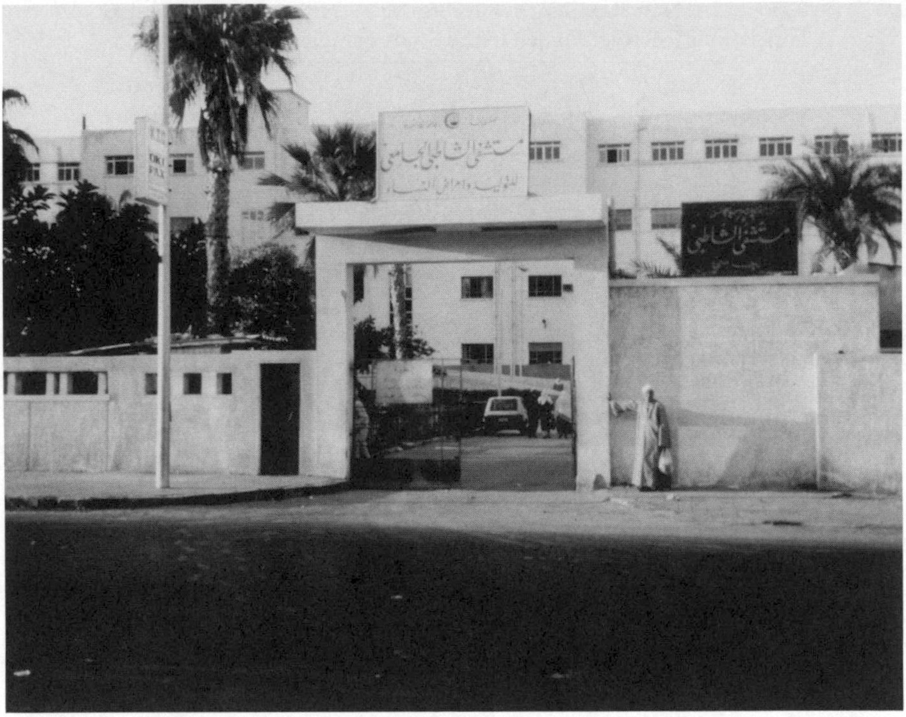

Photograph 10. Shatby Hospital. (Photograph by Marcia Inhorn)

ments indicated impending ovulation either were asked to bring their husbands with them to the hospital for the insemination procedure, or were given special sterile plastic test tubes in which their husbands were expected to ejaculate through masturbation at home on the morning of the procedure. When the supply of these rather expensive test tubes was eventually depleted, women began bringing semen samples from home in various containers.

Worms in an Injection

Semen samples collected in this manner were first identified according to patients' names (written with an indelible felt-tip marker on each test tube). These samples then underwent processes of liquefaction, "washing" with a liquid fertilization medium, centrifugation, and incubation using the laboratory facilities in the small "artificial insemination room" in the hospital—the same room where women underwent the insemination procedure itself.

Thus, as the AIH program became more and more routinized, women who were to be inseminated typically brought their husbands' "samples" to the artificial insemination room between the hours of 8 A.M. and 10 A.M.; underwent follicular scanning, for which they were expected to drink large quantities of water in order to fill their bladders (thus providing the "window" to, or view of, the ovaries when ultrasound monitoring was carried out with an abdominal probe) between the hours of 10 A.M. and noon; purchased special syringes for intrauterine insemination at the nearby pharmacy between the hours of 11 A.M. and noon; and underwent the insemination itself between the hours of noon and 1:30 P.M.

Both the ultrasound follicular scanning and the inseminations themselves were typically unpleasant somatic experiences for women. With respect to the ultrasounds, women were expected to fill their bladders with liquid and then wait, full-bladdered, until their turn at the ultrasound machine arrived. The period between the achievement of a full bladder and one's turn at the ultrasound machine was often more than an hour, during which time many women lost their bladder control and were forced to urinate. Likewise, insemination was often painful for women, especially when performed by an inexperienced physician "without a light touch." Typically, women were called by name for the inseminations, were asked to remove their underwear only, and then were told to lay on their backs on the one gynecological examination table in the laboratory. Women were inseminated with their husbands' sperm using a special needle and syringe inserted through a speculum into the uterus itself. This uterine "injection" was often accompanied by severe pain and cramping—what one woman described as "cutting my body into small pieces with a knife." However, because of the need for rapid turnover, women were allowed to remain on their backs for only a few minutes before being told to replace their undergarments and leave the room in order for other inseminations to take place. Normally, from two to ten inseminations occurred on any given morning.

Despite their fear of pain and becoming "exhausted from down," the vast majority of infertile women who had never been exposed to AIH before coming to the hospital were intrigued by the "injections," viewing them as a modern therapy that could possibly provide the long-awaited solution to their infertility problems. In fact, part of the enthusiasm over a therapy involving an injection directly into the uterus was related to the wider Egyptian preference for injections, which are viewed as a treatment modality superior to oral medications. Thus, women who were undergoing

AIH were thrilled to be receiving an injection instead of, or in addition to, the more familiar oral ovulation-inducing agents.

Local Moral Worlds

Yet, despite this enthusiasm, AIH posed numerous dilemmas for most women, despite their ardent desires to undergo the procedure and thereby end their quests for therapy. These dilemmas were of both a practical and moral nature and presented serious challenges to the moral identities of "good" Muslim women as they attempted to overcome their infertility problems.

Expense

First, AIH was an expensive undertaking for most of the women undergoing the procedure at the hospital, because the majority of these women were poor and the insemination procedure, especially if repeated, was costly. When the AIH program began, women were charged a one-time fee of forty Egyptian pounds (sixteen dollars) for the ultrasound follicular monitoring and an additional forty pounds for the insemination itself—or a total of eighty pounds (thirty-two dollars) for up to six trials of AIH. The forty pounds charged for the insemination process was intended to cover the costs of test tubes, fertilization media, and physicians' time spent in laboratory preparation of semen samples. However, as the months passed and the demand for AIH services grew steadily, hospital administrators decided to levy these charges on a monthly basis. Given that many women were forced to repeat AIH cycles up to six times (and to discontinue AIH if it had failed to produce conception by that point), the cost of therapy amounted to nearly five hundred pounds (two hundred dollars) in some cases—a huge sum for most women. Not surprisingly, given the patient population at this supposedly free university hospital, demand for AIH services declined as the cost of AIH increased, because, for many poor women, AIH became unaffordable.

In particular, women objected to the forty pounds charged monthly for *it-taṣwīr*, the series of ultrasound examinations undertaken to assess ovulation. Even though most women realized that this amount was much less than that charged in private gynecologists' offices (where one ultrasound examination might cost forty pounds), they repeatedly mentioned that monthly payments of forty pounds were beyond their financial means.

As a result, in both resignation and protest, many women stopped coming for AIH when the price of ultrasound monitoring was raised. One such dropout remarked bitterly, "Do they want us to steal? Or do they just want us to wait at home until God gives us [children]?"

In response to patients' complaints and waning demand, hospital administrators eventually decreased the monthly ultrasound charge to twenty-five pounds (ten dollars). But, for many women, this price was also too high. Thus, many women were eliminated as AIH candidates by virtue of economic default.

Coming and Going

For many women, AIH also posed a serious problem of "coming and going." Affordable and accessible transportation was rarely available for those women who lived in poor neighborhoods far from the hospital, as was often the case. Consequently, many women were forced to leave their homes as early as 4 A.M. to reach the hospital by 8 or 9 A.M. In addition, some women, whose therapeutic quests had been limited largely to familiar neighborhoods, were extremely uncomfortable traveling outside their neighborhoods by themselves, and, in many cases, their husbands were even more troubled by this prospect. However, because husbands could rarely leave their jobs without being economically penalized, they were often unable to accompany their wives to the hospital during normal hours of operation. As a result, some women were "allowed" by their husbands to come to the hospital only if accompanied by a relative or friend; for many women, this posed significant difficulties, given the frequency of hospital visits during a typical AIH treatment cycle.

In addition, many husbands, and women themselves, were bothered by the frequency of hospital visits and how the necessity of constant coming and going, often on a daily basis, would be viewed with suspicion by family and community members, who covertly monitored women's movements. Husbands whose wives attended the hospital every day during AIH cycles were legitimately concerned about safeguarding their wives' and their own reputations, given that women who "come and go" are suspected of working as wage laborers, a situation that reflects poorly on men's abilities as breadwinners.

Furthermore, because of the stigma surrounding infertility, women were often reluctant to tell others that their comings and goings were for treatment—especially when the treatment failed to bring results. With respect to treatment results, husbands often complained to their wives that they were "coming and going for nothing"—a complaint that made women's quests for immediate conception more urgent, given their fear that their husbands would eventually fail to support, financially and otherwise, their AIH endeavors.

Women, too, were often irritated by the frequency of hospital visits and of the directives of their physicians, who told them to "come tomorrow" for reasons that were rarely disclosed. In fact, many of the problems of physician-patient communication discussed in Chapter 8 were exacerbated in the AIH treatment setting by the high physician-to-patient ratio. Although women desperately wanted information about the reasons for such frequent attendance and the rationale behind AIH therapy, the few physicians who were responsible for everything from ultrasound monitoring of follicles to preparation of semen to insemination of patients were overloaded with work and, hence, unable to spend adequate time in patient education. As a result, women educated themselves in the hospital corridors, with those women who had already undergone the procedure attempting to spread information about the AIH experience.

Eggs and Worms

Yet, because women who had already undergone AIH served as the major patient educators, women's understandings about the procedure were often incomplete. Few women understood the exact relation of ultrasound follicular monitoring to AIH, given their confusion over the concept of women's "eggs," a problem discussed in Chapters 3 and 8. Because many women did not accept the biomedical notion that women have eggs that contribute to conception, they were at a loss to explain physicians' concerns about the number and size of their *buwaiḍāt* (ova), as assessed by ultrasound. Not surprisingly, questions about eggs, their size, and their role in AIH abounded, and women were often forced to turn to each other in order to obtain information that was less than accurate.[1]

Furthermore, women could only guess as to why AIH was a useful treatment for infertility. Naturally, given the mechanistic nature of the procedure, they viewed it as a solution to various types of mechanical failures of reproduction—either of the husband's "equipment" (an impotent penis or weak fetus-bearing worms) or of the wife's "catching and carrying" uterus and ovaries. Most women believed that AIH was for situations in which "the husband's worms don't reach"—either by virtue of worm weakness or a woman's body rejecting the worms. According to women who had witnessed semen preparation in the small AIH laboratory, this is why "medicine" was added to semen samples in order to "strengthen," "activate," or "clean" the worms, which were kept alive in a machine (namely, an incubator).

Confusion also reigned regarding the location of the AIH injection in the woman's body. Because many women found the intrauterine injection of sperm to be excruciatingly painful, they reasoned that the insemination syringe had bypassed their vaginas to a site deep inside their pelvises. Yet, they were unsure whether sperm had been injected into the uterus, ovaries, or fallopian tubes, given their realization that only women with "open tubes" were candidates for AIH. Furthermore, women who had yet to undergo the procedure tended to confuse AIH mechanics with those of IVF, believing that some product of the woman's body was actually extracted during AIH and then returned with the husband's ejaculated sperm to an internal site in the woman's pelvis.

Coming and Bringing

Male ejaculation—or "bringing," as orgasm is called in Egyptian colloquial Arabic—was also a major source of difficulty for both husbands and wives undergoing AIH. Women who lived within an hour of the hospital were allowed to "collect" their husbands' semen samples at home and bring the ejaculate in a sterile test tube to the hospital. However, "bringing from home," in both senses of that verb, was problematic on a number of scores. First, given the shamefulness of women's requests for sex, women were often extremely uncomfortable asking their husbands to "bring," and especially into a tiny test tube. Second, many husbands' reluctance or inability to "bring on demand" and "by hand" resulted in occasional failures of women to complete the AIH cycle during a given ovulatory period. Third, many husbands were unable to masturbate without the use of creams or lubricants that served to contaminate the semen sample. Fourth, women whose husbands were able to "bring" at home often had great difficulties in thermoregulating (and hiding) transported semen samples, which they tended to keep tucked between their breasts. Finally, many women experienced significant problems in traveling from home to hospital within an hour, the period of maximum viability of the ejaculated semen.

Yet, women were more willing to tolerate these difficulties than were their husbands willing to accompany them to the hospital for the purposes of insemination. In fact, in this study, only 10 percent of husbands regularly accompanied their wives to the hospital. Although 50 percent of the husbands had come at least once, often on the initial AIH visit, the other 50 percent had never attended the hospital with their wives. In other words, for most of these women, coming to the hospital to undergo AIH was a solitary journey, one marked by the lack of active involvement of their husbands.

However, for most husbands, coming to the hospital with their wives was more problematic than "bringing" at home, not only because of work schedules that conflicted with the morning insemination hours, but also because of men's reluctance to attend a women's gynecological hospital for a procedure that they found to be most intimate, embarrassing, and a threat to their virility and masculinity. Obviously, in a patriarchal culture with a strict sexual modesty code, being asked by a biogynecologist at a women's hospital, often in front of numerous female nurses and patient onlookers, to (1) take a test tube to the communal (that is, male and female) bathroom, (2) ejaculate into this test tube by means of masturbation while many other female patients waited outside for bathroom stalls, and (3) return down the busy hallway with sample "in hand" could only be a humiliating, threatening, and alienating experience for most men, many of whom refused to or were physically unable to undertake this procedure even in the privacy of their own homes. Therefore, those few husbands who were willing to accompany their wives to the hospital in order to abide by these directives were truly exceptional, both as men and as supportive husbands to their wives; for "bringing at the hospital" constituted nothing less than a test of the limits of a man's tolerance and the strength of his male ego.

Mixing and Mix-Ups

Men were also known to refuse AIH on another ground: the moral one. Despite Islamic legal opinions on the permissibility of AIH and IVF, which were issued as early as 1980 from Egypt's famed Al-Azhar University (El Hak 1981; Serour, El Ghar, and Mansour 1990), many Egyptian Muslims were still uncertain at the end of the decade as to whether AIH was *ḥarām* (forbidden) or *ḥalāl* (permitted) in the religion, as evident in Table 13. Yet, even though most infertile women had checked on the religious permissibility of both AIH and IVF and were aware that these techniques were allowed as long as they employed only the sperm of the husband, they and their husbands continued to fear the possibilities of both "sperm mixing" and "sperm mix-ups" by unscrupulous or careless physicians.

The primary concern of patients contemplating AIH was that husbands' semen samples might get mixed up with those of other men or that physicians knowingly mixed the samples of "weak-wormed" men with

TABLE 13. Permissibility of the New Reproductive Technologies (NRTs) in Islam: Perceptions of Fifty-four Fertile and Seventy-two Infertile Women in the Study Sample.

	ARTIFICIAL INSEMINATION BY HUSBAND (AIH)	ARTIFICIAL INSEMINATION BY DONOR (AID)	IN VITRO FERTILIZATION (IVF)
Fertile Women			
Permitted (*ḥalāl*)	17%	2%	28%
Forbidden (*ḥarām*)	22%	53%	26%
Don't know	61%	45%	46%
Total	100%	100%	100%
Infertile Women			
Permitted (*ḥalāl*)	84%	0%	76%
Forbidden (*ḥarām*)	12%	96%	19%
Don't know	4%	4%	5%
Total	100%	100%	100%

those of "strong-wormed" ones—resulting, effectively, in artificial insemination by donor (AID). Not only is AID religiously forbidden in Egypt (Serour, El Ghar, and Mansour 1990), but the practice is culturally repugnant to Egyptians, who consider AID equivalent to adultery and the product of AID to be an *ibn ḥarām,* or bastard (literally, a "son of sin").

Women vehemently objected to AID in the same way that most of them objected to adoption, a practice that is illegal in Islam, but that is circumvented in Egypt through permanent legal fostering (qua adoption) arrangements (Inhorn n.d.; Sonbol 1992).[2] Women's objections to AID took a number of forms. First, many women argued that the child of an AID conception would not be their husbands' nor, in their minds, their own; in effect, the child would be like "a stranger" to them and, like an orphan, would be an *ibn ḥarām.* Second, some women argued that motherhood does not entail taking care of "just any child"—that the reason women marry is to have the children *of their husbands* (which, in a monogenetic system, is exactly how children are viewed). Thus, bearing the child of another man would be like "stealing" a child that does not belong to one's husband.

However, the adulterous "betrayal" of one's husband was women's major concern,[3] which they expressed in numerous colorful ways: "It would be like someone jumping in other than my husband"; "It would be like having a lover"; "It would be like sleeping with someone who's not my husband"; "If I were to do this, then why did I marry my husband?"; "Who would accept herself that she gets it from someone else?"; and "It would be better to die than to do this with a man who is not my husband." Many women expressed moral outrage at the mere mention of AID, which they called the "biggest sin" and "one thousand percent wrong." As one woman remarked, "Even if your life depended on having children, you still wouldn't do it!" Others simply stated, "My conscience wouldn't accept it."[4]

These anxieties about unwitting adultery through the "mixing" of sperm were played out in women's behavior as they contemplated AIH at the hospital. First, many women were willing to undergo AIH only after developing feelings of trust toward at least one physician in the AIH program, who could be counted on to inject women with the "correct" sperm. Because several of the physicians in the program had large followings of devoted patients who felt their cases had been well handled, enthusiasm and feelings of confidence spread among patients. For this reason, many patients were willing to entrust physicians in the hospital with their bodies in ways that they might not have had the program and its physicians been less public and highly acclaimed.

Second, women were careful observers of the AIH procedure—paying special attention to how semen samples were handled by physicians. As they noted, women's names were written immediately and carefully on their husbands' test tubes by physicians, and women were later called by these exact names for insemination, giving other observant women great confidence that mistakes were not made. Nevertheless, women often sought to verify the implausibility of rumors they had heard—for example, that all of the husbands' semen samples were mixed together in the hospital in a large container. Indeed, some Christian patients had been told this by Christian private practitioners, who warned that Muslim hospital staff could not be trusted completely. As they pointed out, if sperm were mixed, a Christian woman would most certainly end up giving birth to a Muslim man's child, given the preponderance of Muslims in the country.

Because of such concerns, some bold women asked physicians directly about this possibility of sperm mixing and mix-ups. Physicians' answers further convinced most of them—and their skeptical husbands—that AIH was morally acceptable in every way and that mistakes were never made. However, as one woman with lingering concerns maintained, "We women are usually very doubtful, because how would you know? There are so many tubes, and so many women give their solution [that is, husbands' semen]. How do you really know it's yours?"

Safe, But Effective?

In addition, a nagging question remained in the minds of many women and their husbands: Namely, even if AIH was safe, morally and otherwise, was it effective in causing pregnancy?

For many infertile women, their doubts about the efficacy of AIH grew as the AIH program at the hospital expanded. Little did they realize that, as the number of women being accepted for the AIH program increased, fewer ideal candidates were undergoing the procedure, and, with greater numbers of borderline cases in the program, pregnancy rates fell. Thus, over the months, more and more women underwent AIH but with fewer noticeable successes—leading many women to wonder whether their efforts were all for naught.

To counteract the possibility that this expensive, morally troublesome procedure would "bring no results," women undergoing AIH usually prayed to God at the moment of "injection," asking him to grant their wishes for a child. Yet, women acknowledged that only God could decide whether the act of insemination would lead to a child. As one woman said, "We say the injections cause pregnancy, but it's really God who decides these things."

According to women, nowhere was God's decisive role in human creation more apparent than in the "artificial creation" of test-tube babies—babies "manufactured" by men but ultimately enlivened by God. These God-given "babies of the tubes"—the final hope of so many infertile Egyptian women—are the subject to which we now turn.

11. Babies of the Tubes

Sakina's Story

On a rainy day in late November 1988, Sakina sat weeping on a bench in a corridor of Shatby Hospital. Just told that both of her fallopian tubes were blocked and that the only way for her to achieve pregnancy was through in vitro fertilization (IVF), Sakina was inconsolable. Her worries were many. First, she feared the reaction of her husband, Hany, who was tired of spending his hard-earned money on her infertility therapies and who had told her three times over the past year that he planned to divorce her and remarry "for children" if she did not become pregnant soon. Second, she was concerned about the cost of IVF, given that her first instruction was to purchase two packets of medicine costing £E 350 ($140) each. Having only £E 100 ($40) left after selling her last gold bracelet for £E 300 ($120), Sakina knew that she was definitely unable to afford IVF on her own and that Hany, with his small salary as a laborer in a textile factory, was probably unwilling and unable to finance this expensive therapy. Third, she was worried about the effect of IVF on her body. Although as the daughter of a *dāya* she had already tried many painful ethnogynecological and biogynecological therapies, Sakina heard from other women in the hospital that the IVF doctors "took things from the tubes and put them back" and, frankly, she had no idea which "tubes" they were talking about or whether these tubes were the same ones that the doctor had said were "blocked" in her body. Fourth, as a Muslim woman, Sakina was uncertain about the acceptability of IVF in her religion. Although she suspected that IVF was not forbidden as long as "it's from the husband," she was uninformed about the opinions of religious experts on this subject and feared Hany's interpretation of the religious permissibility of the procedure. Finally, Sakina was extremely concerned about the reaction of her family and neighbors to her bringing home a "tubes baby" — a baby that might face perpetual ostracism if the nature of its creation was made known to the community. Thus, she realized that if she were to undertake IVF, she would have to keep this fact secret from everyone — except, of course, from her sympathetic mother.

However, of all of these concerns, Sakina's financial worries were the most immediate and were the ones that had made her burst into tears in the doctor's office. When the doctor told her to purchase the two packets of expensive medicine, she told him that she could not afford even one packet and would therefore be unable to undertake IVF therapy. He offered to provide one packet of the drug for free if she would agree to participate as a subject in his clinical study of IVF patients. Furthermore, he told her of a government pharmacy in midtown Alexandria where the drug could be purchased for only £E 220 ($88). However, with only £E 100 ($40) to her name, Sakina was still £E 120 ($48) short.

A week after her despairing episode in the hospital, Sakina returned to Shatby, smiling, with a packet of the expensive IVF medication in hand. During the ensuing week, she had received *zakawāt,* or alms, from some upper-class Egyptians to whom she had told her sad story and who, taking pity on her, gave her the remaining £E 120 as a charitable donation. However, this did not solve all of Sakina's problems. For one, she had no refrigerator in which to store the sensitive drugs, and when she told the doctor that she had kept the packet of drugs at room temperature for several days, he admonished her for failing to follow his instructions. Second, she was told that the drugs she had purchased would be good for only "one trial" of IVF and that subsequent attempts to make a "tubes baby" would require additional medication.

Sakina's most serious problem, however, involved delays. Although she and other women with blocked tubes were told that the IVF procedure would begin at the hospital imminently, a month of waiting turned into two months, and then into three, and, eventually, a year. During this interval, Sakina and other women like her were advised by their physicians to resell their expensive medications, lest the drugs lose their therapeutic efficacy and the women lose their money.

Thus, more than a year after that fateful day in November 1988 when Sakina was told about her need for IVF, her dreams for a *ṭifl l-anābīb,* or a "baby of the tubes," were still not realized. For Sakina—and many other poor infertile Egyptian women like her—a test-tube baby was, in fact, not in the making by the end of the 1980s.

Test-Tube Babies on TV

By the end of 1988, when Sakina ventured to Shatby Hospital to learn of her need for IVF, the subject of IVF was familiar to many urban Egyptians, who recognized this assisted reproductive technology by the name *ṭifl l-anābīb,* literally, "baby of the tubes." Following an announcement in *Al-Ahram* newspaper in July 1987 of the first Egyptian "test-tube baby," the Egyptian media began to capitalize on Egypt's newest reproductive technology, in the form of factual discussions of the technique, debates over the religious permissibility of the procedure, and melodramatic television dramas about infertile women undergoing IVF. In fact, in a popular televised *tamsīlīya,* a dramatic, fictional soap opera that aired in 1989, the story was told of a woman who spent thousands of Egyptian pounds undergoing IVF following years of hopeless infertility. Unfortunately, the protagonist was forced to remain in bed throughout her pregnancy—a false representation—and, at four months, she miscarried her "baby of the tubes" in a dramatic twist of fate.

This television show served as the primary means by which the Egyptian public learned about IVF, although the information conveyed about this new reproductive technology was flawed and viewers' understandings were thus extremely incomplete. Suddenly, women who had never before heard of "test-tube babies" were instant experts on the subject, having watched the soap opera and drawn rudimentary information from it. As one woman described it, "They take the *nutfa* from him, his back, and another from her, and they put it in a jar. And they put chemicals in to revive the dead worms, and the worms start to grow in a jar, and it becomes a child—not a jar like pickles, [but] like an aquarium where the child grows for seven to nine months, and they put it in a nursery. The woman has to stay on her back all the time."

Thus, following the airing of the *tamsīlīya,* "*ṭifl l-anābīb*" became a household word in Egypt, although, as apparent in this woman's description, few Egyptians understood much about how "babies of the tubes" were actually created or how many had been born in Egypt.[1] The misleading rumor that many test-tube babies had in fact been born in the country was perpetuated by publicity surrounding the eventual birth in Cairo of IVF quadruplets to a woman who had been infertile for seventeen years.

Although most of the national publicity about IVF in Egypt emanated from Cairo, where the first private IVF center was established in 1986 (Serour, El Ghar, and Mansour 1990), Alexandria, too, became the site of major IVF activity, with the emergence of both a private IVF clinic and a public program at the government's military hospital. However, both of these IVF pilot programs failed to produce any "babies of the tubes" and were discontinued almost immediately.

Nevertheless, having begun a successful AIH program, administrators at Shatby Hospital decided to continue with plans to expand their assisted reproductive technology program to include IVF. Laboratory supplies necessary for IVF were ordered from abroad; extra laboratory personnel were hired; research projects involving IVF were designed; and IVF candidates such as Sakina were selected from the patient population and enlisted in the IVF program. Furthermore, as noted previously, a widely read national newsmagazine called *October*—equivalent to *Time* or *Newsweek* in the United States—announced in a lengthy article that Shatby Hospital had begun its own "baby of the tubes" program. This article alone brought hundreds of women to the hospital hoping to undergo IVF. Some were women who had undergone unsuccessful IVF trials in Cairo or Alexandria; some were women who had discovered that they could not afford the costs associated with IVF in a private center; and some were simply infertile women who thought that a "baby of the tubes" might provide the long-awaited solution to their infertility problems.

Of the hundreds of infertile women who came to Shatby seeking IVF, only a small number (including 15 percent of the infertile women in this study), actually entered the IVF program as candidates. Most of these women were those with confirmed bilateral tubal obstruction, for whom AIH was not possible and IVF was their only real hope for achieving pregnancy.

Women's Concerns

Yet, for these women, most of whom were poor, their eagerness to undergo IVF was tempered by numerous practical and moral concerns, similar to those described for AIH, but of a slightly different order. Their questions about IVF, as we shall see, revolved not only around its expense and religious permissibility, but around the complicated "mechanics" of a new reproductive technology in which the technological imperative of biomedicine is perhaps quintessentially embodied.

What Kind of "Tube"?

Many Egyptians, both men and women alike, were troubled by IVF because of the difficult question of "tubes." As we have seen, many Egyptian women had heard about women's "tubes" (that is, fallopian tubes) and realized that their blockage constituted a major infertility problem. Yet, the structure and function of these tubes and their location in relation to other female reproductive organs were subjects only partially understood by most women, who viewed the uterus and ovaries as the major female reproductive parts. As IVF became popularized in Egypt, however, many women came to realize that "babies of the tubes" were for infertile women with blocked tubes. But were these "tubes" of the same kind?

After seeing the soap opera, many Egyptians came to surmise that the term "baby of the tubes" actually referred to babies conceived and even interned in glass tubes during the course of gestation. Naturally, the thought of babies "artificially produced" in glass test tubes was one most disturbing to Egyptian men and women, whose convictions about the necessity of natural, God-given conception, childbirth, and parent-child ties were extremely strong. As a result, many Egyptians suspected that IVF was most certainly *ḥarām,* or forbidden, as reflected in women's discourse on the subject. As women explained:

> They've just invented test tubes and everything two years ago. I consider a child brought this way not to be my own child. It's not the same as when you carry a child in your body. These artificial ways don't feel the same—the tenderness and love.
>
> It's not the same as when you carry the child inside you and suffer with it. It's as if you're taking it from someone else. It grows outside the womb of the mother, so it's like going and getting it "ready-made."
>
> They say they put a tube into the woman and after nine months, she delivers normally. But what would the father feel? If the father does have a child, will he still love the one of the test tube? This is *ḥarām,* of course, because God stopped your pregnancy, so you come and put in tubes? It's as if you're saying, "God didn't give me, so we'll get her pregnant."

A number of important themes emerge from these and other women's statements. First, women were extremely concerned about the "artificial versus natural" creation of fetuses "outside versus inside" women's bodies. In a Muslim country where adoption is prohibited by Islamic law, parenthood is synonymous with "natural" (that is, biological) parenthood, which, for most Muslims, is tantamount to the gestation *inside a woman's body* of her own husband's fetus. Fetuses that are viewed as being gestated outside the woman's body—even if produced through the conceptive substance(s) of husband and wife—are not only deemed unnatural, but, like orphans, would be viewed as strangers by a husband and wife, who will therefore lack appropriate parental sentiments. In addition, many women feared the unknown aspects of IVF, including the dubious origin of the products of conception used in the procedure (which, unlike AIH, could come from both male and female donors); the excessive experimentation on women's bodies;[2] and the tampering with natural processes best left to God. Indeed, women's ultimate fears were of God himself, whose will would be defied if human beings were to attempt to "play God" through the production of man-made babies.

In addition, as reflected in women's statements, considerable confusion existed over the mechanics of IVF, fueling women's concerns about the artificiality of the process, especially the perplexing aspect of prolonged extracorporeal gestation. Given the lack of disclosure on the part of physicians, even women who were being considered or prepared for the procedure could only speculate as to the technical aspects of IVF, based on what they could deduce from the news media, from the infamous soap opera, or from physicians' veiled comments. Because these sources provided only cursory explanations, most women's understandings about the nature of IVF were superficial at best.

Women who were better informed about the mechanical aspects of IVF understood that the procedure involved the initial creation of the embryo outside of the woman's womb through a process that involved extraction of the woman's reproductive component (although few were sure of what this was) and mixture of this component with the husband's component (either "worms," "fluid," or "spermatic animals") in a glass container, or tube. After some period of time, ranging in women's minds from twenty-four hours to three months, the fetus, kept in a "machine" or "incubator" during this period "outside," was returned to the woman's uterus through a process of "injection," as in AIH.[3]

Yet, even women who understood the basic aspects of the procedure were often misinformed about important details. As one such woman explained, "The first thing, they get the sperm. They take one of the eggs out. They mix it in something that looks like a uterus, a glass or a tube. Then they ask her if she wants a boy or a girl. They choose the right worm, and they put it in the thing that looks like the uterus of the woman, and they leave it for three months. After that, they do a very small operation with two stitches and put it back in her uterus. Then she is pregnant."

Women who had some idea about the technical aspects of IVF were usually less likely to view the procedure as morally or religiously forbidden, as an act "going against God." In fact, these women, most of whom were infertile, were more likely to laud IVF as the best exemplar of medical progress. As one such advocate of high-tech reproductive medicine explained, "Now medicine is very advanced. In the old days, lots of people couldn't have kids. But now we have 'tubes babies.'" Another commented, "We see that infertility was there ever since the Prophet's time, only then they didn't have test tubes and things that they have now. So now a woman can go and plant a child in a test tube and have her own baby, but she couldn't do that long ago. This is because science has become very advanced."

Accepted by Islam?

Because of their superior knowledge of the technical aspects of the IVF procedure — including the use of a husband's sperm and wife's ova — infertile women were also more likely than others to accept IVF as religiously permitted (see Table 13). Although a *fatwā,* or formal Islamic legal opinion, on the permissibility of IVF was issued by the grand *shaikh* of Al-Azhar Mosque, Shaikh Gad El Hak Ali Gad El Hak, as early as March 23, 1980 (El Hak 1981), few Egyptians were aware of the *shaikh*'s pronouncement even by the end of the decade. In his opinion, the *shaikh* clearly specified that IVF was an acceptable line of treatment as long as it was carried out by expert scientists with sperm from a husband and eggs from a wife with "no mixing with other cells from other couples or other species, and . . . the conceptus is implanted in the uterus of the same wife from whom the ova were taken" (Aboulghar, Serour, and Mansour 1990).

Infertile women who were being considered for IVF tended to be best informed about this theological opinion, having sought advice from religious clerics in some cases.[4] Yet, many women, both infertile and fertile, continued to doubt that Islam would permit such a "strange and unnatural" act as the creation by physicians of a "ready-made child" from "outside the womb." As with AIH, women's husbands tended to be even more doubtful, creating problems for women who were thus thrust into the position of convincing their husbands of IVF's religious permissibility.

However, many Egyptians' anxieties about the religious permissibility of IVF were relieved when the popular televised Muslim cleric, Shaikh Muhammad Mitwali al-Shaarawi, condoned the use of IVF (with husbands' sperm and wives' ova) as a last resort for infertile couples. Yet, many Egyptians — and especially the fertile, who were less attuned to such matters — were not aware of Shaarawi's statements, as reflected in the high percentages in Table 13 of those who believed IVF to be *ḥarām* or were unsure of its religious permissibility.

How Successful Is IVF?

In addition to these moral-religious concerns, another major question in the minds of infertile women was whether or not IVF was successful in most cases. For poor women, such information was crucial, given the expense of the procedure. As with AIH, women were usually shocked to learn that IVF was not free, even in a public hospital, and that the major expense revolved around purchasing ovulation-inducing agents that could cost anywhere from five hundred to one thousand Egyptian pounds (two hundred to four hundred dollars) per treatment cycle. This problem of expense was coupled with the problem of availability; as discussed in Chapter 9, "new-age" ovulation-inducing agents necessary for IVF were often obtained from abroad and were not widely available in most Egyptian pharmacies.

When women being prepared for IVF learned that one thousand pounds might purchase them only one trial of IVF—and that up to six trials might be necessary without any guarantee of reproductive success—their enthusiasm for the procedure naturally waned. For this reason, success rates were rarely conveyed by physicians, although women were obviously curious to know whether amounts exceeding one thousand pounds would "buy" them a baby. Women often noted that they would spend all the money they could muster on IVF if only it would guarantee them a pregnancy outcome. What they were rarely told, however, was that pregnancy rates in the world's best IVF centers were often less than 30 percent (Jones 1988), and that success rates in start-up programs, such as the one at this hospital, could be expected to be much less. In essence, then, Egyptian women being prepared for IVF had minimal guarantees of success, although most of them did not realize this.

How Soon, If Ever?

Given that many women with bilateral fallopian tubal blockage came to view IVF as their last resort—their "only hope" in their quest for conception—the realization that the highly touted IVF program had yet to become a reality at the hospital more than a year after its promised inception was also a source of frustration and fear for many women, especially those like Sakina who had promptly purchased expensive IVF drugs in preparation for the procedure. When women who had purchased these drugs were told to "sell them back" to pharmacies before their expiration dates, IVF candidates began to panic, criticizing the hospital for false advertising of its program. Questions that had once been framed by IVF candidates as "how soon?" came to be posed as "will there ever be?" Unfortunately, by the end of the 1980s, IVF had yet to become a reality at Shatby Hospital, because of numerous political, economic, and logistical problems beyond the control of those who had hoped to make the IVF program a success.

* * *

Epilogue

After many delays, the long-awaited inception of the IVF program at Shatby Hospital occurred in the early months of 1991, almost two and a half years after the announcement of the program in *October* magazine. The equipment necessary to run an IVF laboratory was slow in coming to Alexandria, but by early 1991, it had arrived, and soon thereafter the IVF laboratory and an accompanying andrology laboratory for high-tech semen analysis were in place. A team of young physicians, several of whom were trained in IVF in the United States and Great Britain, was assembled to run the assisted reproduction program (both AIH and IVF) in the hospital.

The first delivery of an Alexandrian "baby of the tubes" occurred in early 1992, only ten months after the IVF program's inception. The baby was delivered by cesarean by the gynecology professor who had referred the case, and members of the Egyptian media, including those from the television, radio, newspapers, and magazines, were received during the delivery by the head of the IVF program, who was also the chairman of the University of Alexandria Department of Obstetrics and Gynaecology.

In addition, at the time of this writing, there are five or six ongoing IVF pregnancies at Shatby Hospital, other than those that have ended in spontaneous abortion. However, there have been some problems in following the IVF pregnancies, because many of the infertile women in the program consider it shameful to have become pregnant through IVF and therefore do not return to the hospital when they discover that they are pregnant with a "baby of the tubes."

It is important to point out in closing that, even as IVF has successfully unfolded in Alexandria, many daunting questions about the implementation and future of IVF in Egypt—similar to those raised by concerned feminists in the West[5]—remain. For example, will the focus on IVF divert attention away from the primary prevention of infertility in Egypt, especially among the poor, who are at greatest risk for infertility but who can least afford the NRTs (Henifin 1988; Nsiah-Jefferson and Hall 1989)? Will the commercialization of IVF in Egypt lead to the proliferation of for-profit clinics run by unscrupulous physicians, whose *raison d'être* is financial gain rather than the reproductive success of women (Meyers 1990; Ratcliff 1989b)? Will success rates be inflated and massaged in Egypt as they are elsewhere to boost the spirits of physicians and to encourage persistence among patients (Corea and Ince 1987; Powledge 1988; Rowland 1987)? Will the choice to undergo IVF turn into pressure for Egyptian women, who will be "compelled to try" IVF over and over again and hence become trapped in endless infertility careers (Beck-Gernsheim 1989; Sandelowski 1991)? Will IVF lead to the commodification of life in Egypt, with perfect babies being manufactured and purchased for a significant price only by the affluent (D'Adamo 1988; Rothman 1988; Rowland 1987)? Will IVF reinforce existing patriarchal, pronatalist biases in Egypt, leading to the continuing disenfranchisement of infertile women who have failed in their mandate to reproduce (Modell 1989; Shannon 1988)? Will IVF lead to further untoward manipulation of and experimentation on Egyptian women's bodies, such that embryos become the "leading actors" and women mere "living laboratories" for the products of man-made conception (Laborie 1987; Rowland 1987, 1992)? And, finally, will the effectiveness and safety of IVF be monitored in Egypt, given the current absence of professional or consumer bodies concerned with technology assessment and biomedical ethics (Oakley 1987; Ratcliff 1989b)?

Although the future of IVF in Egypt is quite uncertain, perhaps it is heartening to realize that ethical debates about research in human reproduction have begun to emerge in Egypt and elsewhere in the Muslim world (Anees 1989; Serour 1992), leading to the development of incipient guidelines and standards for the practice of IVF in both research and clinical settings (Serour and Omran 1992). Currently, Egypt leads the way in these efforts to forge a safe path for IVF and the other NRTs in the Muslim world and may very well serve as a model for other Muslim countries attempting to implement these technologies (Serour, El Ghar, and Mansour 1991).[6] As Serour and his Egyptian colleagues note, the total Muslim population in the world is 1.14 billion (1988 estimate), mostly located in developing countries and particularly in Africa and Asia. If one considers that 24 percent of the population of developing countries consists of women of reproductive age and that 10 percent (on average) of all married women of reproductive age experience infertility, then approximately 27 million Muslim women may be currently infertile and may either accept or reject IVF treatment services as they become available (Serour, El Ghar, and Mansour 1991).

Thus, the experiences of poor infertile Egyptian women such as Sakina, as they attempt to grapple with the complex practical and moral dilemmas posed by IVF, may well serve as a guide for the therapeutic journeys of other Muslim women, whose voices and stories have yet to be heard.

12. Futures for the Infertile

Although the new reproductive technologies have come to Egypt and have been hailed as transformative—even revolutionary—in the treatment of infertility, their ability to alter the ambiguous futures of women such as Sakina, Lubna, Maisara, Ghada, Hind and the other poor infertile Egyptian women who have shared their stories of suffering, searching, and hoped-for salvation remains uncertain. Technology alone cannot "cure" infertility (Shannon 1988); at best it can compensate and at worst it can destroy women whose "fertility mandate" has already been impaired (Boddy 1989). Because technological interventions in infertility treatment in Egypt often lead to deleterious outcomes, it is essential to ask, What can be done to prevent infertility in Egyptian women in the first place and to ensure that Egyptian women who are infertile receive appropriate diagnostic and treatment services?

To attempt to answer this multifaceted question requires consideration of the broader spectrum of reproductive health policy in Egypt, including assessment of the major factors impinging on Egyptian women's reproductive careers. The recommendations for reproductive health policy that follow are intended as a step in this direction and may well apply to many other nations (both developed and developing) besides Egypt, where infertility has been seriously trivialized as an issue of public health concern (Schroeder 1988). In addition, these recommendations are intended as calls for future research by medical anthropologists as well as by other social and health scientists interested in human reproduction. That infertility and the childlessness engendered by pregnancy loss have been underprivileged in anthropological and other fields of scholarly discourse is clear. But what is also clear is the need for the scholarly community to turn its gaze to the crisis of childlessness worldwide and to the human suffering experienced by the millions of women and men around the globe who are unable to meet their dreams of building a family.

Recommendation 1: Incorporate Infertility as an Integral Part of Family Planning

The Universal Declaration of Human Rights, adopted by the General Assembly of the United Nations on December 10, 1948, states in Article 16: "Men and women of full age, without any limitation due to race, nationality or religion, have the right to marry and to found a family. . . . The family is the natural and fundamental group unit of society and is entitled to protection by society and the State."

Although the United Nations has enjoined its member nations to consider "founding a family" as a basic human right, too few nations have viewed assisting *wanted* pregnancies as part of their "family planning" missions. This is especially true in the developing nations of the Third World, where exclusive attention is often focused by states *and* by First World development agencies on the prevention and control of purported population problems through family planning programs which are aimed at women but which ignore entirely women's infertility problems (Corea 1988; Nsiah-Jefferson and Hall 1989; Richters 1992). The racist and classist attitudes often pervading population control efforts are especially apparent when infertility is seen exclusively as a problem of (white) affluent women and as a nonissue for poor women (of color), who are deemed entirely "too fertile" and in need of reproductive regulation and surveillance (Corea 1988; Nsiah-Jefferson and Hall 1989; Schroeder 1988). When new reproductive technologies, which are manufactured in the First World, are made available or affordable only to the Third World elite (Rowland 1987; Turshen 1991), these issues of race, class, and gender bias are magnified even further.

Egypt is no exception in this regard. As the first Middle Eastern Muslim nation to initiate a state-sponsored population-control program in the 1960s (Stycos et al. 1988), Egypt has consistently focused its population-control efforts on family planning through the introduction and active promotion of subsidized contraceptive technologies targeted primarily at women. Egyptian women visiting state-run maternal and child health (MCH) centers for biogynecological and pediatric care are actively encouraged to practice *tanẓīm il-usra,* or "organization [control] of the [nuclear] family," by limiting their number of children to two through the use of generally long-term contraceptives.

The irony of this family planning initiative, of course, is that *women* are not deemed the "baby-makers" according to the widely held monogenetic procreation theory found among Egypt's poor. Thus, if culturally sensitive and specific family planning efforts *were* to be enacted in Egypt, they would be directed at men, would encourage the use of male contraceptives (including surgical vasectomy, which is rarely if ever performed), and would challenge the patriarchal ideology of male ascendancy in the procreative realm, as well as the paradox of women's victimization for reproductive failure. However, because Egyptian family planning programs and messages are fashioned with Western development aid (Lane and Rubinstein 1991; Mitchell 1991) and are based on faulty (and probably unexplored) assumptions about the content, magnitude, and tenacity of pronatalist ideologies, they miss the mark—badly, in fact—in convincing the Egyptian public to contracept.

Although the causes of widespread family planning resistance in Egypt are many, part of the reason why poor Egyptian women fail to "control" their family sizes is their fear of the long-term health consequences of contraception, including contraceptive-induced infertility (DeClerque et al. 1986; Fox 1988; Gadalla, Nosseir, and Gillespie 1980; Inhorn 1994a). Although Egyptian women realize that their bodies serve as the site of the state's population-control efforts—including untoward experimentation with long-lasting contraceptives such as Depo-Provera and Norplant (Morsy 1985, 1993, n.d.)—they also realize that their concerns about the health consequences of contraception, including infertility, are not met by the state in public health-care facilities. MCH centers, which are underutilized even by the fertile because of poor service (Abu-Zeid and Dann 1985), rarely provide adequate infertility counseling, screening, or treatment, leading women concerned about their potential infertility to the "outside" world of private, fee-for-service medicine. Because infertility is not prioritized by the Egyptian state, which sees its major problem as one of rampant *hyper*fertility, no coordinated program is in place to meet the needs of the infertile, both women and men, who flock to private, public, and charitable clinics by the thousands and who pay dearly for these mostly unsubsidized services (Abu-Zeid and Dann 1985).

That the management of infertility should be made an integral part of comprehensive, coordinated family planning services in Egypt and elsewhere and that men must be included as interested planners of their families and as partners to their wives in infertility diagnosis and treatment have been noted by numerous scholars and population policymakers (e.g., Baumslag 1985; Gadalla 1978; Lane and Meleis 1991; Omran 1992). Even some Egyptian physicians who treat the infertile advocate the national coordination of infertility services, administered by the state and governed by law. As one such gynecologist in this study argued,

> We need a higher, countrywide program, a sort of organization to say, by law, that people should do this and this. We need to study treatment results and costs and find the best methods. You cannot educate people about infertility in specific areas; you must do it countrywide, because this is the only way we can come up with a program to really meet our problems. This is realistic for Egypt, but, currently, we don't know exactly what our problems are. It's impossible to do a program now because there are no statistics.

Indeed, the need for statistical documentation of the magnitude and causes of the infertility problem in Egypt is apparent. Because of the dearth of national statistics, the extent of the infertility problem in Egypt remains speculative, as described in Chapter 1. If, however, prevalence studies carried out in Egypt demonstrate levels of infertility (*both* male and female) approaching those of Egypt's southern neighbors, perhaps the Egyptian state will begin to take infertility seriously as the public health problem that it represents—one with the potential to threaten the reproduction of Egyptian society at large.

Recommendation 2: Expand the Scope of the Safe Motherhood Initiative

Article 25 of the United Nations' Universal Declaration of Human Rights states: "Motherhood and childhood are entitled to special care and assistance." Part of the recent international effort to care for and assist mothers has been the Safe Motherhood initiative, started at a World Bank-supported conference in 1987 with the goal of "putting the M back in MCH" (Rubinstein and Lane 1990). Between 1987 and 1988 alone, twelve conferences on Safe Motherhood were held in Africa, Asia, Latin America, and the Middle East and were funded by a number of major international development agencies (Rubinstein and Lane 1990).

Although the Safe Motherhood initiative is intended to redress the international health community's neglect of mothers in favor of children, the scope of this initiative as it has developed over the past seven years has been rather narrow; the primary focus has been on the reduction of maternal mortality resulting from unsafe delivery and abortion, and many of the other pressing health needs of women have been effectively ignored. Thus, while applauding the campaign's concern with maternal mortality, many feminist critics have come to question the lack of comprehensiveness of program goals. As Richters (1992:749) points out, "In the global community of women a broader definition of women's health and well-being is therefore called for: a definition that incorporates women's entire lives, the full range of their needs and activities, and all the discomforts and illnesses that they face."

Certainly, the social, psychological, and physical discomfort engendered by infertility — or the failure to achieve "safe motherhood" — is one of the major perceived health problems of women in Egypt, who fear this outcome following marriage and even after the birth of a child. As numerous scholars have noted,[1] motherhood is a cultural imperative for women in Egypt and serves as a highly valued basis of power, especially for women who lack education and employment skills. To fail to become a mother — or to fail to produce enough children for one's husband — is nothing short of a catastrophe for most women. Thus, concern with infertility and with the various ethnogynecological and biogynecological causes of this affliction are major cultural themes and the topic of significant everyday discourse (Early 1985).

Yet, in the rhetoric of Safe Motherhood, infertility is not privileged, nor are the many potential insults to women's reproductive bodies — *in addition to* unsafe delivery and abortion — that prevent women from achieving safely their motherhood goals. To understand such insults — including STDs, undernourishment and obesity, female circumcision, occupational exposures, and various forms of ethno- and bio-iatrogenesis — is to expand the meaning of "safe motherhood" significantly and to make this initiative more responsive to the needs of real women in Egypt and elsewhere.

Unfortunately, because international health program planners have too often failed to listen to Egyptian and other Third World women — particularly poor urban women, who generally constitute a most muted, subaltern group (Pick et al. 1990) — they have often failed to gather information on women's *perceived* health needs, as well as on the many obstacles facing women in their quests to obtain adequate health care. A truly "woman-centered definition of reproductive health" (Turshen 1991) would acknowledge such needs and obstacles and would be used to create comprehensive reproductive health services for women, in which problems such as infertility, reproductive tract infections, and pregnancy loss are effectively addressed and remedied (Dixon-Mueller and Wasserheit 1991).

In addition, an expanded Safe Motherhood initiative would challenge the patriarchal wisdom that women around the world *must* become mothers. If women continue to be valued only for their reproductive capabilities and continue to be targeted solely as reproducers in international health campaigns, then little progress toward expanding women's roles and responsibilities and providing them with valued alternatives to motherhood will be made (Richters 1992). For poor infertile Egyptian women, who often lament their dependency on a maternal role that they are unable to fulfill, the provision of alternatives to motherhood and the subversion of traditional gender norms that perpetuate the "cult of maternity" would be welcome and would initiate women's own activism. Indeed, an expanded—and markedly radicalized—Safe Motherhood initiative in Egypt could be the first step in such salubrious subversion and could lead to infertile women's desperately needed empowerment.

Recommendation 3: Recognize and Integrate the Services of Traditional Healers

The training of traditional midwives in safe (as biomedically defined) birthing practices and the encouragement of traditional midwives to refer difficult obstetric cases to biomedical personnel have been key strategies in the Safe Motherhood initiative. In addition, the World Health Organization (WHO) has supported the training of traditional birth attendants (TBAs), as traditional midwives are often called, as part of the Primary Health Care (PHC) initiative begun under WHO and UNICEF sponsorship at the International Conference on Primary Health Care held at Alma-Ata, Kazakhstan, in 1978 (Belsey 1985; Pillsbury 1982).

Unfortunately, most TBA training programs, including those in Egypt, have failed to recognize the other important roles often played by midwives, including the provision of nonobstetrical women's health care. Furthermore, training programs that are targeted at midwives alone have failed to recognize the host of other traditional healers who provide important health services, including to women, in many countries around the world.

As Pillsbury (1982) has pointed out, despite much laudatory rhetoric about utilizing traditional health practitioners in government-sponsored PHC programs, few countries have actually succeeded in integrating traditional healers into their national health-care systems, and those that have have tended to focus exclusively on TBAs. According to Pillsbury, the reasons for this failure of integration include, among others, the following factors: (1) the cautious and qualified nature of international health resolutions regarding traditional healer incorporation; (2) the small-scale, preliminary nature of most traditional healer training programs; (3) the attempt to convert traditional healers into community health workers (CHWs) rather than to recognize them for their own expertise and skills; (4) the belief that it is easier to train young, inexperienced CHWs than to retrain old traditional healers who are set in their ways; (5) the low priority of traditional healer integration in the context of scarce resources; (6) the political and bureaucratic problems in coordinating such integration at the level of Ministries; and (7) the lack of promising evaluation of traditional healer integration and PHC programs in general.

Egypt is no exception in this regard. Despite the Egyptian ruler Muhammad Ali's historical mission to integrate traditional healers into public health programs, efforts to incorporate healers into national health-care schemes in recent years have been weak and restricted in scope. For example, TBA training programs begun in the early 1980s have been very limited in their geographical coverage and have viewed midwives unidimensionally as the purveyors of obstetric services (Hong 1987). No attempts to incorporate midwives or other traditional healers into Egypt's national health-care system *as ethnogynecologists*—who serve as the primary providers of women's gynecological health care in many cases—have been made. In addition, the numerous categories of ethnomedical specialists described in Chapter 4 are not officially recognized by the Egyptian state or by the medical profession, thus continuing the long, colonially inspired policy of denial and denigration of the existence of traditional practitioners and their healing services in the country (Gallagher 1990; Kuhnke 1990; Pillsbury 1978; Sonbol 1991).

Although calls for the formal recognition, training, and integration of Egypt's numerous traditional healers into the national health-care system have been made by policy analysts (Abu-Zeid and Dann 1985), little progress in this direction has occurred. Much of the problem emanates from Egypt's powerful biomedical establishment, which continues to deny the importance of traditional healers in providing a variety of health-care services (ranging from bonesetting to minor surgery to herbal therapy to psychiatric care) to Egypt's populous but disenfranchised rural and urban masses (Assaad and El Katsha 1981; Millar and Lane 1988; Morsy 1993; Nadim 1980; Pillsbury 1978).

In the realm of women's health, many Egyptian physicians recognize the continuing existence of *dāyāt* but view them mainly as competitors for their obstetric services and as the perpetrators of unsafe birthing practices. Furthermore, most Egyptian biogynecologists, especially those in urban areas, vehemently deny that *dāyāt* or other traditional healers treat women for their infertility problems or that infertile patients, especially in urban areas, could possibly desire the services of such nonbiomedical practitioners. As one such biogynecologist in this study argued, "In the past, there were too many of them [traditional healers], but now their incidence is very low. Because they [patients] read and because of the large number of doctors in the country, all of these traditions are ended now. They [patients] go to the physician directly. *Dāyāt* are mainly for deliveries — not for infertility."

This perception is pervasive in the Egyptian biogynecological community, although it is obviously misinformed. Because so few physicians are aware of the existence and services of their ethnogynecological counterparts, they are reluctant to imagine the integration of these healers into biomedical diagnosis, treatment, and referral networks, including for the care of infertile patients. As shown in Chapter 4, many ethnogynecologists, particularly *dāyāt,* do not view themselves as competing with biogynecologists and would, in fact, welcome being recognized by physicians for their significant referral services. In addition, many ethnogynecologists, who admire the expertise and skills of physicians, would welcome official recognition as ancillary PHC personnel and could be trained to perform simple differential diagnosis of infertility problems and to direct patients' husbands to laboratories for semen analysis.

As it now stands, however, no such integration of ethnogynecologists into the national health service in Egypt has been tried or even contemplated. Furthermore, until Egyptian physicians are encouraged through educational efforts to modify their negative attitudes toward traditional healers, such integration is unlikely to occur.

Recommendation 4: Evaluate and Upgrade Biomedical Health Services

That Egyptian physicians need to be made more responsive to popular health culture, including the existence of traditional healers, has been noted by a number of analysts of the Egyptian health-care system (Abu-Zeid and Dann 1985; El-Mehairy 1984b). El-Mehairy (1984b), for one, has advocated mandatory social science training of Egyptian physicians to help (1) bridge the chasm between physicians' and patients' cultural backgrounds, (2) promote a more productive and communicative relationship between physicians and their patients, (3) increase physicians' understandings of patients' traditional beliefs and the services provided by traditional healers, and (4) make physicians more responsive to the perceived needs of their patients, particularly women, whose illnesses and obstacles to adequate health care have been largely neglected.

According to El-Mehairy, such "resocialization" of physicians must begin in the medical school years, which are crucial, formative ones for the thousands of physicians who graduate each year from fourteen Egyptian medical schools and who proceed into community practice. The other limitations of Egyptian medical education described in Chapter 8 — including overcrowded classrooms, lack of texts, inadequate clinical, research, and subspecialty training, and paternalistic patron-client relations between students and professorial "demigods" — must also be overcome to improve the clinical knowledge and skills of physicians, thereby preventing many of the importunate treatment practices undertaken on unwitting patients. Blizard (1991), for one, has called for the "unfreezing" and "decolonization" of medical education in postcolonial societies such as Egypt, where British-style medical education may be neither appropriate for nor responsive to existing national health-care needs. In Egypt, in particular, such unfreezing would allow medical education to shift its focus from technologically driven curative care to technologically restrained preventive care.

Beyond medical education, numerous structural changes in the Egyptian biomedical system are certainly necessary (Abu-Zeid and Dann 1985; El-Mehairy 1984b; Institute of Medicine 1979; Kandela 1988). These include, *inter alia:* (1) the implementation of continuing medical education programs for physicians to upgrade their knowledge and skills; (2) the formulation of ethical standards for medical research and practice, including the standardization of informed consent procedures; (3) the formalization of a system of medical malpractice through which patients are able to seek redress for injurious treatment; (4) the fair compensation of government-appointed physicians for their services in public health-care facilities, thereby obviating physicians' needs to focus their energies in the private sector; (5) the provision of incentives to help redistribute health manpower to underserved areas, thereby mitigating unhealthy competition in urban areas; (6) the training of qualified paramedical personnel, from medical secretaries to bookkeepers to technicians to nurses; and (7) the improvement of the public health-care infrastructure, including the upgrading of health-care facilities themselves, as well as the enhanced provision of supplies and treatment services.

In addition, Egyptian biomedicine (and biomedicine throughout the Middle East) would benefit from demasculinization, or the reversal of long-term male domination of the biomedical sector, including in health specialties devoted to women (Haddad 1988). Although women are increasingly represented in Egyptian medical school classes (El-Mehairy 1984b), they are infrequently found in the clinically demanding, prestigious specialties of surgery, internal medicine, and obstetrics and gynecology. If more Egyptian women physicians *were* to enter the field of obstetrics and gynecology and were, in fact, able to take over this male-dominated specialty in Egypt, the character of women's health care might change for the better, with biomedically trained Egyptian women healing their fellow women, as has been the practice for centuries in the Egyptian ethnogynecological realm. That this may eventually occur is quite likely, given the growing preference of religiously conservative Muslim women in Egypt to be treated only by female physicians.

Recommendation 5: Promote and Monitor the Use of Appropriate Health Technology

Furthermore, if Egyptian obstetrics and gynecology were to become truly gynocentric, women would have a much greater voice in reproductive decision making, including in decisions regarding the appropriate use of reproductive technologies (Henifin 1988; Ratcliff 1989b). As it now stands in Egypt, women have little input—either as physicians or as patients—into the kinds of reproductive technologies directed at female bodies or into issues surrounding economic equity and fair access to technologies that are useful (Ratcliff 1989b). Furthermore, because of the forces fueling the technological imperative in Egypt, Egyptian women are extremely vulnerable to the inappropriate application of excessive technology, much of which is deemed useless by Egyptian biogynecologists themselves.

Obviously, the promotion of the appropriate use of health technology in Egypt will require the development of a technology assessment profession in which women are involved. The major goals of such technology assessment would be to monitor the importation of technologies (including pharmaceuticals) into the country and to evaluate their safe use in clinical practice.

In addition, physicians' attitudes toward the use of technologies must be changed, given that, in Egypt, medical professionals play a crucial role in technological diffusion and routinization. In Egypt, transforming physicians into technological "change agents" (Bonair, Rosenfield, and Tengvald 1989) will certainly require reorienting medical education, as described above. However, it will also require that physicians upgrade their knowledge and practices through continuing medical education and board certification procedures designed to teach physicians to dispense with the use of outmoded technologies and apply soundly new technologies of the body, including reproductive technologies, of real benefit to women.

Recommendation 6: Redress Political and Economic Problems Impinging on Fertility

Finally, redressing Egypt's infertility problem through the implementation of new directions in reproductive health policy will require, in some cases, far-reaching changes on the political-economic level. As described in Chapter 1, the major underlying risk factors for infertility in Egypt—including sterilizing STDs, iatrogenic ethno- and biogynecological practices, and migration-linked changes in diet and activity levels among poor urban women—are linked to political and economic factors that have metamorphosed Egyptian society since the 1950s. Conditions of widespread impoverishment and class stratification in both the countryside and cities have led to large-scale population movements among the poor, which have indirectly impinged on the fertility of the Egyptian populace. Significant levels of male labor migration in particular have led to long-term absences of husbands from households and to the introduction of STDs, both of which have affected women's fertility adversely. Furthermore, poor urban migrant women trapped in tiny apartments and subsisting on high-starch, high-fat, low-protein diets are experiencing an epidemic of obesity linked to ovulatory infertility problems in many cases. This, coupled with women's frequently iatrogenic encounters in competitively driven, economically pressured biomedical settings, does not bode well for poor urban Egyptian women in terms of their reproductive health and futures.

Yet, little has been done on a policy level to either recognize or rectify the unfortunate political epidemiology of women's infertility in Egypt and the need for primary prevention. Tackling this problem will require state intervention and political will, which are currently absent in the face of Egypt's other pressing political, economic, and health problems. Indeed, the magnitude of the challenge is apparent when one considers that the future mitigation of the infertility problem in Egypt will require nothing less than increased job opportunities for men to obviate the need for male labor migration abroad; improved training, redistribution, and fairer government compensation of health-care personnel to eliminate the injudicious application of profit-driven medical procedures; reversal of colonially produced conditions of dependency on Western technology and know-how; and increased educational and employment opportunities for women, to empower them as health managers and consumers and as individuals with viable options other than motherhood.

Given this daunting agenda, as well as the need for major redirection in Egyptian reproductive health policy, the future for the infertile women of Egypt remains unclear. Both collectively and individually, they face a "medical and emotional road of trials" (Sandelowski, Harris, and Black 1992) — one whose end is certainly not in sight. That they journey down this tortuous road with such fortitude, magnanimity, dignity, and conviction is a testament to their spirit as pilgrims, whose "search for children" holds in store the promise of a better life.

Appendix 1. Fieldwork

This anthropological study is based on ethnographic field research carried out over a fifteen-month period (October 1, 1988, to December 31, 1989) in Alexandria, Egypt. A significant portion of the study took place in the public teaching hospital of the Department of Obstetrics and Gynaecology, University of Alexandria, Egypt. This hospital is popularly known among Alexandrians as "Shatby Hospital." In this book, I have chosen to use the hospital's name, as well as its location in Alexandria, because of the requests of those in the Department of Obstetrics and Gynaecology who permitted me to base my study in the hospital and who wished for its real name to be used.

Fieldwork in Shatby Hospital

Shatby Hospital proved to be an ideal site on which to base a study of infertility among Egyptian women for a number of reasons. First, because of its reputation as the primary university women's hospital, Shatby serves as the major tertiary care center for difficult obstetrical and gynecological cases, including those involving infertility, presenting to physicians within a broad geographical catchment area in the northwestern Nile Delta region of Egypt (and occasionally beyond). In addition to receiving difficult, physician-referred cases, the hospital serves as a primary obstetrical-gynecological (ob-gyn) care center for poor women in the Alexandria vicinity who cannot afford the more prohibitive fees charged by outside, private physicians and private inpatient facilities. Thus, the university hospital attempts to serve the ob-gyn needs of a large population of mostly lower- and lower-middle-class women, including a rather significant population of infertile women. It is these women who served as informants for my study, and it is their interactions within the Shatby Hospital setting that I spent hundreds of hours observing and discussing, in addition to other aspects of my study conducted outside of the hospital.

Second, shortly before I arrived in Egypt, this hospital had instituted an "artificial insemination by husband" (AIH) program, which had received rather wide publicity in the Egyptian media and which was therefore attracting an unusually large number of infertile patients to the hospital. Similarly, the hospital's plans for an in vitro fertilization (IVF) program were revealed in a widely read Egyptian newsmagazine called *October* (the December 4, 1988, issue), and this announcement precipitated an influx into the hospital's infertility program of hundreds of women who might not otherwise have sought care at the hospital. Unfortunately, the IVF program at the hospital never began during my fifteen months in Egypt, because of numerous bureaucratic and fiscal delays. Thus, many of the women hoping to undergo IVF eventually discontinued (at least temporarily) their involvement with the hospital and its staff. Nevertheless, despite the lack of resources associated with its public status, the hospital offered a wide range of other diagnostic and treatment services for infertility — in fact, the most comprehensive services to be offered in any Egyptian hospital outside of Cairo. As a result, large numbers of infertile women — both hospitalized and outpatients — were available at most times for participation in this study.

Third, I had designed this study to include a representative reference, or control, group of fertile women, who were free of infertility problems and had living children. Not only did I hope to learn about societal attitudes toward infertility from these women, but I also hoped to compare them (that is, their behaviors, beliefs, and life problems), both anthropologically and epidemiologically, to the infertile women in this study. In choosing this study site, I realized that such a population of age- and class-matched fertile women could be easily found in the hospital, both as inpatients (for example, undergoing vaginal and cesarean deliveries, various noninfertility-related gynecological operations, and monitoring for various prenatal problems) and as outpatients (for example, receiving contraceptive services and care for various minor gynecological complaints). Interestingly, upon interviewing a significant number of these fertile women, I also discovered that nearly one-third of them had considered themselves to have been infertile at one time, usually early in their marriages when they were unable to conceive immediately. Thus, their knowledge of and interest in infertility were sometimes personal in nature and facilitated our discussions of the subject.

Semistructured Interviewing

Because of such excellent access to populations of both infertile and fertile reproductive-age women, I was able to recruit 190 women — including one hundred infertile cases and ninety fertile controls—for formal participation in this study. Each woman, both infertile and fertile, participated in a confidential, semistructured interview administered by me in the Egyptian dialect of Arabic. Each of these semistructured interviews took place in the hospital, usually in a private room designated for that purpose. The interviews were lengthy (two to twelve hours), and often required several interview sessions to complete. First, many informants were quite talkative by nature and by virtue of the fact that they were allowed to give voice to their realities, frustrations, and anxieties, often for the first time. Second, many women had time to kill—either because they were inpatients who were sitting in bed with nothing to do or outpatients who were waiting, sometimes for hours, for a designated appointment. Third, interviewing took longer because I chose not to tape-record responses, instead using a nearly verbatim shorthand note-taking system I developed when I once worked as a journalist. Like Early (1993), I chose not to tape-record interviews in the hospital setting, because these were my first contacts with informants in a potentially alienating institutional environment, and I did not want a tape recorder, a possible technological barrier, to inhibit women from responding to my questions. (I should note here, however, that as I came to know my informants better, I often tape-recorded informal interviews when alone with them in their homes.) By the end of the fifteen-month period, I had completed the entire semistructured interview with eighty-nine of the one hundred infertile informants (89 percent) and fifty of the ninety fertile ones (56 percent). In the case of the fertile women, my primary goal was to obtain demographic, social, and behavioral information and then, if time and interest permitted, to ask more open-ended "thought" questions at the end of the interview. In the case of my infertile informants, on the other hand, I had hoped to complete the entire interview in every case, and the eleven incomplete interviews reflect the fact that these women discontinued their treatment at the hospital and could not be located for follow-up interviews outside the hospital.

The semistructured interview itself involved oral administration of a ninety-two-page questionnaire that was structured around three sections: (1) demographic and behavioral data, including information on personal history, marital history, menstrual history, hygiene, birth-control history, coital history, pregnancy history, reproductive health, and general health; (2) data on infertility among cases only, including history of biomedical and ethnomedical diagnosis and treatment and social and psychological problems engendered by infertility; and (3) general thought questions on reproduction, the various determinants of fertility outcome, fertility ideals, religious doctrine relating to these areas, and general questions about the infertility problem. Because of my previous fieldwork experience in Egypt and my extensive reading of the Egyptian literature, I felt comfortable designing a draft of the interview schedule before leaving for the field. However, once in Egypt, I modified the interview schedule substantially to reflect the input of Egyptian colleagues. Furthermore, following informal pretesting, I realized that many of the questions were either irrelevant or could not be asked as framed in writing. As a result, the interview became further modified over time, and I tailored my open-ended questioning substantially to reflect the interests and personalities of each informant. All in all, then, the "structure" of these semistructured interviews was not set in stone, and, in fact, the interviews were quite open-ended.

Reciprocity through Education

Through these semistructured interviews, I became painfully aware of the dilemmas of women who had never been informed sufficiently—or at all—of the biomedical cause of their infertility, even though most of them had visited numerous physicians. This lack of knowledge on the part of my informants was extremely troubling to me, especially given the fact that most women desperately wanted to know what was wrong with them and whether their husbands were also implicated in the infertility problem by way of "weak worms." Having gained insight into the magnitude of this problem early on in my fieldwork, I decided that this was an area in which I could be of great service to my informants. Thus, I decided to spend time with each infertile woman in my study reviewing her medical records and explaining them to her.

My ability to review these records was facilitated by my access to patients' charts. As mentioned in Chapter 8, patients are usually given their records—including results of diagnostic procedures, X rays, and prescriptions—which they then carry with them from physician to physician. In the case of infertile women presenting to Shatby Hospital, some of them carried plastic shopping bags literally brimming with the recorded history of their therapeutic searches. I could eventually spot infertile women in the hallways of the hospital by noting whether they carried on their person the telltale, canary-yellow-paper-wrapped, hysterosalpingogram X ray of their fallopian tubes and uterus.

In addition to these patient-carried records, at least two of the physicians with whom I worked at the hospital kept their own records about the infertile patients they were treating, often as part of clinical research projects. The physician who, during the first nine months of my fieldwork, saw the greatest number of infertile patients was willing to review with me the contents of his rather comprehensive records on about half of the infertile patients in my study and also agreed to let me relay as much of this information to patients as I liked, given that he had neither the time nor the support staff to undertake this task (as described in Chapter 8). Thus, for the women in my study, I became the official interpreter of their medical records, a job that I had never anticipated doing, but one that I came to view as extremely important to my study and to the women in it.

I should note here that I, like most medical anthropologists, maintain a healthy skepticism about biomedicine and its explanatory models of disease. Although I do not accept the notion that infertility constitutes a "disease," I do believe in most of the functional explanations of infertility offered by biomedicine. For example, I accept as verifiable fact that problems such as anovulation, blocked fallopian tubes, and low sperm count exist and adversely affect a couple's chances of conceiving. Thus, for me, accepting responsibility for perpetuating the biomedical model of infertility by actually inculcating it in the minds of Egyptian women was not problematic, given my own critical acceptance of the model and, more important, the women's acceptance of the model and their resultant active and enthusiastic participation in the biogynecological system.

My interpretation of women's cases generally involved two parts: first, textual analysis, and then culturally appropriate translation. I use the term "textual analysis" to describe the process of sorting through the stacks of papers and X rays given to me by each woman and then interpreting the findings. Although I have never received any formal biomedical training, my eight years spent as a medical editor and my long-term interests in reproductive health (Inhorn 1986; Millar 1987; Inhorn and Brown 1990; Inhorn and Buss 1993, 1994) served me well in assessing and understanding the findings of the various diagnostic procedures performed on infertile women and their husbands. These included primarily diagnostic laparoscopies and HSGs to assess the status of the fallopian tubes; endometrial biopsies, serum progesterone studies, and ultrasound follicular scanning to determine the existence of ovulation; postcoital tests and cervical mucus smears to look for cervical-factor infertility; and semen analyses to determine whether a male factor is present. In some cases, other diagnostic procedures were performed as well.

In almost every case, the reports of these diagnostic procedures were written in English, as described in Chapter 8. I spent anywhere from ten minutes to half an hour deciphering the scribbled handwriting of the various physicians who had written the results of their diagnoses. When I had difficulty interpreting the records, I consulted one of about five staff physicians who were specializing in infertility, whose opinions I trusted, and who were willing to help me.

Once I felt confident that I understood the biomedical interpretation of the infertility problem, the next step was to impart this information—in Egyptian colloquial Arabic—in a manner acceptable to each woman. Given the minimal schooling of most of the women in my study and the lack of reproductive (and sex) education on the part of even the more educated ones, explaining various infertility problems required a back-to-basics approach. I soon discovered that the easiest way for me to convey such information was to draw for each woman a rudimentary picture of the female reproductive tract and then to explain, first, such important concepts as ovulation, fertilization, menstruation, and basic embryology, including the genetic basis of the sex of the offspring. Once I had explained these concepts slowly and carefully, I attempted to pinpoint for each woman the nature of her infertility problem, most of which involved problems with ovulation, completely or partially blocked fallopian tubes, and/or poor semen quality. For the fertile women in the study, who, in many cases, faced ongoing problems in controlling their fertility, I also provided a similar explanation, but focused instead on how pregnancy is prevented.

Over the course of fifteen months, I became quite skilled at these pictorial explanations in Arabic, which most women found totally absorbing. Several of them specifically requested that I carefully redraw the picture of the reproductive tract on a piece of paper that they could then add to their carry-home medical records. Others told me that my explanation had frankly changed their lives. This was especially true when I was the first to inform the woman that her own reproductive system was healthy and that the infertility problem stemmed from her husband. The first such episode (out of several that followed) occurred during my second month of fieldwork, when I had not yet decided to discuss the women's biomedical records with them. Yet, in this case, the need to relieve this woman of the burden of responsibility and self-blame was so apparent that I could not resist explanation. After completing my interview with the woman in question, I decided to tell her that there was nothing wrong with her and that her husband was the cause of her infertility. She had delivered a child after the first year of marriage, but it had died on the same day. All subsequent tests showed her reproductive tract to be healthy, but she insisted that she was the cause—either because they had left something in her after the cesarean delivery that "needed to come out" or because she was "rejecting" her husband's sperm, which "all flowed out" after sex. I felt sorry for this woman, who had been coming to Shatby for the last five months, whose husband was about to take a second wife because of pressure from his family and who told her that he refused to pay for any additional ultrasounds and artificial inseminations, since they were "without success." Therefore, I decided that I should tell her that there was nothing wrong with her, that her husband was the cause (his "worms were weak"), and that she should talk to one of the doctors about this. I then took her to see her treating physician, who, at my request, reiterated to her the diagnosis of male-factor infertility. Much to our surprise, within a week, her previously uncooperative husband appeared with her at the hospital, where I arranged a meeting for both of them with the treating physician. The woman sat trembling as the physician explained to her and her husband that she was healthy but that he required therapy to improve his semen quality. After several weeks had passed, I saw the woman again, and she told me, beaming, that this series of exchanges had, indeed, changed the course of her marriage. When I ran into her at a tram station shortly before my departure from Egypt, she told me that, although she was not yet pregnant, she was still married, and she thanked me again for helping her.

Not all such attempts at patient education were as rewarding for me. I found it especially difficult to tell women with bilateral fallopian tubal blockage that they would not be able to become pregnant except through IVF—information that was extremely depressing, given the expense of IVF and the delay in the hospital's proposed IVF program, about which I was constantly being questioned by women in my study who required this procedure. However, in one case, I had the pleasure of telling a young rural woman that her fallopian tubes were *not* blocked—a mistaken diagnosis that had been given to her by an incompetent physician who had incorrectly interpreted the findings of her diagnostic laparoscopy. A follow-up diagnostic laparoscopy, the results of which I disclosed to her for the first time, showed that both tubes were patent, or open. The woman went on to become pregnant, although she miscarried in the first trimester. Yet, even after her miscarriage, she told me that she could never thank me enough for my having told her that her "baby tubes were open" and that she could become pregnant.

In addition to discussing women's cases with them, I also found myself playing another important but unintended role: that of liaison between the women in my study and the physicians at the hospital who were treating them. Because these women were mostly poor, uneducated, and socially unempowered, they were often intimidated by the upper-class, educated physicians who treated them, and who, in the case of infertile patients in this study, were exclusively male. These feelings of intimidation were most often transformed into an extreme reluctance on the part of women to speak up and ask questions, even when the doctor's orders were unclear to them. Thus, I found myself being sought out, even by women I did not know, to clarify the meaning of therapeutic encounters that I had not witnessed. In many cases, I ended up taking the woman with me to the physician, where I asked, in English, for clarification, then translated the physician's instructions to the patient.

I also soon became cognizant of the fact that, because I was also a woman, women were able to express to me certain intimate details of their lives that bore upon their infertility situations, but that they felt reluctant to discuss with the male physicians who treated them. This was especially true of women whose infertility problem was either caused by or tied to a sexual problem, most often a husband's impotence. In several cases, women who required a postcoital test or whose treatment involved either timed intercourse or artificial insemination with their husbands' semen admitted to me the panic they—and, in some cases, their husbands—felt about having to perform sexually on the doctor's orders when the husband had been experiencing ongoing sexual performance problems. In most of these cases, cultural modesty had prevented the women from divulging this information to male physicians, most of whom never asked about sexual problems as part of the infertility evaluation. In addition, women who were told by physicians to "go home and have sexual relations with your husband tonight" often came to me, distraught over the fact that this prescription would require them to actually *request* sex from their husbands, a cultural taboo among the poor, as described in Chapter 8.

Thus, I found myself in the delicate position of being the one to relate the more intimate aspects of my informants' lives to their male physicians, most of whom were surprised by this information and apologetic for having overlooked it altogether. For example, during the course of her interview, one of the women in my study explained how her feelings had changed toward her husband, given his ongoing impotence problems. The woman viewed her husband's impotence as the major problem in her life, given what she perceived to be its relationship to her inability to become pregnant. Thus, it occurred to me that so-called timed intercourse, which had been prescribed instead of artificial insemination to overcome this woman's infertility problem, was unlikely to succeed, and I suggested this to her at the conclusion of her interview. She said that she realized this but was embarrassed to tell her doctor. She asked if I might write the problem in English on a piece of paper, which she could then hand to the doctor and "run." Instead, I suggested that we might go together to speak to the physician. She consented, and the doctor, puzzled by her reluctance to divulge this information to him, immediately referred her for artificial insemination.

In other cases, I found myself defending women's positions to physicians, who were sometimes too quick to admonish patients for not following instructions. For example, when an irritated physician chastised a young woman for not refrigerating her expensive IVF medication, I pointed out to him in English that the woman was from a rural area outside Alexandria and had no refrigerator, like many of the other poor patients coming to the hospital. When he learned of this, he began asking all patients whether they would like to store their IVF drugs in the hospital's refrigerator.

However, in serving as a physician-patient cultural broker, a role often played by clinically applied medical anthropologists, I realized that I might be overstepping the boundaries of physician tolerance—as well as unofficial ethical boundaries—since I had never been asked to play this role. Thus, I tried to be sensitive to the problems of the overburdened physicians at the hospital and to avoid taxing them with requests and information. Yet, at times, I simply could not help but play the role of patient advocate, especially when I saw extremely disempowered women with severe personal problems in desperate need of support in the clinical setting. Overall, the physicians involved in treating these patients seemed to appreciate the role I played with their patients, since I was able to answer questions, provide sympathy, and generally take the time with women that these physicians, most of whom openly advocated patient education and counseling, simply could not afford.

Fieldwork in the Community

Partly because of the help I rendered to them in the hospital setting, many of the women in my study took an active interest in my well-being in Egypt, accepting me as a friend and taking me into their homes. Outpatient hospital hours were short (officially 8 A.M.–2 P.M., but unofficially 9 A.M.–1 P.M.), so I had considerable time to spend during afternoons and evenings with informants in their homes. As I had anticipated, many of the infertile women whom I interviewed at the hospital feared that meeting me in their home environments would lead to their inevitable exposure as seekers of infertility treatment, a reality that many preferred to keep hidden from overly inquisitive neighbors. On the other hand, many of the women I met at the hospital expressed an interest in seeing me socially after hospital hours, and, during the course of my fifteen months in Egypt, I spent considerable time in the homes of twenty-five infertile women and six fertile ones. Of these thirty-one women, twelve became close, personal friends, with whom I interacted regularly in their homes and in mine.

I was also invited to the homes of many other women during my stay in Egypt, but I made it a policy to visit only those women who made an actual date with me. I knew that if a woman was persistent enough to set a date, she and her husband felt comfortable having me as a guest and had the economic resources to entertain me. Unfortunately, despite my active protestations and insistence that I ate very little, each woman would go out of her way, at least initially, to prepare an elaborate, Egyptian-style lunch during the late afternoon hours, which inevitably included some form of meat. I knew that meat of all kinds was a luxury item for these poor women and their families and that they rarely ate it. Thus, it bothered me to see women devoting a considerable portion of their husbands' meager monthly earnings toward a food item that meant so little to me. However, to insist that no meat be served would have been a grave insult on my part, and I was usually implored to eat huge quantities of whatever form of meat was being served. I attempted to repay this hospitality by bringing each of my hosts a luxury gift item—such as the more expensive varieties of fruit, chocolates, cosmetic items, and, in a few cases, meat itself—and by taking many photographs, which I later distributed to them.

In these women's homes, which were mostly located in Alexandria's poor, peripherally located neighborhoods or in the smaller, provincial towns outside of Alexandria, I carried out the less formal but equally important aspects of my study, including untold hours of participant observation and informal interviews with the women themselves, their husbands, various family members, and neighbors. It was through these visits that I was also able to accompany women on healing pilgrimages to sacred sites and to meet various traditional healers of infertility, who enacted healing rituals or administered ethnogynecological remedies to my informants in some cases. Over the course of my study, I interacted with thirteen of these healers, including ten *dāyāt* (traditional midwives), two herbalists, and one Bedouin *sitt kabīra* (lay healer) who specialized in various traditional cures, including those for infertility. To each of the midwives—seven of whom lived and practiced in poor neighborhoods in Alexandria and three of whom lived in provincial cities outside of Alexandria—I administered in the Egyptian dialect of Arabic a nine-page semistructured interview, which I designed utilizing ethnomedical knowledge that I had acquired through my work with infertile and fertile women. Interactions with the two herbalists, which took place in their shops in the old market district of Alexandria called Manshiyyah, were less formal and also involved purchasing a number of herbal and mineral substances used in various infertility treatments. During the last month of my research, I also attempted to interview a *munaggima* (female spiritist healer); however, she was extremely busy each time I attempted to meet with her, which, I believe, was a reflection of her reluctance to be held accountable for her unorthodox healing activities.

In addition, in the homes of four of my infertile friends, I conducted more extensive life histories, which I later transcribed verbatim and translated into English. Two such life histories were also conducted in the hospital and were later transcribed and translated in this manner. These life histories, all of infertile women affected by fallopian tubal obstructions, are truly remarkable documents, chronicling the lives of young, lower-class, Egyptian women from childhood through marriage. Much of the content of these life histories revolves around infertility and the kinds of medical, marital, and other social problems these women have encountered as a result of their blocked tubes.

During the final months of my research, I also conducted semistructured interviews in English with seventeen gynecologists who treated infertility. These interviews were intended to supplement the many informal discussions I had had with physicians regarding both biomedical and social aspects of infertility in Egypt. Following these informal interviews, I designed a nine-page, semistructured interview, which I administered to the seventeen gynecologists at various sites around Alexandria, including Shatby Hospital, private offices and hospitals, a maternal and child health (MCH) clinic, an Islamic clinic associated with a mosque, and, in two cases, physicians' homes. Nine of the physicians who participated in these interviews were junior staff members at Shatby Hospital, six of whom were specializing in infertility by virtue of their own clinical research. Three, including one who was also a professor in the Department of Obstetrics and Gynaecology, were physicians specializing in infertility diagnosis and management in their private practices. Three others were well-established community gynecologists, who, as generalists, treated infertility in addition to other problems. And two were recent graduates of the Shatby residency program, who had not yet established their own practices but were working as gynecologists in the community. Only one of the seventeen physicians was a woman, which reflects the male domination of this profession in Egypt, and she was the only Christian of all of the physicians and healers to be interviewed.

Finally, in addition to both formal and informal interviews, life histories, and participant observation, I conducted library research in all of the medical and public health libraries in Alexandria (including the World Health Organization [WHO] library) and at the Ford Foundation and U.S. Agency for International Development libraries in Cairo. In these libraries, I collected as much information as possible pertaining to infertility, fertility, STDs, other aspects of women's reproductive health, and Egyptian women's lives.

Research Assistants and Issues of Language

I conducted all interviews outside the hospital by myself, and, more generally, undertook the bulk of my anthropological research within patients' homes and communities on my own. However, during the semistructured interviewing portion of my fieldwork in the hospital, an Egyptian research assistant was present with me. During my fifteen months in Egypt, I employed four research assistants, all bilingual Egyptian women, who served primarily as translators. All were young (twenty-two to thirty-two), educated, middle- to upper-class women, two of whom were clinicians (a medical student and a nurse) and had worked with this patient population previously. Another was an upper-class woman whom I met at the hospital during her infertility treatment. My primary research assistant, who spent six months working with me, was a graduate student in English literature. She and my medical student assistant were unmarried, whereas the other two women were married and one had children.

I employed these women, all of whom were quite personable, sensitive, and linguistically gifted individuals, to assist me in the interviews when language problems arose. Although I had studied classical Arabic and had some degree of fluency in Egyptian colloquial Arabic from both coursework and previous field experience, I preferred to have an unobtrusive research assistant present during the interviews to assist me should language problems arise. Indeed, they did, for three reasons.

First, Arabic is a notoriously difficult language and is made even more difficult by diglossia, or the presence of a standardized, written classical language and many unstandardized, unwritten colloquial dialects. Although Egyptians have their own distinct dialect of Arabic, it is characterized by many regional variants and accents, some of which I found quite difficult to understand. This was especially true among women whose backgrounds were rural or who came from Upper (southern) Egypt, where accents and even vocabulary differ considerably. My research assistants helped me to make sense of accents that I could not easily understand, although they, too, had difficulty with Egyptian Bedouin Arabic accents.

Second, much of the discussion in these interviews was quite technical, revolving around reproductive, biomedical, and ethnomedical histories. Although I eventually became fairly proficient in expressing myself in this bio- and ethnomedical language—proficient enough to discuss women's medical cases with them—there were constantly unfamiliar terms that arose during interviews, and it required a native Arabic speaker to help me sort out this unfamiliar vocabulary, which, in many cases, was also unfamiliar to them.

Third, although I made great progress in my speaking and comprehension skills during my fifteen months in Egypt, I never achieved complete fluency in the language, perhaps due to the stresses of that period and to my own difficulties with aural language acquisition. I relied on my research assistants to help me in the more standardized, formal interviews in the hospital setting. But, outside of Shatby Hospital, where I conducted significant portions of my fieldwork, I and my Arabic were on our own.

Although I often blundered with the language, my informants were forgiving. For example, early in my research while interviewing a midwife in one of my informant's homes, the midwife asked me, jokingly, whether she was the most beautiful of the women in the room (where a small group had assembled). I attempted to reply, "You are all beautiful" ("*Kullūkum gumāl*"), but, instead, through a simple vowel substitution, I exclaimed, "You are all camels" ("*Kullūkum gimāl*")! Fortunately, following some uncomfortable sideways glances, my informant saved the day, reiterating for me what I had *really* meant.

The Future

Thus, to summarize, the information presented in this book is derived from a number of sources, but comes primarily from lengthy, in-depth interviews conducted by me (sometimes with a research assistant present) with Egyptian women in Shatby Hospital and in their homes, as well as from participant observation in the hospital and in women's homes and home communities. The photographs presented in this book also reflect this fieldwork process, which officially ended on the eve of a new decade—December 31, 1989, when I boarded a plane for home.

It remains to be seen what the 1990s have brought for the poor infertile Egyptian women represented in this study—and what their futures hold in store. Have their quests for conception ended positively? Have their marriages remained intact? Are many of them still "searching for children"? In the summer of 1994—when I intend to return to Egypt with my "new" husband to conduct a study of women's views of IVF—I plan to find out. Meanwhile, here in the United States, I occasionally receive word from my informants, who have taken the time to find a scribe and have spent their little money on an airmail envelope and stamp. They tell me of their hopes and heartaches, their divorces and their continuing marital successes, their hopes for my happiness and fertility. For me, one of the most precious sentiments came in a faded airmail envelope, with a letter written in barely decipherable English. It was from one of the infertile women in my study to whom I had become especially close and for whom I had spent considerable time explaining her five-factor infertility problem. Apparently, she had found someone who was able to translate from colloquial Arabic into broken English her message to me, which was as follows (unedited):

"I hope you are very weel and I hope hapy new year, next you weel have children and so I'm. When I have girl, her name weel be Marsha."

Appendix 2. Informants

One hundred infertile women participated in this study. As this demographic profile and Table A.1 should make clear, they were mostly poor, minimally educated, and unemployed (usually by choice), and, as a group, formed a rather homogeneous population, which can be characterized as follows:

Age

All of the women except one were of reproductive age, mostly between the ages of twenty and forty. Specifically, 41 percent were aged twenty to twenty-nine, and 49 percent were aged thirty to thirty-nine. Only 2 percent were younger than age twenty, and 7 percent were older than forty. One woman, who did not know her date of birth, was most likely older than fifty.

In fact, more than half of the women (58 percent) did not know their exact dates of birth, because they did not have birth certificates. However, most women had a rough idea of their age and/or the year in which they were born. Hence, these figures are approximations of the actual ages of the women in this study.

Rural-Urban Residency

Most of the women in this study currently resided in Alexandria or, in some cases, in one of the smaller provincial cities in the northwestern Nile Delta region. However, their degree of "urbanness" varied, given that the peri-urban neighborhoods in which many of these women resided were very similar to the rural settings from which many of them hailed. In fact, 25 percent of the women had transitional backgrounds, in that they had migrated from rural to urban areas as children with their parents, at the

Table A.1. Demographic Profile of the Study Sample of One Hundred Infertile Egyptian Women.

AGE	15–19 2%	20–29 41%	30–39 49%	40+ 7%	
RESIDENCY	Rural 13%	Urban 87%			
ETHNICITY	Lower Egyptian 64%	Upper Egyptian 32%	Bedouin 2%	Nubian 2%	
RELIGION	Muslim 94%	Coptic Christian 6%			
EDUCATION	None 32%	Primary 43%	Junior High School 4%	Secondary/ Vocational High School 17%	University 4%
LITERACY	Illiterate 51%	Semi-literate 20%	Literate 29%		
EMPLOYMENT	Never 62%	Ever 18%	Current 20%		
COMBINED: ANNUAL INCOME	$0–239 7%	$240–479 30%	$480–959 35%	$960+ 26%	

time of marriage, or after marriage with their husbands. In some cases, they lacked the same amenities (e.g., electricity, running water, plumbing) in both their poor urban neighborhoods and their home villages. Thus, although most women classified themselves as Alexandrians, this characterization was not necessarily synonymous with an urban life-style. Furthermore, 13 percent of the women in the study were currently living in rural areas outside of Alexandria, and, of these thirteen women, ten considered themselves *fallāḥīn,* or peasant farmers.

Household Residency

Overall, 67 percent of the women in the study lived in small apartments, sometimes shared with relatives, while 33 percent lived in single rooms, either in nucleated rural households (14 percent) or in urban apartment buildings with separate rooms for rent (19 percent). Nearly half (45 percent) of the women in this study currently resided in an extended-family household with other relatives, usually those of the husband (in 87 percent of cases). In 45 percent of these cases, related families kept separate but adjacent apartments in the same building, sometimes owned by one or more members of the family (usually the husband's). However, in 55 percent of these cases, relatives actually shared the same apartment or room.

Many women reported their living conditions as cramped and expressed their desires to be living alone with their husbands in their own capacious apartments. However, a widespread housing shortage in Egypt and the expense of procuring an apartment served to prevent many of these women and their husbands from realizing this goal.

Ethnicity

Ethnicity in Egypt is, in some senses, geographically based and reflects ancient divisions between north (so-called Lower Egypt, an area roughly equivalent to the ancient, pharaonic kingdom ruled from a site near present-day Cairo) and south (so-called Upper Egypt, corresponding to the ancient, pharaonic kingdom ruled from Luxor). Although no word exists to describe that section of the Nile Delta north of Cairo, a designation exists for the inhabited region of the Nile River south of it, a region that is known to Egyptians as *Ṣaʿīd*—a name deriving from the Arabic verb "to go up," or in this case, "to go upstream" to Upper Egypt. Individuals who hail from this southern region are known as *Ṣaʿīdīs*, and the region is considered by Lower Egyptians and by Upper Egyptians themselves to be culturally conservative (as reflected in the large repertoire of *Ṣaʿīdī* jokes, which poke fun at the backward mentality of the male inhabitants of this region).

Of the women in this study, 32 percent considered themselves to be of *Ṣaʿīdī* ethnicity, because either they themselves were born in Upper Egypt or their fathers (through whom they traced their ancestry) came from this region. The majority, 64 percent, were Lower Egyptian, but the women themselves never used this term, since it is not a culturally accepted construct. Rather, they spoke of themselves as "Alexandrian" or "Cairene" or "Rashidian" or "Damanhurian," to designate the cities of their birth. In many cases, they simply noted that they or their parents were "from the *fallāḥīn*," the term used to designate the peasant farmers of the northern Nile Delta region of the country.

Thus, in this study, the major ethnic demarcator was a geographic one, based on an invisible boundary across the Nile River south of Cairo. The fact that so many of the women in this study considered themselves to be Upper Egyptian is a reflection of south-to-north internal migration patterns that continue unabated today.

In addition, four of the women in this study were members of Egypt's two major ethnic minority populations. Namely, two women considered themselves to be Bedouin, or Arab, terms that are used interchangeably by Egyptians to designate the once largely nomadic populations living in the vast desert regions of Egypt and the Sinai Peninsula. (Ethnically, most Egyptians do not consider themselves to be Arabs, or descendants of Arabian nomadic tribes, but rather view themselves as heirs of the pharaonic civilizations that existed along the Nile as early as 3,000 B.C.) In both of these cases, the women's ancestry could be traced to the nomadic tribes living in the desert west of Alexandria; however, the women themselves were no longer living a nomadic Bedouin existence. Similarly, two of the women in this study were Nubian, or members of the non-Arabic-speaking, Nilotic tribal population located on the Egyptian-Sudanese border, most of whom were relocated with the construction of the Aswan High Dam-Lake Nasser complex. Although these women both currently lived in Alexandria, they maintained strong ties to Nubian tribal communities in the southernmost region of Egypt near Aswan.

Religion

The majority of the women in this study, 94 percent, were Muslims, specifically Sunni Muslims (as opposed to Shiite Muslims, who do not comprise a religious community in Egypt). The rest, 6 percent, were Coptic Christians, five of whom were Orthodox and one of whom was Catholic. (Nationally, Muslims, almost exclusively Sunni, are said to represent roughly 90 percent of the population and Coptic Christians roughly 10 percent. Copts, who have been persecuted throughout the centuries and continue to be suspicious of Egypt's large Muslim population, believe their numbers are underestimated.)

Among the Muslim women, the degree of religiosity varied considerably. None of the women except two—one whose husband was a religion teacher and the other who was part of the growing Islamist movement in Egypt—had received any formal religious education, which was reflected in a general lack of knowledge of Islamic doctrine. Nonetheless, most of these women considered themselves to be "good Muslims," and the majority prayed regularly (although I have no precise figures on this). However, symbolic expressions of religiosity, as reflected in the dress code (Rugh 1986; MacLeod 1991), varied considerably among these women. Thirty-nine percent were *muḥāgibīn,* or covered by a veil that revealed the face (and one's Muslimness) but concealed the hair completely. Although most of the women had become veiled by choice during the past five years, reflecting a widespread conversion in Egypt to a more Islamic dress code, some indicated that they had begun to veil at the request of their husbands.

Most of the remaining Muslim women, 49 percent, wore loose scarves over their heads—more a traditional sign of modesty among the urban and rural lower classes than of religious faith. The rest, 12 percent, were uncovered, as were all of the Christian women.

Education

Most of the women in this study were minimally educated, given the cultural devaluation of formal schooling for girls and continuing low attendance levels of girls in schools throughout Egypt. Of the women in this study, 32 percent had received no formal education whatsoever, while 43 percent had attended primary (that is, elementary) school, but not necessarily for a full six years. A small percentage of the women had proceeded to the junior high (4 percent) or high school/vocational school (17 percent) levels; however, only 4 percent had gone to a university and all of these women were of lower-middle rather than lower-class backgrounds.

This lack of formal education was clearly reflected in literacy rates. More than half of the women in the study, 51 percent, were completely illiterate, with more than half of these women (59 percent) being unable to sign their own names to the mandatory informed consent form read to them before the semistructured interview. Of the rest of the women, 20 percent were, like me, semiliterate in Arabic, in that they could read individual words, but not well enough to, for example, read the newspaper with ease. Only 29 percent of the women were completely literate, reflecting approximately the national rate of literacy among Egyptian women. Amazingly, considering the difficulty of the Arabic language, some of these literate women had maintained their ability to read and write even though they had been forced to discontinue their educations following the sixth grade. The majority of women who had attended only primary school reported that they had "forgotten everything," including how to read and write.

Employment

Not surprisingly, given the lack of formal education among this group of women, the majority did not work and described themselves as *sittāt il-bait,* or housewives. Specifically, 62 percent of the women in this study had never been employed in any type of formal or informal paid labor. Those who had worked in the past (18 percent) or were currently working (20 percent) were largely employed in positions of unskilled or semiskilled manual labor, mostly in the informal sector, as follows: sewing (10 percent), domestic labor in the homes of the affluent (7 percent), factory labor (6 percent), and paid agricultural labor (2 percent). The remaining 13 percent who currently or had previously held semiskilled, white-collar jobs were employed as clerical workers (9 percent), teachers (2 percent), nurses (1 percent), and agricultural inspectors (1 percent); obviously, all of these women were educated.

Many of the women who did not work expressed an interest in income-generating employment but believed that job opportunities would not be available to them. The most commonly cited obstacles were lack of education (usually construed as "lack of a certificate"), husband's opposition, lack of transportation, and "shamefulness" of women's work. In fact, those women who expressed no desire to work—or had never even considered the possibility—often noted that "among us, women's work is shameful."

Furthermore, a common perception among these women was that whatever work could be found would not pay well enough to make "the exhaustion worthwhile." In fact, among the women workers, including the semiskilled ones, salaries were low—although often no lower than those of their husbands. Of the twelve women who were salaried employees, salaries ranged from £E 35 ($14) to £E 120 ($48) per month, with the average being £E78 ($31) per month. (During the fifteen months in which this study was conducted, the average exchange rate was two-and-a-half Egyptian pounds per U.S. dollar. This is the rate used to calculate all monetary figures in this text.) Thus, annual incomes of these women ranged from approximately $168 to $576, with the average being $372.

Income

Because so few of the women in this study were employed either in the formal or informal sectors, most of them were entirely reliant on their husbands as economic providers. Yet, most of the husbands of the women in this study were also unskilled or semiskilled manual laborers, whose meager incomes reflected their lack of skills and formal education. (Boys in Egypt are often unable to complete their schooling because they are required to assist in agrarian production or to contribute economically in other ways to their families, often beginning at a young age.) Actually, the term "blue-collar workers" would be appropriate to describe most of these men, were it not for the fact that many of them did not dress in Western-style, "collared" clothing (and, therefore, the symbolism is inaccurate).

Specifically, 84 percent of the husbands of these women were employed in the following types of unskilled or semiskilled occupations: factory worker (21 percent, with nearly half of these working in textile companies), driver (8 percent), farmer (6 percent), electrician (5 percent), shopkeeper or worker (5 percent), guard (4 percent), painter (4 percent), baker/candymaker (3 percent), carpenter (3 percent), construction worker (3 percent), salesman (3 percent), sanitation worker (3 percent), ship mechanic/builder (3 percent), loader/carrier (2 percent), medical assistant/first aid (2 percent), plumber (2 percent), porter/doorman (2 percent), waiter/hotel employee (2 percent), policeman (1 percent), tailor (1 percent), and blacksmith (1 percent). Only 16 percent of husbands held skilled or semiskilled, "white-collar" jobs, which included the following occupations: accountant (4 percent), teacher (4 percent), engineer (3 percent), tax collector (1 percent), computer programmer (1 percent), lawyer (1 percent), clerical worker (1 percent), and calendar editor (1 percent).

Monthly combined family incomes were estimated for each woman in the study, based on women's reports of their own wages in a few cases and those of their husbands (which were sometimes estimated by women who were unsure of the exact amount). These incomes were then categorized and percentages were estimated as follows: 7 percent of couples had incomes of £E 0–49 a month ($0–19/month); 30 percent of couples had incomes of £E 50–99 a month ($20–39/month); 35 percent of couples had incomes of £E 100–199 a month ($40–79/month); and 26 percent of couples had incomes exceeding £E 200 a month ($80/month), but usually not in excess of £E 400 a month ($160/month). In two cases, women were unaware of their husbands' salaries.

Thus, the majority of women in this study survived with their husbands (and, in a few cases, child or children) on annual incomes ranging from $240 to $960. Among this group, much of this money went to support infertility treatments and, in many cases, husbands' cigarette habits. Most of the women involved in infertility diagnosis and therapy complained bitterly about their dire financial straits and how being infertile had impoverished them even further. For more than a third of these women, relative poverty had been a lifelong experience, because their natal families had also been poor. However, most women noted that their natal families had been better off financially and that the experience of relative poverty was a postmarital phenomenon, brought on by the high costs of infertility treatment and a worsening Egyptian economy that has made once-adequate salaries insufficient to cover even the most basic costs of living. Thus, for many of these women, life after marriage consisted of a series of adjustments to poverty and childlessness—or the absence of the two "adornments" of earthly life, according to the Qur'an.

Notes

Preface: Hind's Story

1. All names used in this book are pseudonyms.

Chapter 1: The Infertility Problem in Egypt

1. For a detailed discussion of the social problems facing infertile women in Egypt, see my *Missing Motherhood: Infertility, Patriarchy, and the Politics of Gender in Egypt* (University of Pennsylvania Press, forthcoming).

2. Foucault's work on biopower has been criticized for its "gender blindness," or its neglect of the gendered character of the body (Bartky 1988; McNay 1991); for focusing only on the surface, or visible body and thus neglecting medical control and surveillance of the internal body (Bartky 1988); and for viewing the body as docile and passive, thereby failing to account for individuals' (especially women's) agency and resistance (McNay 1991). Despite these limitations, Foucault's theory of biopower is important to discussions of bodily subjectivity under biomedicine and will be used in this analysis.

3. In her article on women's health in the Arab world, Haddad (1988) has pointed to the unfortunate male domination of health care and particularly gynecology throughout this region, domination that has led to a lack of quality control, pharmaceutical "dumping" on women, and the use of inappropriate technologies.

4. Rugh (1982) has pointed to the "falsity of fatalism" in describing Egyptian women's lives, especially in the realm of health-seeking. El-Hamamsy (1972), in an earlier article on Egyptian peasants' health beliefs and practices, described the situation as one of "activism mixed with predestination."

5. Prevalence rates of infertility may vary within Egypt. For example, in an epidemiological study of infertility in rural Assiut Governorate in Upper Egypt, the overall infertility rate was 10.2 percent, of which 54.5 percent was primary and 45.5 percent was secondary infertility (Abdullah, Zarzoor, and Ali 1982). In a survey of villages in Menoufia Governorate in Lower Egypt, both the primary and secondary infertility rates were 7.9 percent (Gadalla 1978). And in a family planning study undertaken in a neighborhood of Alexandria, the childlessness rate (which could include both primary and secondary infertility cases) was 7.3 percent (Gadalla and Hassan 1970).

6. *Fadādīn* is the plural of *faddān*. One *faddān* is equivalent to 1.038 acres or 0.420 hectares.

7. Recent studies of STDs and their prevalences in Egypt include the follow-

ing: O. Ali (1980); Y. Ali (1980); Amer (1987); Basha (1981); El Ghazzawy (1980); Elhefnawy (1985); El Lakany (1988); El-Latiff (1982); Fathalla (1986); Ghamri (1986); Hanafy et al. (1984); Kholeif (1980); Kotkat (1978); Mehanna (1989); and Sallam et al. (1982).

8. For references to infertility in the Middle Eastern fertility literature, see, for example, Brown (1978); El-Hamamsy (1972); Gadalla (1977, 1978); Good (1980); Sebai (1974); and Youssef (1978).

9. References to infertility in the Egyptian social scientific literature can be found in Ammar (1966); Assaad and El Katsha (1981); Biegman (1990); Early (1982, 1988, 1993a, 1993b); el-Aswad (1987); El-Hamamsy (1973); El Malatawy (1985); El-Mehairy (1984b); El-Messiri (1978); el Sendiony (1974); Gilsenan (1982); Harrison et al. (1993); Kennedy (1978a); Khattab (1983); Lane and Meleis (1991); Morsy (1978a, 1978b, 1980a, 1980b, 1982, 1993); Nadim (1980); and Pillsbury (1978). Case studies, stories, and life histories about infertile Egyptian women can be found in Abu-Lughod (1993a); Atiya (1982); Morsy (1993); van Spijk, Fahmy, and Zimmerman (1982); and Watson (1992).

10. Recent major works by feminist scholars focusing on the problems and implications of the new reproductive technologies include Baruch, D'Adamo, and Seager (1988); Corea et al. (1987); Hepburn (1992); Klein (1989a, 1989b); Ratcliff (1989a); Rowland (1992); Stanworth (1987a); and Strathern (1992).

11. Anthropological research on infertility (including that by medical sociologists and historians who use anthropological research methods and publish in medical anthropological journals) includes Becker (1990); Becker and Nachtigall (1991); Early (1993b); Ebin (1982); Farquhar (1991); Katz and Katz (1987); Modell (1989); Sandelowski (1991, 1993); and Sandelowski, Harris, and Black (1992). In addition, a forthcoming subsection of *Social Science & Medicine,* entitled "Interpreting Infertility: Medical Anthropological Perspectives," Marcia C. Inhorn, ed. (1994b), will feature cross-cultural research on infertility from Cameroon, Egypt, India, and the United States.

12. Medical anthropological articles on the Middle East focus on the following topics: (1) children's health (including breastfeeding, weaning, and nutritional beliefs) (Harrison et al. 1993; Myntti 1993; Sukkary-Stolba 1987); (2) culture-bound syndromes (Good and Good 1982; Swagman 1989); (3) cultural construction of biomedicine (Gallagher and Searle 1984, 1985); (4) doctor-patient communication (Creyghton 1977); (5) ethnopharmacology (Sukkary-Stolba 1985); (6) ethnophysiology (Good 1980; Morsy 1980a); (7) female circumcision (Assaad 1980; Boddy 1982; Gruenbaum 1982, 1991; Gordon 1991; Hayes 1975; Inhorn and Buss 1993; Kennedy 1970; Meinardus 1967; van der Kwaak 1992); (8) illness and emotion (Good, Good, and Fischer 1988; Good, Good, and Moradi 1985); (9) illness semantics and narratives (Early 1982, 1985, 1988; Good 1977); (10) medical pluralism and the interaction of medical systems (Assaad and El Katsha 1981; Greenwood 1981; Millar and Lane 1988; Morsy 1988; Myntti 1988a; Nadim 1980; Shiloh 1968; Underwood and Underwood 1980); (11) menstruation (Delaney 1988); (12) midwifery and birth (El-Hamamsy 1973; Hunte 1981; Morsy 1982; Scheepers 1991; Sukkary 1981); (13) political economy of health (Morsy 1981); (14) spirit possession and placation ceremonies (Constantinides 1985; el Sendiony

1974; Fakhouri 1968; Kennedy 1967; Morsy 1978b, 1991; Nelson 1971; Safa 1988); and (15) women's health, women healers, and gender differences in health care (Bakker 1992; Bowen 1985; Early 1993b; Haddad 1988; Lane and Meleis 1991; Lane and Millar 1987; Morsy 1978b, 1980b; Myntti 1988b; Olson 1983).

13. Recent book-length works on the lives of contemporary urban Egyptian women include Atiya (1982); Early (1993a); MacLeod (1991); Rugh (1984, 1986); Sullivan (1986); Watson (1992); and Wikan (1980). Recent book-length works on the lives of Egyptian Bedouin women include Abu-Lughod (1986, 1993a). Recent historical works about Egyptian women include Kader (1987) and Tucker (1985).

14. Abu-Lughod's (1986) own work focuses on the discourses of honor and shame among Egyptian Bedouin women.

Chapter 2: Ancient Alexandria and Its Modern Poor

1. Because there is no comprehensive history of Alexandria extending into the twentieth century, information for this chapter is derived from a number of sources, including: Dols (1984); El-Hamamsy (1985); Elon (1988); Forster (1986); Kuhnke (1990); Mitchell (1988); and Seton-Williams and Stocks (1988).

Chapter 3: Past and Present in Theories of Procreation

1. In the centuries before the advent of Islam, the influence of the Alexandrian medical school, which had been Christianized, waned. The school lasted under the Arabs until the early eighth century A.D., when it was moved to Antioch. However, the medical curriculum of the late Alexandrian school became the basis of professional medical education in the Middle East. Its preparatory course included language and grammar, logic, arithmetic, geometry, the compounding of drugs, astrology, and ethics. The main course used four books on logic and twenty books on medicine, including four by Hippocrates and the "Sixteen Books" of Galen. Completion of this curriculum, particularly Galen's works, became the criterion for the accomplished Arab physician (Dols 1984).

2. In her attempt to prove that Islam has promoted a monogenetic theory of procreation, the anthropologist Delaney (1991) acknowledges but dismisses Musallam's argument that Islam, in fact, promoted duogenesis. Instead, she argues that none of the early procreative theories, including those forwarded by Islamic jurists, were truly duogenetic. As she states in a footnote: "Nowhere have I seen any ancient, medieval, or early modern argument that would qualify as saying that both men and women contribute *equally and the same kind of thing*" (1991:48). In forwarding this thesis, Delaney may have overlooked Islamic scriptural evidence to the contrary, as well as the recent works of other scholars (e.g., Ahmed 1989; Omran 1992) who support Musallam's position. Although Delaney's symbolic analysis of the links between Islamic monotheism and Muslim folk monogenetic theory in Turkey is quite convincing, her seeming dismissal of the *Hadith* sources casts doubt

on her interpretation of the Islamic textual evidence. Weigle (1989), in fact, ties Delaney's thesis about monogenesis and the devaluation of women's procreativity not to Islam, but to Christian tradition, in which the denigration and disregard of women's procreative powers are clearly evident.

3. The practices of cupping and cauterization, which, as will be seen in Chapter 6, are still used in Egypt for the treatment of infertility, were the most common methods employed by pre-Islamic practitioners. However, with the coming of Islam, the Prophet Muhammad is said to have forbidden cauterization, which is quite painful and stigmatizing, and to have recommended the use of hot compresses instead (Ullman 1978).

4. Alternatives to the term "biomedicine" include "allopathic medicine," "cosmopolitan medicine," "modern medicine," and "Western medicine." Biomedicine is the most common term currently used by medical anthropologists.

5. Descriptions and analyses of some of the problems inherent in contemporary Egyptian biomedicine can be found in Abu-Zeid and Dann (1985); Carney (1984); El-Mehairy (1984b); Institute of Medicine (1979); Kandela (1988); Kuhnke (1990); Lane and Millar (1987); Morsy (1980b, 1988); and Sonbol (1991).

6. It also underlies the refusal of Egyptian men to undergo vasectomy as a means of birth control.

7. "To bring," like the English "to come," is the verb popularly used to describe orgasm in Egyptian colloquial Arabic. Men "bring" an ejaculate. Women are also thought to "bring" a comparable orgasmic fluid. Thus, "bringing" the vaginal lubricant that occurs naturally during sexual arousal is viewed by most women as the sign of female orgasm. Because the vast majority of women in this study were circumcised, few of them reported actual orgasmic experiences. Only a handful of women described a "shaking of the whole body" or a "feeling of electricity" that occurred during sexual intercourse with their husbands. When I used these indigenously generated phrases to ask other women about their sexual sensations, the vast majority claimed not to have experienced such feelings.

8. Whereas some women attribute fetal sex determination to men, most attribute it entirely to God, who "does not reveal his secrets." A small number of women in this study were aware of the biomedical concept of X and Y sex chromosomes, but none could fully explain how these operated to determine fetal sex. Other explanations of fetal sex determination were offered, including: (1) relative strength of men's sperm and women's eggs (i.e., stronger sperm leading to boys, stronger eggs to girls); (2) relative profuseness of men's and women's "liquids" (i.e., more profuse male liquid leading to boys, more profuse female liquid to girls); and (3) relative rapidity of presumed orgasm (i.e., the man "bringing" first leading to boys, the woman "bringing" first to girls; however, see the previous footnote on the nature of female orgasm).

Some women also believe that fetal sex can be determined during pregnancy. The most widely accepted view is that a female fetus begins to move at five months and a male at four. Other women claim that a male fetus makes his pregnant mother become ugly and jaundiced, while a female fetus produces beauty and radiance. The majority of women, however, claim to know no such predictive features, stating that "a pregnant belly is just like a watermelon—you can never tell what's inside."

9. The Qur'an describes menstrual blood as polluting and suggests sexual abstinence until the menses is ended and the woman is "purified." Of 180 women questioned in this study, only three said that they had ever engaged in sexual intercourse during their menses. More than one-third of women, 38 percent, said that sex during the menses is considered sinful in Islam, while the vast majority, 83 percent, contended that sex during menses is to be avoided lest sickness and fatigue befall the man (65 percent), the woman (6 percent), both of them (28 percent), or the child conceived from this union (1 percent).

10. Many women are aware that recurrent, light bleeding occasionally occurs during pregnancy on a monthly basis, perhaps due to "extra blood." Such a pregnancy is called *ḥamla ghizlāni,* or a "gazelle-like pregnancy."

11. Occasionally, other terms are substituted for these component parts. Thus, both men and women are sometimes said to have "eggs" or "sperm" or "worms." Nevertheless, both men and women must have the "fluid" containing these elements.

12. In her book devoted to the implications of procreative theory in rural Turkey, Delaney (1991) explores in great depth the instantiation of the monogenetic theory in the everyday realities of village social life, and particularly in the symbolic representations of the gender system. Yet, she is little concerned with procreative *disruptions*—with the consequences engendered by seeds and fields that fail to produce life. Although, in passing, she attributes infertility to "barren fields"—that is, to women and not to men and their "seeds"—she does not examine villagers' conceptions of infertility (including whether men's seeds can be "spoiled") and the repercussions of infertility on gender relations.

Chapter 4: Healers, Herbalists, and Holy Ones

1. Not all biomedical practices are condoned by Egypt's religious establishment. For example, during the period of this study, Egypt's Shaikh Muhammad Mitwali al-Shaarawi, a popular televised Muslim cleric, announced his opposition to renal dialysis, a statement that led to an uproar in the biomedical community. Furthermore, as we shall see in Chapters 10 and 11, some of the new reproductive technologies—primarily those involving male donors and female surrogates—are viewed as religiously forbidden and have been legislated against by Egypt's religious leaders. Nevertheless, historically, Egypt's religious establishment, as well as Islamist groups such as the Muslim Brotherhood, have done much to support "modern medicine" and public health in the country (Gallagher 1990; Morsy 1988; Musallam 1983).

2. Morsy (1993) has also noted the growing reaction against popular medical traditions in Egypt, which she attributes to the "etatisation" of medical culture as promoted through formal education and the mass media.

3. Around the world, women are typically responsible for domestic health management and serve as informal healers and advisers in domestic contexts (McClain 1989). This pattern has been reported for the Middle East as well (Early 1982, 1985, 1988, 1993a, 1993b; Good 1980; Lane and Meleis 1991; Lane and Millar 1987; Morsy 1993). Furthermore, gender is extremely significant to some healing discourses, with women serving as the primary healers of other women (Bakker 1992;

Constantinides 1985; McClain 1989). Such is the case with *kabsa* healing, to be described in Chapter 5.

4. In this study, for example, seven of ten *dāyāt* interviewed had inherited their profession from female family members or in-laws.

5. Although traditional midwifery has been a significant topic of scholarly discourse in Egypt (Assaad and El Katsha 1981; El-Hamamsy 1973; El Malatawy 1985; Morsy 1982; Nadim 1980; Pillsbury 1978; Sukkary 1981), the roles of *dāyāt* in healing the infertile have been poorly investigated. Brief references to their ethnogynecological healing roles can be found in Assaad and El Katsha (1981); El-Hamamsy (1973); El Malatawy (1985); Gadalla (1978); Khattab (1983); Nadim (1980); and Shiloh (1968). Hunte (1981) also mentions the ethnogynecological role of midwives in urban Afghanistan.

6. The largest sum reportedly charged by a *dāya* in this study was one hundred Egyptian pounds (forty dollars) for a three-month regimen of treatment.

7. *Munaggim* comes from the Arabic verb, *najjam,* which means to observe the stars or to predict the future from the stars. Thus, strictly speaking, *munaggim* means "astrologer." Very few contemporary *munaggimīn* are actually astrologers, basing their divinational practices on celestial observation. Nevertheless, the term *munaggimīn* has become accepted in urban Egypt as the term of reference for this class of practitioners. According to Morsy (1993), who conducted fieldwork in a rural Delta village in the early 1970s, these healers were called *rawḥaniya,* or spiritualist healers (from the root, *rūḥ,* meaning spirit). This term was never used by the urban Egyptians in my study. Occasionally, participants in my study referred to *munaggimīn* as *ʿarrāfīn,* meaning "diviners" or "fortune-tellers" (from the Arabic verb, *ʿarafa,* "to know" or "to perceive").

Reference to such healers and, in some cases, descriptions of their practices can be found in the following sources. For Egypt, see Atiya (1982); Early (1988); El-Messiri (1978); Kennedy (1967); Morsy (1993); Pillsbury (1978); and Rugh (1984). For other regions of the Middle East, see Bakker (1992); Creyghton (1977); Greenwood (1981); Myntti (1988a); and Swagman (1989).

8. Perhaps for these reasons, *munaggimīn* proved elusive as participants in my study, and the infertile women who had visited *munaggimīn* demonstrated considerable reluctance to introduce me to these healers (as opposed to *dāyāt,* with whom they felt quite comfortable). Thus, interactions with *munaggimīn* were described by women in this study, but no *munaggimīn* were interviewed or observed by me. When I finally reached the home of one such person—a *munaggima* who had agreed prior to my visit to speak with me—she canceled our meeting at the last minute for fear that I would report her practices to governmental authorities. Although I spent considerable time attempting to explain my innocent intentions to her educated son, and my Egyptian friends who had brought me also vouched for my integrity, the *munaggima* would not change her mind.

Chapter 5: Kabsa and Threatened Fertility

1. In this study, the term *kabsa* was used much more frequently by informants than the term *mushāhara,* which is why *kabsa* is used here. However, these terms

were recognized as interchangeable by the vast majority of informants, who also used the terms *makbūsa* and *mitshāhara* interchangeably. However, in a few cases, women made distinctions between these terms, noting that (1) *makbūsa* refers to the one who causes *kabsa* and *mitshāhara* to the one who suffers it, or (2) *makbūsa* is the colloquial term and *mitshāhara* is the classical Arabic one.

2. Whether the *kabsa* complex is found among peoples of the Upper Nile or among people in other parts of the Middle East is not clear. Suggestive reports of similar practices in the Middle East (but not by the name of *kabsa* or *mushāhara*) can be found in Bourdieu (1977) for tribal Algerians; Darity (1965) for Palestinians; and Delaney (1991) for rural Anatolian Turks.

3. In her recent book, *Gender, Sickness, & Healing in Rural Egypt,* Morsy (1993) does not include *kabsa* as one of the culturally constructed illness categories covered in her chapter on "Medical Taxonomy." Given that gender, sickness, and healing is the topic of the book, this would seem to be a significant lacuna, especially since Morsy reported the belief in *kabsa* among rural Egyptian villagers in previous works (1980a, 1982) and described an anecdote pertaining to *kabsa* (but not by this name) in her book. Early (1993a), on the other hand, describes the "infertility syndrome of *mushāhara*" in her recent book *Baladi Women of Cairo,* and she notes in a previous work that "the theme of *mushāhara* (infertility or insufficient lactation) permeates both formal and informal performance in baladi culture" (Early 1985:177).

4. Passing references to or brief descriptions of *kabsa* (*mushāhara*) in Egypt can be found in: Abu-Lughod (1993a); Ammar (1966); Atiya (1982); Early (1985, 1988, 1993b); El-Hamamsy (1973); El-Mehairy (1984b); El-Messiri (1978); Harrison et al. (1993); Morsy (1980a, 1982); Nadim (1980); Pillsbury (1978); and van Spijk, Fahmy, and Zimmerman (1982).

5. The Muslim calendar is based on the lunar cycle. Thus, unlike the Gregorian calendar, the beginning of a given lunar month falls eleven to twelve days earlier each year (Harrison et al. 1993).

6. *Kabsa* does not affect adult males. However, according to some Egyptian women, *kabsa* can affect infants, including infant males, making them fretful, colicky, and unwilling to breastfeed. Others believe that juvenile males may suffer eventual male infertility as a result of postcircumcision *kabsa*. However, the predominant view is that *kabsa* is an exclusively female affliction.

7. For additional information on the normative forty-day postpartum rest period and its contemporary lack of observance in the Middle East, see Forman et al. (1990); Morsy (1980b, 1993); and Pillsbury (1978).

8. Virtually all of the women in this study had undergone so-called female circumcision (Inhorn and Buss 1993). About half had undergone clitoridectomy, in which the clitoris or the prepuce of the clitoris had been removed, while the rest had undergone excision, in which the clitoris and part or all of the labia minora had been removed.

9. Of the reproductively related events, only abortions are not culturally or religiously condoned in Egypt and are, in fact, illegal. Nevertheless, illegal biomedical abortions are available in Egypt, as are traditional methods of abortion. Women resort to illegal abortions for various reasons, including poverty. Because abortions cause women to be "open," women who have undergone an abortion are liable to suffer the effects of infertility-producing *kabsa*.

10. Most authors have translated the effect of *kabsa* as that of reproductive "binding," given that rituals to overcome *kabsa* are referred to as "unbinding" or "untying" the problem. In fact, women occasionally refer to *kabsa* as being like "a knot." However, Morsy (1980a), and Abu-Lughod (1993a) following her, describe *kabsa* as an "obstruction." Among urban Lower Egyptian women, *kabsa* is not perceived as an obstruction, given that obstructions and blockages occur to fallopian tubes. Rather, *kabsa* is a member of the culturally constructed illness taxon involving "tying," "binding," and "locking" problems.

11. In Egypt, women practice extensive depilation of body hair using a sticky, homemade, sugar-and-lemon substance called *ḥalāwa*. Leg, arm, underarm, pubic, and sometimes facial hair are removed. At least initially, the process is often painful and may draw blood.

12. The metaphorical analogy between birth/death and womb/tomb has been noted by Delaney (1991) and el-Aswad (1987). El-Aswad also describes the defilement of death in rural Egypt.

13. Black eggplants may, in fact, be *kabsa*-producing for two reasons: (1) their symbolic association with death, and (2) their symbolic association with brides, who can cause *kabsa* to other brides. The former is reaffirmed by the fact that *green* eggplants, also a popular vegetable in Egypt, are never thought to cause *kabsa,* nor are they used in *kabsa* healing rituals.

14. Individuals who are thought to behave in a tyrannical fashion are often called "pharaohs" by other Egyptians.

15. Although the vast majority of *kabsa* rituals occur during the Friday noon prayer hour, other Friday prayer times are occasionally substituted. For example, the second most popular time for the performance of *kabsa* rituals is during the Friday midafternoon prayer, followed in frequency by rituals undertaken during the Friday dawn prayer. Rarely, women suggest that these rituals be carried out between or after, rather than during, prayer times. Despite this variation, women always carry out these rituals on Friday, which in Egypt and in the rest of the Muslim world is observed as a day of Sabbath.

16. The historical origin of *kabsa* beliefs and practices is unknown, although placenta rituals, part of the *kabsa* complex, are believed to derive from ancient Egypt (Davidson 1985). The contemporary degree of cultural entrenchment of *kabsa* beliefs and practices among poor urban Egyptian women suggests that these beliefs and practices have existed for centuries, and, given the nature of Egyptian medical traditions, probably predate Islam.

17. Some women disagree about increased vulnerability to *kabsa* in the hospital. As one woman explained, "In the hospital, there's no *kabsa* because *she* is the one who is entering the operating room, and the *doctor* [who is newly shaved] is the one who is delivering." Another woman argued that "women don't become *makbūsīn* in the hospital, because they're all urinating on the same place" (thereby unbinding each others' *kabsa* effects). Another woman, skeptical of all *wasfāt baladī,* including *kabsa* rituals, stated, "It's nonsense. Here in the hospital, I deliver and another woman delivers, all in the same room, and nothing happens."

Despite such skepticism on the part of a few women, numerous new mothers in Alexandria's Shatby Hospital wore *kabsa* bracelets as a preventive measure—to ensure both their future fertility and ability to lactate. However, most obstetricians either had never noticed these bracelets or had never bothered to ask their patients why they wore them. Only one of seventeen obstetrician-gynecologists participating as informants in this study had ever heard of *kabsa*—an indication of the great cultural and communicative chasm existing between mostly upper-middle- and upper-class male physicians and their mostly lower-middle- and lower-class female patients.

18. Small Muslim cemeteries, especially those in rural settings, are often located on an elevated mound of land, but are not walled. Women visiting these cemeteries for *kabsa* healing rituals are instructed to "walk around" inside the cemetery to make the effects of *kabsa* vanish. Likewise, Christian women say that they go to Muslim cemeteries for *kabsa* healing rituals, because their own cemeteries have only one door and thus cannot be properly exited. Muslim women, on the other hand, occasionally mention the necessity of walking over Christian bones in order to unbind themselves; therefore, they may visit a deserted Christian cemetery for this purpose.

19. Given that most poor urban Egyptian women are mildly to severely obese and black eggplants are relatively soft, sitting on eggplants without destroying them is probably impossible.

20. Bourdieu (1977) mentions the symbolic significance of crossroads, or intersections, in his analysis of ritual praxis in Algeria.

21. Pearls may serve a dual purpose. Like gold and diamonds, they are precious gems, unaffordable to poor women who are liable to become polluted by them. But, in addition, they come from genitalia-resembling oysters in the sea and, like clamshells, may be effective in unbinding the effects of sexual pollution.

22. The use of palm fronds, usually with seven "leaves," is a distinctly Upper Egyptian variant. Women of Upper Egyptian background occasionally mentioned *kabsa* healing rituals involving palm fronds. However, these are not commonly performed by the women of Alexandria.

23. The perception that menstrual blood and postpartum discharges, including the placenta, have powerful polluting effects has been described by a number of authors working in the Middle East, including Constantinides for Sudan (1985); Delaney (1988) for Turkey; Good (1980) for Iran; Morsy (1980b, 1993) for Egypt; and Pillsbury (1978) and Shiloh (1968) for the Middle East in general. Musallam (1983), however, has noted that, historically, menstrual and postpartum blood were incorporated into traditional contraceptives in the Muslim Middle East. Such incorporation may, in fact, have been tied to *kabsa* beliefs—namely, that blood entering a woman's reproductive passageway pollutes her, rendering her temporarily infertile.

Chapter 6: From Humidity to Sorcery

1. Other brief descriptions of *ruṭūba* and/or *ṣūwaf* therapy in Egypt can be found in Atiya (1982); Early (1993b); El-Hamamsy (1973); Lane and Meleis (1991); Morsy (1993); Nadim (1980); Pillsbury (1978); and Walker (1934).

Musallam (1983) also describes the historical use of vaginal suppositories and tampons in traditional contraceptives.

2. The plural form, *ṣūwaf,* appears to be a colloquialized version of the proper form, *aṣwāf,* in classical Arabic. Both mean "wool."

3. All information on common English and Latin plant names and the history of medicinal use of these herbs is derived from Bedevian (1936); Manniche (1989); Niazi (1988); and Tackholm and Drar (1950).

4. Unusual patterns include the use of one *ṣūfa* each Friday over three consecutive weeks and the use of one *ṣūfa* every other day for three days.

5. For purposes of comparison, in Morocco, infertility is thought to be a "cold" illness and is treated similarly. Greenwood (1981) notes: "But in both sexes barrenness, associated as it often is with pelvic pain and discharge—the consequence of abortion and venereal disease—is a cold illness that can be sexually transmitted either way. It has a place in the pattern of hot and cold symbolism in reproduction. Barrenness is treated with hot medicines or pessaries to 'heat up' the sex organs: the Berber Bride, at her wedding, crouches over smoking 'hot' incense to heat her womb and make her fertile" (1981:227). In Sudan, prospective brides take "smoke baths," in which they sit, covered by a blanket, over a hole in the floor which is filled with fragrant, burning woods (Boddy 1989); this process of purification is intended to remove dead skin.

6. It is said that if a pregnant woman is beaten in the back she will miscarry, but not if she is beaten in the belly. Or, as a *dāya* put it, "Isn't your uterus hanging on your back? You can see this when you butcher an animal."

7. Cautery is reportedly practiced in Morocco (Bakker 1992); Sudan (Boddy 1989); Yemen (Myntti 1988a; Swagman 1989; Underwood and Underwood 1980); Jordan (Pillsbury 1978); and among Palestinian Bedouins in Israel (Rosenberg et al. 1988). Although cupping has been reported for other parts of the Middle East as well (Bakker 1992; Pillsbury 1978), it is described much more frequently than cautery in reports on Egypt (Dols 1984; Early 1993b; El-Hamamsy 1973; Nadim 1980; Walker 1934).

8. Brief descriptions of the role of *khaḍḍa* in illness causation in Egypt can be found in Ammar (1966); Atiya (1982); Early (1982, 1988); el-Aswad (1987); El-Hamamsy (1973); Kuhnke (1990); Nadim (1980); Pillsbury (1978); and Walker (1934). For a more complete account of fright illness, or *tarba,* in rural Egypt, see Morsy (1993).

9. Some women view men as "unshockable" and, hence, unsusceptible to *khaḍḍa*-induced infertility. Similarly, some women discount the role of *khaḍḍa* in *causing* female infertility, although they believe *khaḍḍa* may be useful in overcoming it.

10. Morsy (1993) describes the role of cautery on the lower back in overcoming fright illnesses in rural Egypt. Swagman (1989) reports that hot-iron "branding," usually on the back of the patient's neck, is the most common cure for fright illnesses among both men and women in Yemen.

11. An early, colorful account and photograph of the *ṭast it-tarʿba,* called the "fear cup" by the author, can be found in Walker (1934). For a more recent description, see Morsy (1993).

12. Although thirteen types of *shīḥ* (*Artemisia* genus) exist, only seven types are available in Egypt, according to those with herbal expertise.

13. For Egypt, descriptions of sorcery can be found in Ammar (1966); Atiya (1982); Early (1993a); el-Aswad (1987); El-Mehairy (1984b); el Sendiony (1974); Kennedy (1967, 1978a); Morsy (1978a, 1993); Nadim (1980); Pillsbury (1978); van Spijk, Fahmy, and Zimmerman (1982); and Walker (1934). For other parts of the Middle East, see Bakker (1992); Boddy (1989); Greenwood (1981); Swagman (1989); and Underwood and Underwood (1980).

14. It is also said that an infertile woman whose husband is pressuring her to have children may have an *ʿamal* made against him, thereby "tying" him and making him impotent.

15. The *Hans Wehr Dictionary of Modern Written Arabic* also defines *qarīna* as a "female demon haunting women, specifically, a childbed demon" (Cowan 1976:760).

16. This is why women say "God's name on you and your brother" when they pick a baby girl off the floor, and "God's name on you and your sister" when the baby is a boy.

17. For information on spirit possession and the *zār* cult in Egypt, see Atiya (1982); Biegman (1990); Early (1982, 1988, 1993b); Fakhouri (1968); Kennedy (1967, 1978b); Morsy (1978a, 1978b, 1993); Nelson (1971); Pillsbury (1978); Rugh (1984); and Walker (1934). For other parts of the Middle East, see Boddy (1989); Constantinides (1985); Crapanzano (1973); Greenwood (1981); Pillsbury (1978); Safa (1988); Shiloh (1968); Swagman (1989); and Underwood and Underwood (1980).

18. For information on cross-cultural evil-eye beliefs and theories to explain them, see Dundes (1992); Elworthy (1986); Maloney (1976); and Siebers (1983). For information on the health-demoting consequences of the evil eye in the Middle East (other than Egypt), see Greenwood (1981); Shiloh (1968); Swagman (1989); and Underwood and Underwood (1980).

19. In this study, only one woman had ever contemplated a connection between her infertility and *ḥasad*, which she speculated might have occurred due to her exceptional beauty on her wedding day. This woman was, by all standards, pulchritudinous and was probably the subject of continuous envy for this reason.

Chapter 7: Divinity, Profanity, and Pilgrimage

1. Although the ethnographic work on women's religious experience in the Middle East is sparse, recent examples include Abu-Lughod (1993b); Betteridge (1983, 1989, 1992); Bowen and Early (1993); Delaney (1991); Dwyer (1978); Early (1993a); Mernissi (1977); Tapper (1990); Tapper and Tapper (1987); and Young (1993).

2. Although none of the women in this study knew the exact translation of this and other relevant Qur'anic verses, a few had an approximate idea. The vast majority professed—and often apologized for—their lack of knowledge of the Qur'an and their religion in general. A few who did not know this and other Qur'anic passages

argued that God would not have concerned himself with matters as trivial as infertility in his most important text.

3. Very few women in this study knew the stories of these religious figures at all or had only partial or inaccurate information about them. Some women were able to cite the story of Maryam (Mary), to whom God gave Jesus as an example of God's ability to cause miracles.

4. For brief descriptions of healing pilgrimages to saints' tombs, see Atiya (1982); Bakker (1992); Early (1985, 1993a, 1993b); El-Messiri (1978); Morsy (1993); Myntti (1988a); Pillsbury (1978); Shiloh (1968); and van Spijk, Fahmy, and Zimmerman (1982).

5. Information on these pilgrimage centers is derived from Biegman (1990) and Seton-Williams and Stocks (1988).

6. As Biegman (1990) notes, there are many commonalities between Muslim and Christian pilgrimage and shrine visitation traditions in Egypt, with Muslims and Christians visiting each other's shrines in many cases.

7. Information on the Shrine of Saint Mena is derived from Biegman (1990), Forster (1986), Grossman (1986), and Seton-Williams and Stocks (1988).

Chapter 8: Biomedical Bodies

1. It is important to note that the first international conference on "Bioethics in Human Reproduction Research in the Muslim World" was held December 10–13, 1991, in Cairo. The conference was organized in large part by a medical anthropologist, Sandra Lane, then of the Ford Foundation in Cairo. For details of the conference and the ethical guidelines that resulted from it, see Serour (1992) and Serour and Omran (1992).

2. Critical examinations of biomedicine by medical anthropologists and other social scientists working in the Middle East include: Bowen (1985); Creyghton (1977); Darity (1965); Gallagher and Searle (1984, 1985); Lane and Millar (1987); Morsy (1988); and Underwood and Underwood (1980).

3. According to the World Health Organization (1989), so-called male factors are thought to occur in about 40 percent of cases of infertility; various female factors in another 40 percent of cases; and unknown factors, perhaps involving immunological incompatibility between partners, in 20 percent of cases.

4. Despite the fact that many Egyptian biogynecologists acknowledge the relationship between obesity and infertility, very few encourage their infertile patients to lose weight or provide strategies for weight reduction. In this study, for example, the majority of the infertile women in the sample suffered from mild to severe obesity. However, only two of one hundred women had been encouraged by physicians to lose weight. These women assumed that "fat on the stomach or ovaries" was causing their infertility.

5. In a leading 1922 monograph on *Sterility and Conception* (Child 1922), uterine "displacements," including anteflexion and retroflexion, and the "infantile uterus," are considered to be major causes of female sterility, and are ideas that appear to have emerged with the beginning of obstetrics and gynecology as a specialty in the

nineteenth century (Speert 1958, 1980). The late nineteenth century and early twentieth century were called, retrospectively, "the dark ages of operative furor," because of the many surgical procedures devised for the purported cure of uterine retroversion (Speert 1973; Roy 1990). In modern gynecology textbooks (e.g., Aiman 1984; Carr and Blackwell 1993), however, references to these uterine "conditions" are either altogether absent or are dismissed as insignificant causes of infertility.

6. Although none of the seventeen physicians participating as informants in this study believed in the relationship between consanguinity and infertility, studies among other highly inbred populations show that couples married to cousins have longer intervals from marriage to the birth of each child, as well as smaller family sizes (Ober et al. 1988). This may be due to shared human leukocyte antigens (HLAs), which serve to reduce fertility.

Among this study sample of Egyptian women and their husbands, analysis of mean inbreeding coefficients showed that infertile women (without tubal-factor infertility) were significantly more likely than fertile controls to be related to their spouses. Thus, inbreeding may be a significant risk factor for infertility, probably of the immunological variety, among Egyptian couples (Inhorn and Buss 1994).

7. The practice of postcoital douching in Egypt has also been noted by El-Messiri (1978).

8. Occasionally, infertile women express the belief that diagnostic laparoscopy is therapeutic and is intended to "open the tubes" or "enlarge the uterus."

9. Problems of doctor-patient communication in the Middle East have also been reported by Assaad and El Katsha (1981); Creyghton (1977); Darity (1965); El-Mehairy (1984b); El-Messiri (1978); Gallagher and Searle (1985); Good (1980); Mernissi (1977); and Morsy (1993).

10. Racy (1969) also describes the reluctance of Arab physicians to deliver negative diagnostic information to patients and their families, given that such disclosure reflects poorly on their curative omnipotence.

11. Early (1985) describes how poor Egyptian women are "cut short" by doctors when they launch into their explanatory illness narratives.

12. Because of lack of disclosure on the part of *both* physicians and husbands, many women assume their husbands' semen analyses to be "good" (and are quick to report this), when, in fact, male factors are present.

Chapter 9: Untherapeutic Therapeutics

1. In this study, most infertile women embarked on their biogynecological quests early in their marriages—46 percent within the first six months and 79 percent within the first year. Virtually every woman had visited at least one biogynecologist within the first five years of marriage, and, in most cases, women had visited many more.

2. The attitude of some Egyptian biogynecologists is that women too poor to pay for infertility diagnosis and treatment are too poor to be bringing children into the world. Therefore, it does not bother them to charge fees that are difficult for many women to afford.

3. In this study, average total estimated expenses for biogynecological infertility services were £E 1,660 ($664) among the fifty women who provided this information.

4. In this study, 38 percent of the infertile women had visited between one and four biogynecologists; 27 percent between five and nine; 20 percent between ten and fifteen; and 15 percent more than fifteen. In one case, a woman estimated that she had seen approximately sixty biogynecologists during the course of her marriage and had yet to be given a diagnosis. In yet another case, a woman counted nearly 150 visits to different physicians, including four during the course of one month.

5. Egyptian women's doctor shopping has also been described by Early (1988) and Morsy (1980a).

6. Because of Shatby Hospital's reputation, infertile women are also referred or taken there by husbands, relatives, neighbors, or acquaintances who work there.

7. During the period of my study and much to my surprise, I developed a reputation in Alexandria as a "good *duktūra* from America" who had come to Egypt to start an infertility clinic! As a result, women would occasionally seek me out at Shatby Hospital to ask me when my private clinic was opening. In addition, women in my study occasionally told me that they wished I was the one who was treating them, since they had become "fed up" with other doctors. Of course, I could offer nothing to these women in the way of treatment. See Appendix 1, however, for a discussion of my role as patient educator and liaison.

8. In this study, for example, 88 percent of the infertile women had taken ovulation-inducing agents at some time in the past and, in most cases, for periods lasting longer than five years.

9. In this study, for example, 22 percent of infertile women had taken oral contraceptives, usually obtained over the counter in pharmacies, in an attempt to become pregnant.

10. Because "new-generation" ovulation-inducing drugs are expensive, powerful, and require careful monitoring (by ultrasound and hormonal assays), very few Egyptian physicians prescribe them regularly or at all. Those who do so tend to be urban-based biogynecologists specializing in infertility.

11. In this study, for example, twenty-seven of fifty women (54 percent) who were prescribed clomiphene citrate suffered from blurred vision. As one woman described it, "it looked as though the television was jumping up and down."

12. The problem of gynecological iatrogenesis in the West has been noted by a number of scholars, including Barger-Lux and Heaney (1986); Beck-Gernsheim (1989); Corea (1988); and Ratcliff (1989b).

13. Discussions of men's technological control over procreation can be found in, among others, Baruch (1988); Corea (1988); Henifin (1988); Mies (1987); Morsy (n.d.); Oakley (1987); Rapp (1988); Ratcliff (1989b); Rowland (1987); Ruddick (1988); and Stanworth (1987b).

14. It is interesting to note that the use of electricity in infertility therapy began in the late 1800s in the West and was widely applied for a variety of infertility-related conditions, including salpingitis, fibroids, primary amenorrhea, and uterine "displacements" (Speert 1980).

15. In this study, women who underwent one or more episodes of cervical electrocautery were at 2.1 times greater risk of cervical-factor infertility than were women who were never electrocauterized, a result that was statistically significant (Inhorn and Buss 1994).

16. In this study, tubal insufflation appeared to be a significant independent risk factor for tubal-factor infertility (TFI), with the risk of TFI increasing with repetitive insufflations (Inhorn and Buss 1993).

17. At the time of this study, the only recognized gynecological microsurgery and laparoscopic surgery center in Egypt was in Cairo's Al-Azhar University (Serour et al. 1988, Serour et al. 1989).

Chapter 10: The Injection of Spermatic Animals

1. During the period of my fieldwork, women in my study and women whom I did not even know often sought me out to interpret their ultrasound records, which they carried with them. These records contained information about women's follicular development, especially their "egg size," during given menstrual cycles.

2. Not only is adoption officially illegal in Islamic family law, but it is culturally unacceptable to most poor urban Egyptians on a number of grounds. These include the distrust of illegitimacy in general and of illegitimate children in particular; the fear that biological parents may intervene later in a child's life; the belief that adoptive parents cannot feel as much toward adopted children as toward biological ones; the concern over potentially sinful relations between adopted children and their adoptive family members; the concern over potential incest between siblings adopted into different families and then reunited as spouses later in life; the stigmatization of adopted children in the community; the stigmatization of adoptive parents; and the belief that only the wealthy can afford to adopt. For a more detailed discussion of these attitudes toward adoption, see Inhorn (n.d.).

3. According to Savage (1992), reactions to AID in Yaoundé, Cameroon, were similar to those reported here. Major concerns of Cameroonians revolved around issues of unknown genitor and the fear of incest among the AID children of different mothers.

4. Nevertheless, four infertile women in this study said they were willing to undergo AID clandestinely without telling their husbands. To them, but certainly not to their husbands, achieving motherhood was more important than ensuring paternity.

Chapter 11: Babies of the Tubes

1. Given varying levels of knowledge and understanding about IVF, women disagreed about whether the procedure was more or less successful than AIH and whether IVF was widely available in Egypt. Some women argued that many "babies of the tubes" had been born in Egypt, while others contended that the procedure was only widely available abroad, especially in the United States and Saudi Arabia.

Some women, especially fertile ones, were poorly informed about either AIH or IVF and had "no idea" about these issues.

2. One woman argued that scientific experimentation is always directed at women's bodies, because "the woman is like a rabbit exactly, and science always makes tests on rabbits."

3. The standard IVF protocol involves nine steps, occurring over four weeks (Harkness 1992), as follows: (1) a woman's current menstrual cycle is halted with gonadotropin-releasing hormone (GnRH) agonists; (2) ovulation is then induced through the administration of fertility drugs for eight to twelve days; (3) ultrasounds and blood tests are performed to monitor the development of ovarian follicles over a six- to twelve-day period; (4) serum progesterone levels are measured to assess the growth of the uterine lining; (5) mature eggs (usually at least four) are retrieved from the woman vaginally through ultrasound-guided aspiration of the follicles; (6) ova and sperm (obtained through the male partner's masturbation) are prepared in the laboratory and then combined for fertilization and cell division over a period of about forty-eight hours; (7) embryos emerging through the fertilization process are transferred (injected by a catheter) into the woman's uterus through the cervix within two days of egg retrieval; (8) the woman receives hormonal support, usually progesterone, for the first eight to ten weeks of pregnancy or until menstruation occurs; and (9) a pregnancy test is usually performed ten to twelve days after an IVF transfer.

4. Women who were part of the growing Islamist movement in Egypt said they consulted their sisters and brothers at the mosque about such matters of religious permissibility.

5. Because of the Eurocentric focus in the feminist literature on the new reproductive technologies, very few scholars have examined the emerging practice of IVF in the Third World. Dos Reis's (1987) content analysis of Brazilian newspaper reports on IVF is a notable exception. Despite the dearth of cross-cultural scholarship, many of the criticisms of feminist scholars concerning the dangers of the NRTs also apply overseas.

6. IVF centers have been established in a number of other Middle Eastern Muslim countries, including Saudi Arabia, Kuwait, Jordan, and, by the time of this writing, probably Morocco (Serour, El Ghar, and Mansour 1990).

Chapter 12: Futures for the Infertile

1. The importance of motherhood in Egypt has been noted by, among others, Abu-Lughod (1993a); Ammar (1966); Early (1993b); El-Hamamsy (1972); El-Mehairy (1984b); Gadalla (1978); Lane and Meleis (1991); Morsy (1978b, 1980a, 1980b, 1982, 1993); Rugh (1984); Sukkary-Stolba (1985); van Spijk, Fahmy, and Zimmerman (1982); and Watson (1992). See Inhorn (n.d.) for a more in-depth discussion of the motherhood mandate and the social consequences of infertility.

Glossary of Arabic Terms

abū kabīr: lit. "old father," as in an unidentified herbal substance used in folk remedies.

'adwā: infection.

agsām muḍādda: lit. "anti-bodies," as in antisperm antibodies.

'a'ila: extended family.

akh taḥt il-arḍ (pl.: *ikhwān taḥt il-arḍ*): spirit-brother under the ground.

'amal: lit. "work," "making," "doing," as in sorcery.

'amalīya (pl.: *'amalīyāt*): surgical operation.

amrāḍ nisā': lit. "diseases of women," as in obstetrics and gynecology.

anābīb: tubes, as in fallopian tubes.

anābīb masdūd: blocked fallopian tubes.

'aqm: infertility.

'aranful: clove.

arasiya (a.k.a. *sha'ar hindī*): herbal substance used in folk remedies.

arḍ: soil, land.

armūt: fish used in sorcery nullification, renowned for its ability to avoid capture.

'arrāf(a) (pl.: *'arrāfīn*): diviner, fortune-teller; an alternative term for *munaggim.*

'asmah: vegetable-glue plant.

aṭrūn (a.k.a. *naṭrūn*): mineral substance from salt lakes of Egypt's al-Wadi Naṭrūn, northwest of Cairo.

'aṭṭār (pl.: *'aṭṭārīn*): herbalist.

'ayyina min il-mahbal: lit. "a specimen from the vagina," as in cervical mucus analysis.

'ayyina min il-mahbal ba'd il-iktimā': lit. "a specimen from the vagina after sexual intercourse," as in postcoital test (PCT).

'ayyina min ir-raḥim: lit. "a specimen from the uterus," as in premenstrual endometrial biopsy.

baiḍa (pl.: *buwaiḍāt*): egg, ovum.

bait: house.

bait il-wilid: lit. "house of the child," as in womb, uterus.

bakhūr: incense.

baladī: traditional, native, folk, indigenous.
baqshīsh (pl.: *baqāshīsh*): tip, gratuity.
baraka: divine blessing.
bārnūf: plowman's spikenard.
baṣal: onions.
bil bang: under anesthesia.
bizra: lit. "seed," as in sperm.
brūstata: prostatitis.
daggāl(a) (pl.: *daggālīn*): quack, charlatan; a pejorative term for *munaggim.*
dagl: deceit, quackery.
dahr maftūḥ: open back.
dam al-akhawain: lit. "blood of the two brothers," as in a resinous substance derived from the dragon tree, *Dracaena draco.*
daura: period, cycle, as in the menstrual period or cycle.
dāya (pl.: *dāyāt*): traditional midwife.
dhahab bundu'i: lit. "nutty gold," as in twenty-four-karat, nut-shaped gold, typically from Sudan.
dhakar: male.
dhakar in-nakhl: male date palm.
dibla: wedding ring.
dūda (pl.: *dīdān*): lit. "worm," used to refer to sperm.
dukhla: lit. "entrance," as in the wedding night (penetration).
duktūra: female physician, sometimes used to refer to any woman with an advanced degree.
faddān (pl.: *fadādīn*): an area of land equivalent to 1.038 acres or 0.420 hectares.
fag'a: see *khaḍḍa.*
fakka: to unbind, untie, or unfasten something.
fallāḥīn: peasants, farmers.
fasūkh: an unidentified herbal substance used in vapor sitz baths.
fatla: twining (the open back).
fatwā: formal Islamic legal opinion.
fil hawā' sawa: lit. "in the air together," as in "we're all in the same boat."
gallābīya: a long, loose, caftan-like garment worn by many Egyptian men.
galsāt kahraba: lit. "sessions of electricity," as in shortwave (infrared) therapy.
ganaina: fetus, embryo.
gidi: billy goat.
ḥabbit il-baraka: black cumin.

hadīya: GIFT (gamete intrafallopian transfer).
hajj: Islamic pilgrimage to Saudi Arabia.
ḥakīma (pl.: *ḥakīmāt*): nineteenth-century Egyptian woman physician; now used to refer to government-trained nurse-midwives.
ḥalāl: allowed, permitted (usually referring to Islam).
ḥalāwa: a homemade, sugar-and-lemon substance used by women for depilation.
ḥallāq aṣ-ṣiḥḥa (pl.: *ḥallāqīn aṣ-ṣiḥḥa*): health-barber, barber-surgeon.
ḥamla ghizlāni: lit. "gazelle-like pregnancy," as in a pregnancy with monthly recurrent bleeding.
ḥammām: bath; see *tabwīkha.*
ḥanẓal: colocynth.
ḥarām: forbidden, prohibited (usually referring to Islam).
ḥasad: envy, the evil eye.
ḥayawānāt il-minawī: lit. "spermatic animals," as in sperm.
ḥigāb (pl.: *ḥugub*): amulet.
hormōn (pl.: *hormōnāt*): hormone.
ḥu'an: lit. "injections," as in artificial insemination.
ḥu'an fir-raḥim: lit. "injections in the uterus," as in hydrotubation.
ḥulba: fenugreek.
ḥulw: sweet.
ḥummuṣ: chickpeas.
ibn ḥarām: lit. "son of sin," as in a bastard.
i'fāl: locking or closing (the open back).
ʿifrīt(a) (pl.: *ʿafārīt*): see *jinnī.*
ifsantīn: see *shīḥ rūmī.*
iltihāb (pl.: *iltihābāt*): inflammation.
iltiṣāqāt: pelvic adhesions.
ʿirq id-dhahab: long pepper.
ʿirq il-ganāḥ (a.k.a. *'irfa*): cinnamon.
Iskandarīyyīn: the people of Alexandria, Egypt.
jāhilīya: lit. "age of ignorance," as in pre-Islamic times.
jinn: collective term for spirits capable of causing harm.
jinnī(ya) (a.k.a. *ʿifrīt[a]*): mischievous spirit capable of causing harm.
Kaʿba: stone in Mecca, Saudia Arabia, which is circumambulated by Muslim pilgrims.
kabsa (a.k.a. *mushāhara*): the polluting entrance of an individual into a vulnerable woman's room, causing reproductive binding.
kāfūr: camphor.

kaḥt: lit. "scraping," as in curettage of the uterus.
kammūn armanī (a.k.a. *kahramān*): common caraway.
ka'sāt hawā': lit. "cups of air"; see *kasr.*
kasr (a.k.a. *ka'sāt hawā'*): cupping.
kathīrā': astragal.
katīr: a lot.
kawī: traditional cautery; see *kayy.*
kayy (a.k.a. *kawī*): cervical electrocautery; traditional cautery.
khaḍḍa (a.k.a. *fag'a, tar'ba*): shock, fright.
khallafa: to have followers, offspring, or descendants; to leave someone behind.
khawagāt: foreigners.
khuzāmā: lavender.
labānna: white, "milky" bead in a *mushāharāt* necklace.
lissa: still, not yet, waiting.
lubān dhakar: frankincense.
madhbaḥ: slaughterhouse.
mafgū'(a) (pl.: *mafgū'īn*): pained, afflicted, distressed; see *makhḍūḍ.*
mafīsh khair: lit. "there is no goodness [anymore]," used to refer to difficult (economic) circumstances.
maḥlab: mahaleb.
makbūsa (a.k.a. *mitshāhara*): the condition of a woman affected by *kabsa.*
makhḍūḍ(a) (pl.: *makhḍūḍīn*) (a.k.a. *mafgū'[a], matrū'b[a]*): shocked, frightened, terrorized.
makwa: ironing, sometimes used to refer to *kayy* (*kawī*).
malaka (pl.: *malaika*): angel.
malbūs(a) (pl.: *malbūsīn*): lit. "worn," as in spirit-possessed.
manẓar: lit. "view," as in diagnostic laparoscopy.
maraḍ (pl.: *amrāḍ*): disease.
marbūṭ(a) (pl.: *marbūṭīn*): lit. "tied" or "bound," as by sorcery.
mashākil id-dīdān: lit. "problems of the worms," as in male infertility.
mashākil ir-raḥim: problems of the uterus.
mashākil wirāthī: hereditary problems.
matrū'b(a) (pl.: *matrū'bīn*): frightened, terrified, afraid; see *makhḍūḍ.*
mibyaḍ (pl.: *mibāyiḍ*): ovary.
mibāyiḍ da'īf: weak ovaries.
mirwad: lit. "little stick," as in vaginal stick used to widen or clean the vagina and uterus.
mistika: mastic.

mitshāhara: see *makbūsa.*
mufti: religious cleric.
muḥāgiba (pl.: *muḥāgibīn*): Islamically veiled with a scarf that covers the hair completely but not the face.
mūlid (pl.: *mawālid*): saint's day celebration.
munaggim(a) (pl.: *munaggimīn*): lit. "astrologer," as in spiritist healer.
murr: myrrh.
mushāhara: see *kabsa.*
mushāharāt: ritual appurtenances used in unbinding the effects of *kabsa.*
nafq: tubal insufflation.
nutfa: sperm, semen.
qarḥa: cervical erosion.
qarīn(a): subterranean spirit-counterpart.
rabṭ: lit. "tying," as by sorcery.
raḥim: uterus.
raḥim ḍayyiʾ: "tight" uterus.
rūḥ: spirit, soul.
ruṭūba: humidity, moisture, wetness.
ruzz bil-laban: rice pudding.
saḥḥār(a) (pl.: *saḥḥārīn*): sorcerer, magician; a pejorative term for *munaggim.*
Ṣaʿid: Upper Egypt.
Ṣaʿīdī(ya): Upper Egyptian.
sāʾil: fluid, as in seminal fluid.
ṣalāh (pl.: *ṣalāwāt*): prayer.
salīkha: cassia.
samna: clarified animal fat used as cooking oil.
sayyid: direct descendant of the Prophet Muhammad.
shahr: new moon, month.
shaikh(a) (pl.: *shuyūkh*): religious leader; also a title of respect given to a spiritist healer.
shaikh bil-baraka (pl.: *shuyūkh bil-baraka*): blessed *shaikh;* a living healer or dead saint with divine blessing.
shīḥ: wormwood.
shīḥ rūmī (a.k.a. *ifsantīn*): Byzantine wormwood.
shirk: polytheism; association of other beings with God.
shīsha: a large, standing waterpipe used for smoking tobacco.
sitt il-bait (pl.: *sittāt il-bait*): housewife.
sitt kabīra (pl.: *sittāt kabira*): elderly woman who is a lay infertility specialist.

ṣūfa (pl.: *ṣūwaf*): vaginal suppository, often made of sheep's wool, cotton, or gauze.
Ṣūfī: Islamic mystic, member of a *Ṣūfī* brotherhood.
sukkar an-nabāt: rock candy, sugar candy.
ṣūra ashi‘‘a bi ṣibghā: lit. "an X ray by dye," as in hysterosalpingography (HSG).
tabwīḍ: ovulation.
tabwīkha (a.k.a. *ḥammām*): vapor sitz bath.
taḥlīl agsām muḍādda: analysis of antibodies.
taḥlīl id-dam: blood analysis, as in serum hormonal assays.
taḥlīl l-guz: lit. "analysis of the husband," as in semen analysis.
taḥlīl l-hormōnāt: hormonal analysis.
talqīḥ iṣṭinā‘ī: artificial insemination.
tamsīlīya: televised soap opera.
tanẓīf: lit. "cleaning," as in dilatation and curettage of the uterus.
tanẓīm il-usra: lit. "organization [control] of the [nuclear] family," as in family planning.
ṭast it-tar‘ba: pan of shock.
tar‘ba: see *khaḍḍa.*
taṣwīr: lit. "photography," as in ultrasound.
tausī‘ wi kaḥt: lit. "widening and scraping," as in dilatation and curettage (D & C).
ṭibb il-‘arabī: Arab or Bedouin medicine.
ṭifl l-anābīb: lit. "baby of the tubes," as in a test-tube baby via in vitro fertilization.
ukht taḥt il-arḍ (pl.: *akhawāt taḥt il-arḍ*): spirit-sister under the ground.
Umm Il-Ghayyib: lit. "mother of the missing one"; the *kunya,* or term of address for an infertile woman.
unbūba (pl.: *anābīb*): tube, as in fallopian tube.
‘unq ir-raḥim: lit. "neck of the uterus," as in cervix.
waṣfāt baladī: folk cures, traditional remedies.
Yūnānī: Greek.
za‘farān: saffron.
zaghlala: blurred vision.
zangabīl: ginger.
zār: spirit placation ceremony for the possessed.
zarāwind: birthwort.
zakawāt: alms to the poor.
ziyāra (pl.: *ziyārāt*): visit, pilgrimage.

References

Abdullah, S. A., A. Zarzoor, and M. Y. Ali

1982 "Epidemiological Study of Infertility in Some Villages of Assiut Governorate." *Assiut Medical Journal* 6:266–74.

Aboulghar, M. A., G. I. Serour, and R. Mansour

1990 "Some Ethical and Legal Aspects of Medically Assisted Reproduction in Egypt." *International Journal of Bioethics* 1:265–68.

Abu-Lughod, Janet

1985 "Recent Migrations in the Arab World." In *Arab Society: Social Science Perspectives,* ed. Nicholas S. Hopkins and Saad Eddin Ibrahim, 177–88. Cairo: American University in Cairo Press.

Abu-Lughod, Lila

1986 *Veiled Sentiments: Honor and Poetry in a Bedouin Society.* Berkeley: University of California Press.

1989 "Zones of Theory in the Anthropology of the Arab World." *Annual Review of Anthropology* 18:267–306.

1993a *Writing Women's Worlds: Bedouin Stories.* Berkeley: University of California Press.

1993b "Islam and the Gendered Discourses of Death." *International Journal of Middle East Studies* 25:187–205.

Abu-Zeid, Hassan A. H., and William M. Dann

1985 "Health Services Utilization and Cost in Ismailia, Egypt." *Social Science & Medicine* 21:451–61.

Adamson, P. B.

1973 "The Influence of Alexander the Great on the Practice of Medicine." *Episteme* 7:222.

Ahmed, Leila

1989 "Arab Culture and Writing Women's Bodies." *Feminist Issues* 9:41–55.

Aiman, James

1984 "A History of Human Fertility." In *Infertility: Diagnosis and Management,* ed. James Aiman, 1–16. New York: Springer-Verlag.

Ali, Omer Tameim El Dar

1980 "Prevalence of Gonorrhoea among Married Females Presenting with Leucorrhoea." Master's thesis, High Institute of Public Health, Alexandria, Egypt.

Ali, Y.

1980 "Non Specific Urethritis Due to *Chlamydia trachomatis.*" Master's thesis, Faculty of Medicine, Alexandria University, Alexandria, Egypt.

Alubo, S. Ogoh

1987 "Power and Privileges in Medical Care: An Analysis of Medical Services in Post-Colonial Nigeria." *Social Science & Medicine* 24:453–62.

1990 "Debt Crisis, Health and Health Services in Africa." *Social Science & Medicine* 31:639–48.

Amer, Amira Fathi

1987 "*Chlamydia trachomatis* and *Neisseria gonorrhoeae* in the Cervices of Women of the Child Bearing Age from the Egyptian Rural Community." Master's thesis, Faculty of Medicine, University of Alexandria, Alexandria, Egypt.

Ammar, Hamed

1966 *Growing Up in an Egyptian Village*. New York: Octagon.

Anees, Munawar Ahmad

1989 *Islam and Biological Futures: Ethics, Gender and Technology*. London: Mansell.

Ansari, Hamied

1986 *Egypt: The Stalled Society*. Albany: State University of New York Press.

Aral, Sevgi O., and Willard Cates

1983 "The Increasing Concern with Infertility: Why Now?" *Journal of the American Medical Association* 250(17):2327–31.

Ardener, Shirley

1978 *Defining Females: The Nature of Women in Society*. New York: John Wiley.

Assaad, Marie

1980 "Female Circumcision in Egypt: Social Implications, Current Research, and Prospects for Change." *Studies in Family Planning* 11:3–16.

Assaad, Marie, and Samiha El Katsha

1981 "Formal and Informal Health Care in an Egyptian Delta Village." *Contact* 65:1–13.

Atiya, Nayra

1982 *Khul-Khaal: Five Egyptian Women Tell Their Stories*. Syracuse, NY: Syracuse University Press.

Azziz, Ricardo

1993 "Reproductive Endocrinology of Female Obesity." In *Textbook of Reproductive Medicine*, ed. Bruce R. Carr and Richard E. Blackwell, 389–407. Norwalk, CT: Appleton & Lange.

Bakker, Jogien

1992 "The Rise of Female Healers in the Middle Atlas, Morocco." *Social Science & Medicine* 35:819–29.

Barger-Lux, M. Janet, and Robert P. Heaney

1986 "For Better and Worse: The Technological Imperative in Health Care." *Social Science & Medicine* 22:1313–20.

Bartky, Sandra Lee

1988 "Foucault, Femininity, and the Modernization of Patriarchal Power." In *Feminism & Foucault: Reflections on Resistance*, ed. Irene Diamond and Lee Quinby, 61–86. Boston: Northeastern University Press.

Baruch, Elaine Hoffman

1988 "A Womb of His Own." In *Embryos, Ethics, and Women's Rights: Exploring the New Reproductive Technologies,* ed. Elaine Hoffman Baruch, Amadeo F. D'Adamo, Jr., and Joni Seager, 135–39. Special issue of *Women & Health* 13 (1/2). New York: Haworth Press.

Baruch, Elaine Hoffman, Amadeo F. D'Adamo, Jr., and Joni Seager, eds.

1988 *Embryos, Ethics, and Women's Rights: Exploring the New Reproductive Technologies.* Special issue of *Women & Health* 13 (1/2). New York: Haworth Press.

Basha, N. M. K.

1981 "*Chlamydia trachomatis* Infection of the Cervix with Contraceptive Pills and Intrauterine Devices." Master's thesis, Faculty of Medicine, Alexandria University, Alexandria, Egypt.

Bates, G. William

1984 "The Hypothalamus: Physiology and Pathophysiology." In *Infertility: Diagnosis and Management,* ed. James Aiman, 31–49. New York: Springer-Verlag.

Bates, G. William, and Winfred L. Wiser

1984 "Uterine Function and Abnormalities Causing Infertility." In *Infertility: Diagnosis and Management,* ed. James Aiman, 143–60. New York: Springer-Verlag.

Baumslag, Naomi

1985 "Women's Status and Health: World Considerations." In *Advances in International Maternal and Child Health,* vol. 5, ed. D. B. Jelliffe and E. F. Patrice Jelliffe, 1–26. Oxford: Clarendon.

Becker, Gay

1990 *Healing the Infertile Family.* New York: Bantam Books.

Becker, Gay, and Robert D. Nachtigall

1991 "Ambiguous Responsibility in the Doctor-Patient Relationship: The Case of Infertility." *Social Science & Medicine* 32:875–85.

Beck-Gernsheim, Elisabeth

1989 "From the Pill to Test-Tube Babies: New Options, New Pressures in Reproductive Behavior." In *Healing Technology: Feminist Perspectives,* ed. Kathryn Strother Ratcliff, 23–40. Ann Arbor: University of Michigan Press.

Bedevian, Armenag K.

1936 *Illustrated Polyglottic Dictionary of Plant Names in Latin, Arabic, Armenian, English, French, German, Italian and Turkish Languages Including Economic, Medicinal, Poisonous and Ornamental Plants and Common Weeds.* Cairo: Argus & Papazian Presses.

Belsey, Mark A.

1976 "The Epidemiology of Infertility: A Review with Particular Reference to Sub-Saharan Africa." *Bulletin of the World Health Organization* 54:319–41.

1985 "Traditional Birth Attendants: A Resource for the Health of Women." *International Journal of Gynecology and Obstetrics* 23:247–48.

Belsey, Mark A., and Helen Ware
1986 "Epidemiological, Social and Psychological Aspects of Infertility." In *Infertility: Male and Female,* ed. Vaclav Insler and Bruno Lunenfeld, 631–47. Edinburgh: Churchill Livingstone.

Bentley, J.
1989 *Need for Strengthening Managerial, Administrative and Supervisory Capabilities of Midwives in District.* WHO Report EM/CNS.TBA. VLG/9.

Berman, Ruth
1989 "From Aristotle's Dualism to Materialist Dialectics: Feminist Transformation of Science and Society." In *Gender/Body/Knowledge: Feminist Reconstructions of Being and Knowing,* ed. Alison M. Jaggar and Susan R. Bordo, 224–55. New Brunswick, NJ: Rutgers University Press.

Betteridge, Anne H.
1983 "Muslim Women and Shrines in Shiraz." In *Mormons and Muslims,* ed. Spencer J. Palmer, 127–38. Provo, UT: Religious Studies Center, Brigham Young University.
1989 "The Controversial Vows of Urban Muslim Women in Iran." In *Unspoken Worlds: Women's Religious Lives in Non-Western Cultures,* ed. Nancy Aver Falk and Rita M. Gross, 102–11. Belmont, CA: Wadsworth.
1992 "Specialists in Miraculous Action: Some Shrines in Shiraz." In *Sacred Journeys: The Anthropology of Pilgrimage,* ed. Alan Morinis, 189–210. Westport, CT: Greenwood Press.

Biegman, Nicolaas
1990 *Egypt: Moulids, Saints, Sufis.* London: Kegan Paul.

Blizard, Peter J.
1991 "International Standards in Medical Education or National Standards/Primary Health Care—Which Direction?" *Social Science & Medicine* 33:1163–70.

Boddy, Janice
1982 "Womb as Oasis: The Symbolic Context of Pharaonic Circumcision in Rural Northern Sudan." *American Ethnologist* 9:682–98.
1989 *Wombs and Alien Spirits: Women, Men, and the* Zar *Cult in Northern Sudan.* Madison: University of Wisconsin Press.

Bolton, Pamela, Carl Kendall, Elli Leontsini, and Corrine Whitaker
1990 *The Impact of Health Technologies on Women in the Developing World.* The Johns Hopkins University School of Hygiene and Public Health Institute for International Programs, Occasional Paper No. 11.

Bonair, Ann, Patricia Rosenfield, and Karin Tengvald
1989 "Medical Technologies in Developing Countries: Issues of Technology Development, Transfer, Diffusion and Use." *Social Science & Medicine* 28:769–81.

Bouhdiba, Abdelwahab
1985 *Sexuality in Islam.* London: Routledge & Kegan Paul.

Bourdieu, Pierre
1977 *Outline of a Theory of Practice.* Translated by Richard Nice. New York: Cambridge University Press.
Bowen, Donna Lee
1985 "Women and Public Health in Morocco: One Family's Experience." In *Women and the Family in the Middle East: New Voices of Change,* ed. Elizabeth Warnock Fernea, 134–44. Austin: University of Texas Press.
Bowen, Donna Lee, and Evelyn A. Early, eds.
1993 *Everyday Life in the Muslim Middle East.* Bloomington: Indiana University Press.
Bradshaw, Karen D., and Bruce R. Carr
1993 "Modern Diagnostic Evaluation of the Infertile Couple." In *Textbook of Reproductive Medicine,* ed. Bruce R. Carr and Richard E. Blackwell, 443–52. Norwalk, CT: Appleton & Lange.
Brown, K. L.
1978 "The Campaign to Encourage Family Planning in Tunisia and Some Responses at the Village Level." Paper presented at the Workshop on Religions and Population Dynamics, University of Ghana at Legon, January 2–5, 1978.
Browner, Carole H., and Carolyn F. Sargent
1990 "Anthropology and Studies of Human Reproduction." In *Medical Anthropology: A Handbook of Theory and Method,* ed. Thomas M. Johnson and Carolyn F. Sargent, 215–29. New York: Greenwood Press.
Buckley, Thomas, and Alma Gottlieb
1988 "A Critical Appraisal of Theories of Menstrual Symbolism." In *Blood Magic: The Anthropology of Menstruation,* ed. Thomas Buckley and Alma Gottlieb, 3–50. Berkeley: University of California Press.
Bürgel, J. Christoph
1976 "Secular and Religious Features of Medieval Arabic Medicine." In *Asian Medical Systems: A Comparative Study,* ed. Charles Leslie, 44–62. Berkeley: University of California Press.
Byrd, William
1993 "Fertilization, Embryogenesis, and Implantation." In *Textbook of Reproductive Medicine,* ed. Bruce R. Carr and Richard E. Blackwell, 1–15. Norwalk, CT: Appleton & Lange.
Caldwell, John C., and Pat Caldwell
1983 "The Demographic Evidence for the Incidence and Cause of Abnormally Low Fertility in Tropical Africa." *World Health Statistical Quarterly* 36:2–34.
CAPMAS
1988 *Statistical Yearbook: Arab Republic of Egypt.* Cairo: Central Agency for Public Mobilisation and Statistics (CAPMAS).
Carney, Kim
1984 "Health in Egypt." *Journal of Public Health Policy* 5:131–42.
Carr, Bruce R., and Richard E. Blackwell, eds.
1993 *Textbook of Reproductive Medicine.* Norwalk, CT: Appleton & Lange.

Cates, W., T. M. M. Farley, and P. J. Rowe
1985 "Worldwide Patterns of Infertility: Is Africa Different?" *The Lancet* (September 14):596–98.
Chang, R. Jeffrey
1993 "Anovulation of CNS Origin: Anatomic Causes." In *Textbook of Reproductive Medicine,* ed. Bruce R. Carr and Richard E. Blackwell, 265–80. Norwalk, CT: Appleton & Lange.
Child, Charles Gardner, Jr.
1922 *Sterility and Conception.* New York: D. Appleton.
Collet, M., J. Reniers, E. Frost, R. Gass, F. Yvert, A. Leclerc, C. Roth-Meyer, B. Ivanoff, and A. Meheus
1988 "Infertility in Central Africa: Infection Is the Cause." *International Journal of Gynecology and Obstetrics* 26:423–28.
Constantinides, Pamela
1985 "Women Heal Women: Spirit Possession and Sexual Segregation in a Muslim Society." *Social Science & Medicine* 21:685–92.
Corea, Gena
1988 "What the King Can Not See." In *Embryos, Ethics, and Women's Rights: Exploring the New Reproductive Technologies,* ed. Elaine Hoffman Baruch, Amadeo F. D'Adamo, Jr., and Joni Seager, 77–93. Special issue of *Women & Health* 13 (1/2). New York: Haworth Press.
Corea, Gena, and Susan Ince
1987 "Report of a Survey of IVF Clinics in the US." In *Made to Order: The Myth of Reproductive and Genetic Progress,* ed. Patricia Spallone and Deborah Lynn Steinberg, 133–45. Oxford: Pergamon.
Corea, Gena, Renate Duelli Klein, Jalna Hanmer, Helen B. Holmes, Betty Hoskings, Madhu Kishwar, Janice Raymond, Robyn Rowland, and Roberta Steinbacher
1987 *Man-Made Women: How New Reproductive Technologies Affect Women.* Bloomington: Indiana University Press.
Cowan, J. Milton, ed.
1976 *The Hans Wehr Dictionary of Modern Written Arabic.* 3d ed. Ithaca, NY: Spoken Languages Services.
Crapanzano, Vincent
1973 *The Hamadsha: A Study in Moroccan Ethnopsychiatry.* Berkeley: University of California Press.
Creyghton, Marielouise
1977 "Communication Between Peasant and Doctor in Tunisia." *Social Science & Medicine* 11:319–24.
D'Adamo, Amadeo F., Jr.
1988 "Reproductive Technologies: The Two Sides of the Glass Jar." In *Embryos, Ethics, and Women's Rights: Exploring the New Reproductive Technologies,* ed. Elaine Hoffman Baruch, Amadeo F. D'Adamo, Jr., and Joni Seager, 9–30. Special issue of *Women & Health* 13 (1/2). New York: Haworth Press.
Darity, William A.
1965 "Some Sociocultural Factors in the Administration of Technical Assistance and Training in Health." *Human Organization* 24:78–82.

Dash, Vaidya B.
1978 *Fundamentals of Ayurvedic Medicine.* New Delhi: Bansal.
Davidson, J. R.
1985 "The Shadow of Life: Psychosocial Explanations for Placenta Rituals." *Culture, Medicine, and Psychiatry* 9:77–92.
DeClerque, Julia, Amy Ong Tsui, Mohammed Futuah Abul-Ata, and Delia Barcelona
1986 "Rumor, Misinformation and Oral Contraceptive Use in Egypt." *Social Science & Medicine* 23:83–92.
Delaney, Carol
1986 "The Meaning of Paternity and the Virgin Birth Debate." *Man* (NS) 21:494–513.
1987 "Seeds of Honor, Fields of Shame." In *Honor and Shame: The Unity of the Mediterranean,* ed. David Gilmore, 35–48. Washington, DC: American Anthropological Association.
1988 "Mortal Flow: Menstruation in Turkish Village Society." In *Blood Magic: Explorations in the Anthropology of Menstruation,* ed. Thomas Buckley and Alma Gottlieb, 83–106. Berkeley: University of California Press.
1991 *The Seed and the Soil: Gender and Cosmology in Turkish Village Society.* Berkeley: University of California Press.
Dixon-Mueller, Ruth, and Judith Wasserheit
1991 *The Culture of Silence: Reproductive Tract Infections among Women in the Third World.* International Women's Health Coalition Report.
Dols, Michael W.
1984 *Medieval Islamic Medicine: Ibn Ridwan's Treatise "On the Prevention of Bodily Ills in Egypt."* Berkeley: University of California Press.
dos Reis, Ana Regina Gomez
1987 "IVF in Brazil: The Story Told by the Newspapers." In *Made to Order: The Myth of Reproductive and Genetic Progress,* ed. Patricia Spallone and Deborah Lynn Steinberg, 120–31. Oxford: Pergamon.
Douglas, Mary
1966 *Purity and Danger.* New York: Praeger.
Doyal, Lesley
1979 *The Political Economy of Health.* Boston: South End Press.
Doyle, Michael B., and Alan H. DeCherney
1993 "Diagnosis and Management of Tubal Disease." In *Textbook of Reproductive Medicine,* ed. Bruce R. Carr and Richard E. Blackwell, 507–16. Norwalk, CT: Appleton & Lange.
Dundes, Alan
1992 *The Evil Eye: A Casebook.* Madison: University of Wisconsin Press.
Dwyer, Daisy Hilse
1978 "Women, Sufism, and Decision-Making in Moroccan Islam." In *Women in the Muslim World,* ed. Lois Beck and Nikki Keddie, 585–98. Cambridge, MA: Harvard University Press.
Early, Evelyn A.
1982 "The Logic of Well Being: Therapeutic Narratives in Cairo, Egypt." *Social Science & Medicine* 16:1491–97.

1985 "Catharsis and Creation in Informal Narratives of Baladi Women of Cairo." *Anthropological Quarterly* 58:172–81.

1988 "The Baladi Curative System of Cairo, Egypt." *Culture, Medicine, and Psychiatry* 12:65–83.

1993a *Baladi Women of Cairo: Playing with an Egg and a Stone.* Boulder, CO: Lynne Rienner.

1993b "Fertility and Fate: Medical Practices among *Baladi* Women of Cairo." *Everyday Life in the Muslim Middle East,* ed. Donna Lee Bowen and Evelyn A. Early, 102–8. Bloomington: Indiana University Press.

Ebin, V.

1982 "Interpretations of Infertility: The Aowin People of Southwest Ghana." In *Ethnography of Fertility and Birth,* ed. Carol P. MacCormack, 147–59. London: Academic Press.

Eddy, Carlton A.

1984 "The Fallopian Tube: Physiology and Pathology." In *Infertility: Diagnosis and Management,* ed. James Aiman, 161–76. New York: Springer-Verlag.

Egypt National Population Council

1989 *Egypt Demographic and Health Survey 1988: Preliminary Report.* Demographic and Health Surveys Institute for Resource Development. New York: Westinghouse.

Ehrenreich, John

1978 "Introduction: The Cultural Crisis of Modern Medicine." In *The Cultural Crisis of Modern Medicine,* ed. John Ehrenreich, 1–35. New York: Monthly Review Press.

Eickelman, Dale F.

1976 *Moroccan Islam: Traditions and Society in a Pilgrimage Center.* Austin: University of Texas Press.

1982 "The Study of Islam in Local Contexts." *Contributions to Asian Studies* 17:1–16.

1989 *The Middle East: An Anthropological Approach.* 2d ed. Englewood Cliffs, NJ: Prentice-Hall.

Eickelman, Dale F., and James Piscatori

1990a "Social Theory in the Study of Muslim Societies." In *Muslim Travellers: Pilgrimage, Migration, and the Religious Imagination,* ed. Dale F. Eickelman and James Piscatori, 3–25. Berkeley: University of California Press.

1990b *Muslim Travellers: Pilgrimage, Migration, and the Religious Imagination,* ed. Dale F. Eickelman and James Piscatori. Berkeley: University of California Press.

el-Aswad, el-Sayed

1987 "Death Rituals in Rural Egyptian Society: A Symbolic Study." *Urban Anthropology* 16:205–41.

El Ghazzawy, Eman Fathy

1980 "Isolation of *Herpes simplex* Virus from the Cervix of Normal Females." Master's thesis, Faculty of Medicine, Alexandria University, Alexandria, Egypt.

El Hak, Gad El Hak Ali Gad

1981 *Medically Assisted Reproduction. Fatwā*. Cairo: Al-Azhar University.

El-Hamamsy, Laila

1972 "Belief Systems and Family Planning in Peasant Societies." In *Are Our Descendants Doomed?*, ed. H. Brown and E. Hutchings, Jr., 335–57. New York: Viking Press.

1973 *The Daya of Egypt: Survival in a Modernizing Society*. Pasadena: California Institute of Technology.

1985 "The Assertion of Egyptian Identity." In *Arab Society: Social Science Perspectives*, ed. Nicholas S. Hopkins and Saad Eddin Ibrahim, 39–63. Cairo: American University in Cairo Press.

Elhefnawy, Azza Mahmoud Mohamed

1985 "Characterization of *Neisseria gonorrhoeae* Isolated from Cases of Urethritis." Master's thesis, Faculty of Medicine, Alexandria University, Alexandria, Egypt.

El Lakany, Hayam Mahmoud Sameh

1988 "Prevalence of Genital Mycoplasmas and Chlamydiae in Infertile, Pregnant and Aborted Women." Ph.D. thesis, Faculty of Medicine, Alexandria University, Alexandria, Egypt.

El-Latiff, Sohair Saad Abd

1982 "Non Specific Urethritis in Males Due to *Herpes simplex* Virus." Master's thesis, Faculty of Medicine, University of Alexandria, Alexandria, Egypt.

El Malatawy, Amira

1985 *Daya Training Programme in Egypt*. Cairo: UNICEF.

El-Mehairy, Theresa

1984a "Attitudes of a Group of Egyptian Medical Students Towards Family Planning." *Social Science & Medicine* 19:131–34.

1984b *Medical Doctors: A Study of Role Concept and Job Satisfaction, The Egyptian Case*. Leiden: E. J. Brill.

El-Messiri, Sawsun

1978 *Ibn Al-Balad: A Concept of Egyptian Identity*. Leiden: E. J. Brill.

El-Mouelhy, Mawaheb T.

1990 "Family Planning and Maternal Health Care in Egypt." *Women and Therapy* 10:55–60.

Elon, Amos

1988 "Letter from Alexandria." *The New Yorker* (July 18) 64:42–53.

El Saadawi, Nawal

1980 *The Hidden Face of Eve: Women in the Arab World*. Boston: Beacon Press.

el Sendiony, M. F.

1974 "The Problem of Cultural Specificity of Mental Illness: The Egyptian Mental Disease and the *Zar* Ceremony." *Australian and New Zealand Journal of Psychiatry* 8:103–7.

El-Sokkari, Myrette Ahmed

1984 "Basic Needs, Inflation and the Poor of Egypt, 1970–1980." *Cairo Papers in Social Science* 7(2):1–103.

Elworthy, Frederick Thomas
1986 *The Evil Eye: An Account of This Ancient and Widespread Superstition.* New York: Julian Press.

Esposito, John L.
1982 *Women in Muslim Family Law.* Syracuse, NY: Syracuse University Press.
1991 *Islam: The Straight Path.* New York: Oxford University Press.

Fakhouri, Hani
1968 "The *Zar* Cult in an Egyptian Village." *Anthropological Quarterly* 41: 49–56.
1972 *Kafr El-Elow: An Egyptian Village in Transition.* New York: Holt, Rinehart and Winston.

Faour, Muhammad
1989 "Fertility Policy and Family Planning in the Arab Countries." *Studies in Family Planning* 20:254–63.

Farley, T. M. M., and E. M. Belsey
1988 *The Prevalence and Aetiology of Infertility.* Paper presented at the International Union for the Scientific Study of the Population, African Population Conference, Dakar, Senegal, November 1988.

Farquhar, Judith
1991 "Objects, Processes, and Female Infertility in Chinese Medicine." *Medical Anthropology Quarterly* (NS)5:370–99.

Fathalla, Eisa Ahmed
1986 "Study of Different Risk Factors for the Development of Pelvic Inflammatory Disease." Master's thesis, Faculty of Medicine, University of Alexandria, Alexandria, Egypt.

Fernea, Elizabeth Warnock, and Basima Qattan Bezirgan
1985 " 'A'ishah bint Abi Bakr: Wife of the Prophet Muhammad." In *Middle Eastern Muslim Women Speak,* ed. Elizabeth Warnock Fernea and Basima Qattan Bezirgan, 27–36. Austin: University of Texas Press.

Fernea, Robert A., and Elizabeth W. Fernea
1972 "Variation in Religious Observance among Islamic Women." In *Scholars, Saints, and Sufis: Muslim Religious Institutions since 1500,* ed. Nikki R. Keddie, 385–401. Berkeley: University of California Press.

Festinger, Leon
1957 *A Theory of Cognitive Dissonance.* Evanston, IL: Row, Peterson.

Forman, Michele R., Gillian L. Hundt, D. Towne, B. Graubard, Barbara Sullivan, Heinz W. Berendes, Baria Sarov, and Lechaim Naggan
1990 "The Forty-Day Rest Period and Infant Feeding Practices among Negev Bedouin Arab Women in Israel." *Medical Anthropology* 12:207–16.

Forster, E. M.
1986 *Alexandria: A History and a Guide.* London: Michael Haag.

Foucault, Michel
1977 *Discipline & Punish: The Birth of the Prison.* Translated by Alan Sheridan. New York: Vintage.

Fox, Karen F. A.
1988 "Social Marketing of Oral Rehydration Therapy and Contraceptives in Egypt." *Studies in Family Planning* 19:95–108.

Gadalla, Fawzy R. A., and Mahmoud Hassan
1970 *Different Role of Husband and Wife in Birth Control and Family Planning (Bab Shark District, Alexandria)*. Research Monograph No. 1. Alexandria, Egypt: Alexandria University Press.

Gadalla, Saad M.
1977 "The Influence of Reproductive Norms on Family Size and Fertility Behavior in Rural Egypt." In *Arab Society in Transition,* ed. Saad Eddin Ibrahim and Nicholas S. Hopkins, 323–42. Cairo: American University in Cairo Press.
1978 *Is There Hope? Fertility and Family Planning in a Rural Egyptian Community.* Cairo: American University in Cairo Press.

Gadalla, Saad, James McCarthy, and Oona Campbell
1985 "How the Number of Living Sons Influences Contraceptive Use in Menoufia Governorate, Egypt." *Studies in Family Planning* 16:164–69.

Gadalla, Saad, Nazek Nosseir, and Duff G. Gillespie
1980 "Household Distribution of Contraceptives in Rural Egypt." *Studies in Family Planning* 11:105–13.

Gadalla, Saad, and Hanna Rizk
1988 *Population Policy and Family Planning Communications Strategies in the Arab States Region*. Vol. 2 of *State of the Art in the Arab World.* UNESCO.

Galal, Osman
1992 "Obesity in Egypt: An Emerging Health and Cultural Issue." Paper presented at the 26th Annual Meeting of the Middle East Studies Association, Portland, Oregon.

Gallagher, Eugene B., and C. Maureen Searle
1984 "Cultural Forces in the Formation of the Saudi Medical Role." *Medical Anthropology* 8:210–21.
1985 "Health Services and the Political Culture of Saudi Arabia." *Social Science & Medicine* 21:251–62.

Gallagher, Nancy E.
1990 *Egypt's Other Wars: Epidemics and the Politics of Public Health.* Syracuse, NY: Syracuse University Press.

Gellner, Ernest
1969 *Saints of the Atlas.* London: Weidenfeld and Nicolson.

George, Susan
1977 *How the Other Half Dies: The Real Reasons for World Hunger.* Montclair, NJ: Allanheld, Osmun.

Ghamri, Lubna Abdullah
1986 "Isolation of Microbial Agents from Adult Females Suffering from Salpingo-oophoritis." Master's thesis, Faculty of Medicine, Alexandria University, Alexandria, Egypt.

Gilsenan, Michael
1973 *Saint and Sufi in Modern Egypt: An Essay in the Sociology of Religion.* Oxford: Clarendon Press.
1982 *Recognizing Islam: Religion and Society in the Modern Arab World.* New York: Pantheon Books.

Ginsburg, Faye, and Rayna Rapp
1991 "The Politics of Reproduction." *Annual Review of Anthropology* 20: 311–43.

Goffman, Erving
1963 *Stigma: Notes on the Management of Spoiled Identity.* Englewood Cliffs, NJ: Prentice-Hall.

Good, Byron J.
1977 "The Heart of What's the Matter: The Semantics of Illness in Iran." *Culture, Medicine, and Psychiatry* 1:25–58.

Good, Byron J., and Mary-Jo DelVecchio Good
1982 "Toward a Meaning-Centered Analysis of Popular Illness Categories: 'Fright-Illness' and 'Heart Distress' in Iran." In *Cultural Conceptions of Mental Health and Therapy,* ed. Anthony J. Marsella and Geoffrey M. White, 141–66. Dordrecht: D. Reidel.

Good, Byron J., Mary-Jo DelVecchio Good, and Robert Moradi
1985 "The Interpretation of Iranian Depressive Illness and Dysphoric Affect." In *Culture and Depression: Studies in the Anthropology and Cross-Cultural Psychiatry of Affect and Disorder,* ed. Arthur Kleinman and Byron Good, 369–428. Berkeley: University of California Press.

Good, Mary-Jo DelVecchio
1980 "Of Blood and Babies: The Relationship of Popular Islamic Physiology to Fertility." *Social Science & Medicine* 14B:147– 56.

Good, Mary-Jo DelVecchio, Byron J. Good, and Michael M. J. Fischer, eds.
1988 "Emotion, Illness and Healing in Middle Eastern Societies." Special issue of *Culture, Medicine, and Psychiatry* 12(1).

Gordon, Daniel
1991 "Female Circumcision and Genital Operations in Egypt and the Sudan: A Dilemma for Medical Anthropology." *Medical Anthropology Quarterly* (NS)5:3–14.

Gordon, Deborah R.
1988 "Tenacious Assumptions in Western Medicine." In *Biomedicine Examined,* ed. Margaret Lock and Deborah Gordon, 19–56. Dordrecht: Kluwer Academic.

Gottlieb, Alma
1988 "Menstrual Cosmology among the Beng of Ivory Coast." In *Blood Magic: The Anthropology of Menstruation,* ed. Thomas Buckley and Alma Gottlieb, 55–74. Berkeley: University of California Press.

Gramsci, Antonio
1971 *Selections from the Prison Notebooks.* London: Lawrence and Wishart.

Gran, Peter
1979 "Medical Pluralism in Arab and Egyptian History: An Overview of

Class Structures and Philosophies of the Main Phases." *Social Science & Medicine* 13B:339–48.

Green, Beverly B., Noel S. Weiss, and Janet R. Daling
1988 "Risk of Ovulatory Infertility in Relation to Body Weight." *Fertility and Sterility* 50:721–26.

Greenwood, Bernard
1981 "III(a) Perceiving Systems: Cold or Spirits? Choice and Ambiguity in Morocco's Pluralistic Medical System." *Social Science & Medicine* 15B:219–35.

Grossman, Peter
1986 *Abu Mina: A Guide to the Ancient Pilgrimage Center.* Cairo: Fotiadis & Co. Press.

Gruenbaum, Ellen
1982 "The Movement Against Clitoridectomy and Infibulation in Sudan: Public Health Policy and the Women's Movement." *Medical Anthropology Quarterly* 13:4–12.
1991 "The Islamic Movement, Development, and Health Education: Recent Changes in the Health of Rural Women in Central Sudan." *Social Science & Medicine* 33:637–45.

Haas, Gilbert G., Jr., and Phillip C. Galle
1984 "The Cervix in Reproduction." In *Infertility: Diagnosis and Management,* ed. James Aiman, 123–41. New York: Springer-Verlag.

Haddad, May
1988 "Women and Health in the Arab World." In *Women of the Arab World: The Coming Challenge,* ed. Nahid Toubia, 93–97. London: Zed Books.

Hafez, Ghada
1989 *Regional Overview of Maternal and Infant Morbidities and Mortalities.* WHO Report EM/CNS.TBA.VLG/5.

Hammami, Reza, and Martina Rieker
1988 "Feminist Orientalism and Orientalist Marxism." *New Left Review* 170:93–106.

Hammond, Mary G.
1984 "Anovulation and Ovulation Induction." In *Infertility: Diagnosis and Management,* ed. James Aiman, 101–21. New York: Springer-Verlag.

Hanafy, N. M., S. Zaki, R. Malaty, A. Awaad, and A. S. Mourad
1984 "Isolation of *Chlamydia trachomatis* from Cases of Cervicitis." *The Journal of the Egyptian Public Health Association* 59:453–64.

Harkness, Carla
1992 *The Infertility Book: A Comprehensive Medical & Emotional Guide.* Berkeley, CA: Celestial Arts.

Harrison, Gail G., Sahar S. Zaghloul, Osman M. Galal, and Azza Gabr
1993 "Breastfeeding and Weaning in a Poor Urban Neighborhood in Cairo, Egypt: Maternal Beliefs and Perceptions." *Social Science & Medicine* 36:1063–69.

Hart, George
1990 *The Legendary Past: Egyptian Myths.* Austin: University of Texas Press.

Hartz, Arthur J., Peter N. Barboriak, Alton Wong, K. Paul Katayama, and Alfred A. Rimm
1979 "The Association of Obesity with Infertility and Related Menstrual Abnormalities in Women." *International Journal of Obesity* 3:57–73.

Hayes, Rose Oldfield
1975 "Female Genital Mutilation, Fertility Control, Women's Roles, and the Patrilineage in Modern Sudan: A Functional Analysis." *American Ethnologist* 2:617–33.

Henifin, Mary Sue
1988 "Introduction: Women's Health and the New Reproductive Technologies." In *Embryos, Ethics, and Women's Rights: Exploring the New Reproductive Technologies,* ed. Elaine Hoffman Baruch, Amadeo F. D'Adamo, Jr., and Joni Seager, 1–7. Special issue of *Women & Health* 13 (1/2). New York: Haworth Press.

Hepburn, Lorraine
1992 *Ova-dose? Australian Women and the New Reproductive Technology.* Sydney: Allen and Unwin.

Holbrook, Sarah M.
1990 "Adoption, Infertility, and the New Reproductive Technologies: Problems and Prospects for Social Work and Welfare Policy." *Social Work* 35:333–37.

Honea, Kathryn L.
1993 "Understanding Unexplained Infertility." In *Textbook of Reproductive Medicine,* ed. Bruce R. Carr and Richard E. Blackwell, 537–45. Norwalk, CT: Appleton & Lange.

Hong, Sawon
1987 *Review of Training Programmes for Traditional Birth Attendants in Selected Countries.* New York: UNICEF.

Hunte, Pamela A.
1981 "The Role of the *Dai* (Traditional Birth Attendant) in Urban Afghanistan: Some Traditional and Adaptational Aspects." *Medical Anthropology* 5:17–25.

Ibrahim, Ezzeddin
1976 *An-Nawawi's Forty Hadith: An Anthology of the Sayings of the Prophet Muhammad.* Translated by Ezzeddin Ibrahim and Denys Johnson-Davies. Beirut: The Holy Koran Publishing House.

Inhorn, Marcia C.
1986 "Genital Herpes: An Ethnographic Inquiry into Being Discreditable in American Society." *Medical Anthropology Quarterly* 17:59–63.
1991 "*Umm Il-Ghayyib,* Mother of the Missing One: A Sociomedical Study of Infertility in Alexandria, Egypt." Ph.D. thesis, University of California, Berkeley.
1994a "Population, Poverty, and Gender Politics: Motherhood Pressures and Marital Crises in Poor Urban Egyptian Women's Lives." In *Popu-*

lation, Poverty, and Politics: Middle East Cities in Crisis, ed. Michael E. Bonine. Gainesville: University Press of Florida, forthcoming.

1994b *Interpreting Infertility: Medical Anthropological Perspectives,* ed. Marcia C. Inhorn. Special issue of *Social Science & Medicine,* forthcoming.

n.d. *Missing Motherhood: Infertility, Patriarchy, and the Politics of Gender in Egypt.* Philadelphia: University of Pennsylvania Press, forthcoming.

Inhorn, Marcia C., and Peter J. Brown

1990 "The Anthropology of Infectious Disease." *Annual Review of Anthropology* 19:89–117.

Inhorn, Marcia C., and Kimberly A. Buss

1993 "Infertility, Infection, and Iatrogenesis in Egypt: The Anthropological Epidemiology of Blocked Tubes." *Medical Anthropology* 15:1–28.

1994 "Ethnography, Epidemiology, and Infertility in Egypt." *Social Science & Medicine,* forthcoming.

Institute of Medicine

1979 *Health in Egypt: Recommendations for U.S. Assistance.* Prepared for Agency for International Development, Washington, DC.

Ismail, Edna

1989 *Training and Performance of TBAs and Midwives in the EMR.* WHO Report EM/CNS.TBA.VLG/6.

Janzen, John M.

1978 *The Quest for Therapy in Lower Zaire.* Berkeley: University of California Press.

1987 "Therapy Management: Concept, Reality, Process." *Medical Anthropology Quarterly* (NS)1:68–84.

Jones, Howard W., Jr.

1988 "Recent Advances in In Vitro Fertilization (IVF)." In *Human Reproduction: Current Status/Future Prospect,* ed. R. Iizuka and K. Semm, 65–79. Amsterdam: Elsevier.

Jordan, Brigitte

1987 "Crosscultural Theories of Conception, Gestation, and the Newborn: The Achievement of Personhood." Unpublished manuscript.

1993 *Birth in Four Cultures: A Crosscultural Investigation of Childbirth in Yucatan, Holland, Sweden, and the United States.* 4th ed. Prospect Heights, IL: Waveland Press.

Kader, Soha Abdel

1987 *Egyptian Women in a Changing Society, 1899–1987.* Boulder, CO: Lynne Rienner.

Kandela, Peter

1988 "Egypt: Medical Care, Public and Private." *The Lancet* (July 2):34–35.

Katz, Sydney S., and Selig H. Katz

1987 "An Evaluation of Traditional Therapy for Barrenness." *Medical Anthropology Quarterly* (NS)1:394–405.

Keddie, Nikki R.

1979 "Problems in the Study of Middle Eastern Women." *International Journal of Middle East Studies* 10:225–40.

Kelsey, Jennifer L., W. Douglas Thompson, and Alfred S. Evans
1986 *Methods in Observational Epidemiology.* New York: Oxford University Press.
Kennedy, John G.
1967 "Nubian Zar Ceremonies as Psychotherapy." *Human Organization* 26:185–94.
1970 "Circumcision and Excision in Egyptian Nubia." *Man* 5:175–91.
1978a "*Mushāhara:* A Nubian Concept of Supernatural Danger and the Theory of Taboo." In *Nubian Ceremonial Life: Studies in Islamic Syncretism and Cultural Change,* ed. John G. Kennedy, 125–50. Berkeley: University of California Press.
1978b *Nubian Ceremonial Life: Studies in Islamic Syncretism and Cultural Change,* ed. John G. Kennedy. Berkeley: University of California Press.
1987 *The Flower of Paradise: The Institutionalized Use of the Drug Qat in North Yemen.* Dordrecht: D. Reidel.
Khattab, Hind Abou Seoud
1983 "The Daya: Knowledge and Practice in Maternal-Child Health Care." Report for Newborn Care Project, Cairo, Egypt.
Kholeif, Laila Hussein
1980 "*Chlamydia trachomatis* in Cervices of Women in Late Pregnancy." Master's thesis, Faculty of Medicine, Alexandria University, Alexandria, Egypt.
Kirmayer, Laurence J.
1988 "Mind and Body as Metaphors: Hidden Values in Biomedicine." In *Biomedicine Examined,* ed. Margaret Lock and Deborah Gordon, 57–93. Dordrecht: Kluwer Academic.
Kissebah, Ahmed H., David S. Freedman, and Alan N. Peiris
1989 "Health Risks of Obesity." *Medical Clinics of North America* 73:111–38.
Klein, Renate D.
1989a *Infertility: Women Speak Out About Their Experiences of Reproductive Medicine.* London: Pandora Press.
1989b *The Exploitation of a Desire: Women's Experiences with In Vitro Fertilisation—An Exploratory Survey.* Women's Studies Summer Institute, Deakin University, Australia.
Kleinman, Arthur M.
1992 "Local Worlds of Suffering: An Interpersonal Focus for Ethnographies of Illness Experience." *Qualitative Health Research* 2:127–34.
Koenig, Barbara A.
1988 "The Technological Imperative in Medical Practice: The Social Creation of a 'Routine' Treatment. In *Biomedicine Examined,* ed. Margaret Lock and Deborah Gordon, 465–96. Dordrecht: Kluwer Academic.
Kotkat, Amira Mahmoud Saad Ahmed
1978 "A Study of the Prevalence of *Trichomonas vaginalis* among Gynaecological Patients Attending Shatby Hospital." Master's thesis, High Institute of Public Health, Alexandria, Egypt.

Kuhnke, LaVerne
1990 *Lives at Risk: Public Health in Nineteenth-Century Egypt.* Berkeley: University of California Press.

Laborie, Francoise
1987 "Looking for Mothers You Only Find Fetuses." In *Made to Order: The Myth of Reproductive and Gender Progress,* ed. Patricia Spallone and Deborah Lynn Steinberg, 48–57. Oxford: Pergamon.

Lamb, Michael E., ed.
1987 *The Father's Role: Cross-Cultural Perspectives.* Hillsdale, NJ: Lawrence Erlbaum.

Lane, Sandra D., and Afaf I. Meleis
1991 "Roles, Work, Health Perceptions and Health Resources of Women: A Study in an Egyptian Delta Hamlet." *Social Science & Medicine* 33:1197–1208.

Lane, Sandra D., and Marcia Inhorn Millar
1987 "The 'Hierarchy of Resort' Reexamined: Status and Class Differentials as Determinants of Therapy for Eye Disease in the Egyptian Delta." *Urban Anthropology* 16:151–82.

Lane, Sandra D., and Robert A. Rubinstein
1991 "The Use of *Fatwās* in the Production of Reproductive Health Policy in Egypt." Paper presented at the 90th Annual Meeting of the American Anthropological Association, Chicago.

Leake, Chauncey D.
1952 *The Old Egyptian Medical Papyri.* Lawrence: University of Kansas Press.

Liu, James H.
1993 "Anovulation of CNS Origin: Functional and Miscellaneous Causes." In *Textbook of Reproductive Medicine,* ed. Bruce R. Carr and Richard E. Blackwell, 281–95. Norwalk, CT: Appleton & Lange.

Lock, Margaret
1988 "Introduction." In *Biomedicine Examined,* ed. Margaret Lock and Deborah Gordon, 3–10. Dordrecht: Kluwer Academic.

Lock, Margaret, and Deborah R. Gordon
1988a "Relationships Between Society, Culture, and Biomedicine: An Introduction to the Essays." In *Biomedicine Examined,* ed. Margaret Lock and Deborah Gordon, 11–16. Dordrecht: Kluwer Academic.
1988b *Biomedicine Examined.* Margaret Lock and Deborah Gordon, eds. Dordrecht: Kluwer Academic.

Lock, Margaret, and Nancy Scheper-Hughes
1990 "A Critical-Interpretive Approach in Medical Anthropology: Rituals and Routines of Discipline and Dissent." In *Medical Anthropology: A Handbook of Theory and Method,* ed. Thomas M. Johnson and Carolyn F. Sargent, 47–62. New York: Greenwood Press.

Longrigg, James
1981 "Superlative Achievement and Comparative Neglect: Alexandrian

Medical Science and the Modern Historical Research." *History of Science* 19:155–200.

MacCormack, Carol P.
1989 "Technology and Women's Health in Developing Countries." *International Journal of Health Services* 19:681–92.

MacLeod, Arlene Elowe
1991 *Accommodating Protest: Working Women, the New Veiling, and Change in Cairo.* New York: Columbia University Press.

Mai, Francois M.
1978 "The Diagnosis and Treatment of Psychogenic Infertility." *Infertility* 1:109–25.

Maloney, Clarence, ed.
1976 *The Evil Eye.* New York: Columbia University Press.

Manniche, Lise
1989 *An Ancient Egyptian Herbal.* Austin: University of Texas Press.

Martin, Emily
1987 *The Woman in the Body: A Cultural Analysis of Reproduction.* Boston: Beacon Press.
1991 "The Egg and the Sperm: How Science Has Constructed a Romance Based on Stereotypical Male-Female Roles." *Signs* 16:485–501.

Mausner, Judith S., and Shira Kramer
1985 *Epidemiology—An Introductory Text.* Philadelphia: W. B. Saunders.

McClain, Carol Shepherd
1989 "Reinterpreting Women in Healing Roles." In *Women as Healers: Cross-Cultural Perspectives,* ed. Carol Shepherd McClain, 1–19. New Brunswick, NJ: Rutgers University Press.

McConnell, John D.
1993 "Diagnosis and Treatment of Male Infertility." In *Textbook of Reproductive Medicine,* ed. Bruce R. Carr and Richard E. Blackwell, 453–68. Norwalk, CT: Appleton & Lange.

McFalls, J. A., Jr., and M. H. McFalls
1984 *Disease and Fertility.* Orlando, FL: Academic Press.

McKinlay, John B., ed.
1984 *Issues in the Political Economy of Health Care.* New York: Tavistock.

McNay, Lois
1991 "The Foucauldian Body and the Exclusion of Experience." *Hypatia* 6:125–39.

McShane, Patricia M.
1988 "*In Vitro* Fertilization, GIFT and Related Technologies—Hope in a Test Tube." In *Embryos, Ethics, and Women's Rights: Exploring the New Reproductive Technologies,* ed. Elaine Hoffman Baruch, Amadeo F. D'Adamo, Jr., and Joni Seager, 31–46. New York: Haworth Press.

Mehanna, Mohammed Taha Riad
1989 "Prevalence of *Chlamydia trachomatis* Infection among Cases of Tubal Infertility and Tubal Ectopic Pregnancy." Master's thesis, Faculty of Medicine, University of Alexandria, Alexandria, Egypt.

Meinardus, Otto

1967 "Mythological, Historical and Sociological Aspects of the Practice of Female Circumcision among the Egyptians." *Acta Ethnographica Academiae Scientiarum Hungaricae* 16:387–97.

Mernissi, Fatima

1977 "Women, Saints, and Sanctuaries." *Signs* 3:101–12.

Meyers, David W.

1990 *The Human Body and the Law.* Stanford, CA: Stanford University Press.

Mies, Maria

1987 "Why Do We Need All This? A Call Against Genetic Engineering and Reproductive Technology." In *Made to Order: The Myth of Reproductive and Genetic Progress,* ed. Patricia Spallone and Deborah Lynn Steinberg, 34–47. Oxford: Pergamon.

Millar, Marcia Inhorn

1987 "Genital Chlamydial Infection: A Role for Social Scientists." *Social Science & Medicine* 25:1289–99.

Millar, Marcia Inhorn, and Sandra D. Lane

1988 "Ethno-ophthalmology in the Egyptian Delta: An Historical Systems Approach to Ethnomedicine in the Middle East." *Social Science & Medicine* 26:651–57.

Mitchell, Tim

1988 *Colonising Egypt.* Cambridge: Cambridge University Press.

1991 "America's Egypt: Discourse of the Development Industry." *Middle East Report* 21(2):18–36.

Modell, Judith

1989 "Last Chance Babies: Interpretations of Parenthood in an In Vitro Fertilization Program." *Medical Anthropology Quarterly* (NS) 3:124–38.

Morinis, Alan

1992 Introduction. In *Sacred Journeys: The Anthropology of Pilgrimage,* ed. Alan Morinis, 1–28. Westport, CT: Greenwood Press.

Morsy, Soheir A.

1978a "Sex Differences and Folk Illness in an Egyptian Village." In *Women in the Muslim World,* ed. Lois Beck and Nikki Keddie, 599–616. Cambridge, MA: Harvard University Press.

1978b "Sex Roles, Power, and Illness in an Egyptian Village." *American Ethnologist* 5:137–50.

1979 "The Missing Link in Medical Anthropology: The Political Economy of Health." *Reviews in Anthropology* 6:349–63.

1980a "Body Concepts and Health Care: Illustrations from an Egyptian Village." *Human Organization* 39:92–96.

1980b "Health and Illness as Symbols of Social Differentiation in an Egyptian Village." *Anthropological Quarterly* 53:153–61.

1981 "Towards a Political Economy of Health: A Critical Note on the Medical Anthropology of the Middle East." *Social Science & Medicine* 15B:159–63.

1982 "Childbirth in an Egyptian Village. In *An Anthropology of Human Birth,* ed. Margarita A. Kay, 147–74. Philadelphia: F. A. Davis.

1985 "The Social Dimension of NORPLANT Use in Assiut: Report of a Preliminary Inquiry." Report to the Population Council and the Department of Obstetrics and Gynaecology, Faculty of Medicine, Assiut University.

1988 "Islamic Clinics in Egypt: The Cultural Elaboration of Biomedical Hegemony." *Medical Anthropology Quarterly* (NS)2:355–69.

1990 "Political Economy in Medical Anthropology." In *Medical Anthropology: A Handbook of Theory and Method,* ed. Thomas M. Johnson and Carolyn F. Sargent, 26–46. New York: Greenwood Press.

1991 "Spirit Possession in Egyptian Ethnomedicine: Origins, Comparison and Historical Specificity." In *Women's Medicine: The Zar-Bori Cult in Africa and Beyond,* ed. I. M. Lewis, Ahmed Al-Safi, and Sayyid Hureiz, 189–208. Edinburgh: Edinburgh University Press.

1993 *Gender, Sickness, & Healing in Rural Egypt: Ethnography in Historical Context.* Boulder, CO: Westview Press.

n.d. "Biotechnology and the International Politics of Population Control: Long-term Contraception in Egypt." Unpublished ms.

Mtimavalye, L. A., and M. A. Belsey

1987 *Infertility and Sexually Transmitted Disease: Major Problems in Maternal and Child Health and Family Planning.* Technical background paper prepared for the International Conference on Better Health for Women and Children Through Family Planning, Nairobi, Kenya, October 1987.

Muir, D. G., and M. A. Belsey

1980 "Pelvic Inflammatory Disease and Its Consequences in the Developing World." *American Journal of Obstetrics and Gynecology* 138:913–28.

Musallam, B. F.

1983 *Sex and Society in Islam: Birth Control Before the Nineteenth Century.* Cambridge: Cambridge University Press.

Myntti, Cynthia

1988a "Hegemony and Healing in Rural North Yemen." *Social Science & Medicine* 27:515–20.

1988b "The Social, Economic and Cultural Context of Women's Health and Fertility in Rural North Yemen." In *Micro Approaches to Demographic Research,* ed. V. Hill and A. Hill. London: Routledge Paul.

1993 "Social Determinants of Child Health in Yemen." *Social Science & Medicine* 37:233–40.

Nadim, Nawal El Messiri

1980 *Rural Health Care in Egypt.* Ottawa: International Development Research Centre.

Nelson, Cynthia

1971 "Self, Spirit Possession and World View: An Illustration from Egypt." *International Journal of Social Psychiatry* 17:194–209.

Niazi, N. M.
1988 *The Egyptian Prescription.* Cairo: Elias Modern Press.
Nichter, Mark
1991 "Ethnomedicine: Diverse Trends, Common Linkages." Commentary. *Medical Anthropology* 13:137–71.
Nsiah-Jefferson, Laurie, and Elaine J. Hall
1989 "Reproductive Technology: Perspectives and Implications for Low-Income Women and Women of Color." In *Healing Technology: Feminist Perspectives,* ed. Kathryn Strother Ratcliff, 93–117. Ann Arbor: University of Michigan Press.
Oakley, Ann
1987 "From Walking Wombs to Test-Tube Babies." In *Reproductive Technologies: Gender, Motherhood and Medicine,* ed. Michelle Stanworth, 36–56. Cambridge: Polity Press.
Ober, C., S. Elias, E. O'Brien, D. D. Kostyu, W. W. Hauck, and A. Bombard
1988 "HLA Sharing and Fertility in Hutterite Couples: Evidence for Prenatal Selection Against Compatible Fetuses." *American Journal of Reproductive Immunology and Microbiology* 18:111–15.
Olson, Emelie A.
1983 "Situational and Attitudinal Factors in Fertility Limitation in Turkey." *Medical Anthropology* 7:47–66.
Omran, Abdel Rahim
1992 *Family Planning in the Legacy of Islam.* London: Routledge.
Omran, Abdel Rahim, and Farzaneh Roudi
1993 "The Middle East Population Puzzle." *Population Bulletin* 48(1) (July):1–40.
Osherson, Samuel, and Lorna Amarasingham
1981 "The Machine Metaphor in Medicine." In *Social Contexts of Health, Illness and Patient Care,* ed. E. Mishler, 218–49. Cambridge: Cambridge University Press.
Pick, W. M., M. N. Hoffman, J. E. Myers, J. M. L. Klopper, and D. Cooper
1990 "Women, Health and Urbanisation." *South African Medical Journal* 77:553–54.
Pillsbury, Barbara L. K.
1978 *Traditional Health Care in the Near East.* Washington, DC: USAID.
1982 "Policy and Evaluation Perspectives on Traditional Health Practitioners in National Health Care Systems." *Social Science & Medicine* 16:1825–34.
Powledge, Tabitha
1988 "Reproductive Technologies and the Bottom Line." In *Embryos, Ethics, and Women's Rights: Exploring the New Reproductive Technologies,* ed. Elaine Hoffman Baruch, Amadeo F. D'Adamo, Jr., and Joni Seager, 203–9. Special issue of *Women & Health* 13 (1/2). New York: Haworth Press.
Preston, James J.
1992 "Spiritual Magnetism: An Organizing Principle for the Study of Pil-

grimage." In *Sacred Journeys: The Anthropology of Pilgrimage,* ed. Alan Morinis, 31–46. Westport, CT: Greenwood Press.

Racy, John
1969 "Death in Arab Culture." *Annals of the New York Academy of Science* 164:871–80.

Rapp, Rayna
1988 "Moral Pioneers: Women, Men and Fetuses on a Frontier of Reproductive Technology." In *Embryos, Ethics, and Women's Rights: Exploring the New Reproductive Technologies,* ed. Elaine Hoffman Baruch, Amadeo F. D'Adamo, Jr., and Joni Seager, 101–16. Special issue of *Women & Health* 13 (1/2). New York: Haworth Press.

Ratcliff, Kathryn Strother
1989a *Healing Technology: Feminist Perspectives.* Kathryn Strother Ratcliff, ed. Ann Arbor: University of Michigan Press.
1989b "Health Technologies for Women: Whose Health? Whose Technology?" In *Healing Technology: Feminist Perspectives,* ed. Kathryn Strother Ratcliff, 173–98. Ann Arbor: University of Michigan Press.

Rebar, Robert W.
1993 "Assessment of the Female Patient." In *Textbook of Reproductive Medicine,* ed. Bruce E. Carr and Richard E. Blackwell, 247–63. Norwalk, CT: Appleton & Lange.

Reeves, Edward B.
1990 *The Hidden Government: Ritual, Clientelism, and Legitimation in Northern Egypt.* Salt Lake City: University of Utah Press.

Renaud, Marc
1978 "On the Structural Constraints to State Intervention in Health." In *The Cultural Crisis of Modern Medicine,* ed. John Ehrenreich, 101–20. New York: Monthly Review Press.

Richters, Annemiek
1992 Introduction. *Social Science & Medicine* 35:747–51.

Rosenberg, Lior, Amiram Sagi, Nador Stahl, Baruch Greber, and Patrick Ben-Meir
1988 "*Maqua* (Therapeutic Burn) as an Indicator of Underlying Disease." *Plastic and Reconstructive Surgery* 82:277–80.

Rothman, Barbara Katz
1988 "Reproductive Technology and the Commodification of Life." In *Embryos, Ethics, and Women's Rights: Exploring the New Reproductive Technologies,* ed. Elaine Hoffman Baruch, Amadeo F. D'Adamo, Jr., and Joni Seager, 95–100. Special issue of *Women & Health* 13 (1/2). New York: Haworth Press.

Rowland, Robyn
1987 "Of Women Born, but for How Long? The Relationship of Women to the New Reproductive Technologies and the Issue of Choice." In *Made to Order: The Myth of Reproductive and Genetic Progress,* ed. Patricia Spallone and Deborah Lynn Steinberg, 67–83. Oxford: Pergamon.
1992 *Living Laboratories: Women and Reproductive Technologies.* Bloomington: Indiana University Press.

Roy, Judith M.

1990 "Surgical Gynecology." In *Women, Health and Medicine in America: A Historical Handbook,* ed. Rima D. Apple, 173–95. New York: Garland.

Rubinstein, Robert A., and Sandra D. Lane

1990 "International Health and Development." In *Medical Anthropology: A Handbook of Theory and Method,* ed. Thomas M. Johnson and Carolyn F. Sargent, 367–90. New York: Greenwood Press.

Ruddick, William

1988 "A Short Answer to 'Who Decides?'" In *Embryos, Ethics, and Women's Rights: Exploring the New Reproductive Technologies,* ed. Elaine Hoffman Baruch, Amadeo F. D'Adamo, Jr., and Joni Seager, 73–76. Special issue of *Women & Health* 13 (1/2). New York: Haworth Press.

Rugh, Andrea B.

1982 Foreword to *Khul-Khaal: Five Egyptian Women Tell Their Stories,* by Nayra Atiya, vii–xxii. Syracuse, NY: Syracuse University Press.

1984 *Family in Contemporary Egypt.* Syracuse, NY: Syracuse University Press.

1986 *Reveal and Conceal: Dress in Contemporary Egypt.* Cairo: American University in Cairo Press.

Safa, Kaveh

1988 "Reading Saedi's *Ahl-e Hava:* Pattern and Significance in Spirit Possession Beliefs on the Southern Coasts of Iran." *Culture, Medicine, and Psychiatry* 12:85–112.

Sallam, Hassan N.

1989 *The Problem of Infertility in Theory and Practice.* Alexandria, Egypt: University of Alexandria.

Sallam, S. A., M. N. Hassan, O. T. Ali, and E. Fares

1982 "Epidemiology of Gonorrhoea among Married Females Presenting with Leucorrhoea." *The Bulletin of the High Institute of Public Health* 12:65–80.

Sandelowski, Margarete

1991 "Compelled to Try: The Never-Enough Quality of Conceptive Technology." *Medical Anthropology Quarterly* (NS) 5:29–47.

1993 *With Child in Mind: Studies of the Personal Encounter with Infertility.* Philadelphia: University of Pennsylvania Press.

Sandelowski, Margarete, Betty G. Harris, and Beth Perry Black

1992 "Relinquishing Infertility: The Work of Pregnancy for Infertile Couples." *Qualitative Health Research* 2:282–301.

Sandwith, F. M.

1905 *The Medical Diseases of Egypt.* London: Kimpton.

Savage, Olayinka Margaret Njikam

1992 "Artificial Donor Insemination in Yaounde: Some Socio-Cultural Considerations." *Social Science & Medicine* 35:907–13.

Scheepers, Lidwien M.

1991 "*Jidda:* The Traditional Midwife of Yemen?" *Social Science & Medicine* 33:959–62.

Scheper-Hughes, Nancy, and Margaret M. Lock
1987 "The Mindful Body: A Prolegomenon to Future Work in Medical Anthropology." *Medical Anthropology Quarterly* 1:6–41.
Schiffer, Robert L.
1988 "The Exploding City." *Populi* 15:49–54.
Schroeder, Patricia
1988 "Infertility and the World Outside." *Fertility and Sterility* 49:765–67.
Sebai, Zohair A.
1974 "Knowledge, Attitudes and Practice of Family Planning: Profile of a Bedouin Community in Saudi Arabia." *Journal of Biosocial Science* 6:453–61.
Seibel, Michelle M.
1993 "Ovarian Dysfunction and Anovulation." In *Textbook of Reproductive Medicine,* ed. Bruce R. Carr and Richard E. Blackwell, 355–69. Norwalk, CT: Appleton & Lange.
Seifelnasr, Ahmad
1986 *Regional Development and Determinants of Internal Migration in Egypt: An Empirical Investigation.* Dokki, Egypt: The Population Council.
Serour, Gamal I., ed.
1992 *Proceedings of the First International Conference on "Bioethics in Human Reproduction Research in the Muslim World."* Cairo: International Islamic Center for Population Studies & Research, Al-Azhar University.
Serour, G. I., M. H. Badraoui, H. M. El Agizi, A. F. Hamed, and F. Abdel-Aziz
1989 "Laparoscopic Adhesiolysis for Infertile Patients with Pelvic Adhesive Disease." *International Journal of Gynecology and Obstetrics* 30:249–52.
Serour, G. I., M. El Ghar, and R. T. Mansour
1990 "In Vitro Fertilization and Embryo Transfer, Ethical Aspects in Techniques in the Muslim World." *Population Sciences* 9:45–54.
1991 "Infertility: A Health Problem in Muslim World." *Population Sciences* 10:41–58.
Serour, G. I., A. F. Hamed, H. Al-Agazi, M. Sultan, and M. Hegab
1988 "Al-Azhar Experience with Microsurgery." *Journal of the Egyptian Society of Obstetrics and Gynecology* 14:9–16.
Serour, Gamal I., and A. R. Omran
1992 *Ethical Guidelines for Human Reproduction Research in the Muslim World.* Cairo: International Islamic Center for Population Studies & Research, Al-Azhar University.
Seton-Williams, Veronica, and Peter Stocks
1988 *Blue Guide: Egypt.* London: A & C Black.
Shannon, Thomas A.
1988 "*In Vitro* Fertilization: Ethical Issues." In *Embryos, Ethics, and Women's Rights: Exploring the New Reproductive Technologies,* ed. Elaine Hoffman Baruch, Amadeo F. D'Adamo, Jr., and Joni Seager, 155–65. Special issue of *Women & Health* 13 (1/2). New York: Haworth Press.
Shiloh, Ailon
1968 "The Interaction Between the Middle Eastern and Western Systems of Medicine." *Social Science & Medicine* 2:235–48.

Siebers, Tobin
1983 *The Mirror of Medusa.* Berkeley: University of California Press.
Simons, Ronald C., and Charles C. Hughes, eds.
1985 *The Culture-Bound Syndromes: Folk Illnesses of Psychiatric and Anthropological Interest.* Dordrecht: D. Reidel.
Singer, A., and J. A. Jordan
1976 "The Anatomy of the Cervix." In *The Cervix,* ed. J. A. Jordan and A. Singer, 13–36. Philadelphia: W. B. Saunders.
Sonbol, Amira el Azhary
1991 *The Creation of a Medical Profession in Egypt, 1800–1922.* Syracuse, NY: Syracuse University Press.
1992 "Adoption in Islamic Society: A Historical Survey." Paper presented at the 26th Annual Meeting of the Middle East Studies Association, Portland, Oregon.
Speert, Harold
1958 *Obstetric and Gynecologic Milestones: Essays in Eponymy.* New York: Macmillan.
1973 *Iconographia Gyniatrica: A Pictorial History of Gynecology and Obstetrics.* Philadelphia: F. A. Davis.
1980 *Obstetrics and Gynecology in America: A History.* Chicago: The American College of Obstetricians and Gynecologists.
Stanworth, Michelle
1987a *Reproductive Technologies: Gender, Motherhood and Medicine.* Michelle Stanworth, ed. Cambridge: Polity Press.
1987b "Reproductive Technologies and the Deconstruction of Motherhood." In *Reproductive Technologies: Gender, Motherhood and Medicine,* ed. Michelle Stanworth, 10–35. Cambridge: Polity Press.
Steinkampf, Michael P., and Richard E. Blackwell
1993 "Ovulation Induction." In *Textbook of Reproductive Medicine,* ed. Bruce R. Carr and Richard E. Blackwell, 469–80. Norwalk, CT: Appleton & Lange.
Stokes, C. Shannon, Wayne A. Schutjer, and John R. Poindexter
1983 "A Note on Desired Family Size and Contraceptive Use in Rural Egypt." *Journal of Biosocial Science* 15:59–65.
Stradtman, Earl W., Jr.
1993 "Thyroid Dysfunction and Ovulatory Disorders." In *Textbook of Reproductive Medicine,* ed. Bruce R. Carr and Richard E. Blackwell, 297–321. Norwalk, CT: Appleton & Lange.
Strathern, Marilyn
1992 *Reproducing the Future: Anthropology, Kinship, and the New Reproductive Technologies.* New York: Routledge.
Stycos, J. Mayone, Hussein Abdel Aziz Sayed, Roger Avery, and Samuel Fridman
1988 *Community Development and Family Planning: An Egyptian Experiment.* Boulder, CO: Westview Press.
Sukkary, Soheir
1981 "She Is No Stranger: The Traditional Midwife in Egypt." *Medical Anthropology* 5:27–34.

Sukkary-Stolba, Soheir

1985 "Indigenous Fertility Regulating Methods in Two Egyptian Villages." In *Women's Medicine: A Cross-Cultural Study of Indigenous Fertility Regulation,* ed. Lucile F. Newman, 77–97. New Brunswick, NJ: Rutgers University Press.

1987 "Food Classifications and the Diets of Young Children in Rural Egypt." *Social Science & Medicine* 25:401–4.

Sullivan, Earl L.

1986 *Women in Egyptian Public Life.* Cairo: American University in Cairo Press.

Swagman, Charles F.

1989 "Fijaʿ: Fright and Illness in Highland Yemen." *Social Science & Medicine* 28:381–88.

Tackholm, Vivi, and Mohammed Drar

1950 *Flora of Egypt.* Vol. 2. Cairo: Fouad I University Press.

Tapper, Nancy

1990 "*Ziyaret:* Gender, Movement, and Exchange in a Turkish Community." In *Muslim Travellers: Pilgrimage, Migration, and the Religious Imagination,* ed. Dale F. Eickelman and James Piscatori, 236–55. Berkeley: University of California Press.

Tapper, Nancy, and Richard Tapper

1987 "The Birth of the Prophet: Ritual and Gender in Turkish Islam." *Man* (NS)22:69–92.

Trostle, James

1986 "Early Work in Anthropology and Epidemiology: From Social Medicine to the Germ Theory, 1840 to 1920." In *Anthropology and Epidemiology: Interdisciplinary Approaches to the Study of Health and Disease,* ed. Craig R. Janes, Ron Stall, and Sandra M. Gifford, 35–57. Dordrecht: D. Reidel.

Tucker, Judith E.

1985 *Women in Nineteenth-Century Egypt.* Cambridge: Cambridge University Press.

Turner, Victor W.

1964 *Betwixt and Between: The Liminal Period in* Rites de Passage. American Ethnological Society Proceedings (1964):4–20.

1969 *The Ritual Process.* Ithaca, NY: Cornell University Press.

1974 *Dramas, Fields, and Metaphors.* Ithaca, NY: Cornell University Press.

Turshen, Meredeth

1984 *The Political Ecology of Disease in Tanzania.* New Brunswick, NJ: Rutgers University Press.

1991 "Taking Women Seriously: Toward Democratic Health Care in Africa." In *Women and Health in Africa,* ed. Meredeth Turshen, 205–20. Trenton, NJ: Africa World Press.

Ullman, Manfred

1978 *Islamic Medicine.* Edinburgh: Edinburgh University Press.

Underwood, Peter, and Zdenka Underwood
1980 "New Spells for Old: Expectations and Realities of Western Medicine in a Remote Tribal Society in Yemen, Arabia." In *Changing Disease Patterns and Human Behavior,* ed. N. F. Stanley and R. A. Joske, 271–97. London: Academic Press.

UNICEF
1985 *"Review and Analysis" of Daya Training Programme in Egypt.* Cairo: UNICEF.

United Nations
1991 *The World's Women, 1970–1990: Trends and Statistics.* New York: United Nations.

U.S. Congress, Office of Technology Assessment
1988 *Infertility: Medical and Social Choices.* OTA-BA-358. Washington, DC: U.S. Government Printing Office.

Valsiner, Joan
1989 *Human Development and Culture.* New York: Lexington Books.

van der Kwaak, Anke
1992 "Female Circumcision and Gender Identity: A Questionable Alliance?" *Social Science & Medicine* 35:777–87.

Van Gennep, A.
1960 *The Rites of Passage.* Chicago: University of Chicago Press.

van Spijk, Marileen van der Most, Hoda Youssef Fahmy, and Sonja Zimmerman
1982 *Remember to Be Firm: Life Histories of Three Egyptian Women.* Leiden: Research Centre Women and Development, State University of Leiden.

Walker, John
1934 *Folk Medicine in Modern Egypt: Being the Relevant Parts of the* Tibb al-Rukka *or* Old Wives' Medicine *of ʿAbd Al-Raḥmān Ismāʿīl.* London: Luzac.

Watson, Helen
1992 *Women in the City of the Dead.* London: Hurst.

Weigle, Marta
1989 *Creation and Procreation: Feminist Reflections on Mythologies of Cosmogony and Parturition.* Philadelphia: University of Pennsylvania Press.

Wikan, Unni
1980 *Life Among the Poor in Cairo.* London: Tavistock.

Winkel, Craig A.
1993 "Diagnosis and Treatment of Uterine Pathology." In *Textbook of Reproductive Medicine,* ed. Bruce R. Carr and Richard E. Blackwell, 481–505. Norwalk, CT: Appleton & Lange.

World Bank
1984 *World Development Report 1984.* Washington, DC: World Bank.

World Health Organization
1975 *The Epidemiology of Infertility: Report of a WHO Scientific Group.* World Health Organization Technical Report Series No. 582.

1987a "Infections, Pregnancies, and Infertility: Perspectives on Prevention." *Fertility and Sterility* 47:964–68.

1987b *WHO Laboratory Manual for the Examination of Human Semen and Semen-Cervical Mucus Interaction*. Cambridge: Cambridge University Press.

1989 *Guidelines on Diagnosis and Treatment of Infertility*. Copenhagen: World Health Organization Regional Office for Europe.

Young, William C.

1993 "The Ka'ba, Gender, and the Rites of Pilgrimage." *International Journal of Middle East Studies* 25:285–300.

Youssef, Nadia Haggag

1978 "The Status and Fertility Patterns of Muslim Women." In *Women in the Muslim World*, ed. Lois Beck and Nikki Keddie, 69–99. Cambridge, MA: Harvard University Press.

Zander, Josef

1988 "History of Human Reproduction Science." In *Human Reproduction: Current Status/Future Prospect*, ed. R. Iizuka and K. Semm, 3–18. Amsterdam: Elsevier.

Index

Abortion: and Safe Motherhood, 348–49; as iatrogenic, 19–20, 255; by midwives, 81, 86; illegal, 385 n.9; punishment for, 217. See also *Kabsa*
Abu Dardar, 226
Abu-Lughod, Janet, 17
Abu-Lughod, Lila, 27, 37, 381 n.14, 386 n.10
Acquired immune deficiency syndrome (AIDS), 13, 18, 231
Adoption, 5, 331, 338, 393 n.2
Adultery, artificial insemination by donor as, 331–32
Africa, 13, 18
Ahmed, Leila, 60
Al-Azhar University, 330, 340, 390 n.1
Alexander the Great, 42–43, 55–56
Alexandria: Arab invasion of, 44; as an Egyptian city, 35; as a pilgrimage center, 225–26; economic conditions in, 42; Europeanization of, 45; foreigners in, 45–46; harbor of, 46; history of, 42–46, 381 n.1; history of medicine in, 52; infertility services in, 278, 281, 310; Islamic revival in, 47; medical school in, 43–44, 55, 57, 381 n.1; Mouseion of, 43; Muhammad Ali's rule over, 45; Ottoman control of, 44; pharmacies in, 299; population trends in, 18, 46; Ptolemaic period in, 43–44; qualities of, 46–47; Roman Empire in, 44
al-Ghazali, 59
Al-Suyuti, 61
Alubo, S. Ogoh, 301
Amulets: against the evil eye, 131; as infertility therapy, 99, 179, 203, 244; in prophetic medicine, 61; in sorcery nullification, 194–95; made by blessed *shaikh*s, 110, 220, 224
Anal therapies, for infertility, 82, 99, 188–89
Angels, in infertility causation, xxiii, 196–98, 213
Anglo-Egyptian treaty, 45
Animals: and male-factor infertility, 190; and shock, xxiii, 160, 184–85; and sorcery, 192, 194; as sperm, 68–69; in spirit appeasement, 202–4; pilgrimages to, 234–38; selling of, 291. See also *Kabsa*
Ansari, Hamied, 15, 17
Antisperm antibodies, 261–62, 275, 277
Arabic: and diglossia, 369; informants' literacy in, 372, 375–76; medical terminology in, 64–65, 68, 248, 254, 280, 284, 296–97, 369; use of in fieldwork, 32, 285, 359, 362, 367, 369
Arab medicine, 61, 177, 318. *See also* Bedouin
Aristotle: as teacher of Alexander the Great, 43, 56; on menstrual blood, 57, 71; on monogenesis, 52, 56–57, 59, 63, 73
Artificial insemination by donor (AID): in Cameroon, 393 n.3; performed clandestinely, 99, 107, 195, 393 n.4; religious prohibitions against, 322, 331; women's opposition to, 331–33. *See also* Adultery
Artificial insemination by husband (AIH): as a new reproductive technology, 7, 245; cost of, 326–27; description of, 323–25; efficacy of, 333; indications for, xxvi, 322–23, 333; moral dilemmas of, 320–21, 326, 330–33; pain of, 325, 329; participation of husbands in, 329–30; practical dilemmas of, 326–30; semen preparation in, 324, 328–29, 332–33; women's enthusiasm for, 325–26; women's experiences of, 88–89, 242, 288–89, 317–20, 325, 364–65; women's understandings of, 328–29, 393 n.1. *See also* Injections; Shatby Hospital; Technologies, new reproductive
Astragal, in infertility therapy, 189
Autopsies, 64

Baby of the tubes. *See* In vitro fertilization
Back, and pregnancy, 71, 168, 173, 388 n.6. *See also* Open back

This book has been set in Linotron Galliard. Galliard was designed for Mergenthaler in 1978 by Matthew Carter. Galliard retains many of the features of a sixteenth-century typeface cut by Robert Granjon but has some modifications that give it a more contemporary look.